Public Health: Global Perspectives

Public Health: Global Perspectives

Edited by **Abby Calvin**

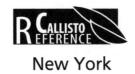

New York

Published by Callisto Reference,
106 Park Avenue, Suite 200,
New York, NY 10016, USA
www.callistoreference.com

Public Health: Global Perspectives
Edited by Abby Calvin

International Standard Book Number: 978-1-63239-776-8 (Hardback)

Printed in the United States of America.

Contents

Preface

Every book is a source of knowledge and this one is no exception. The idea that led to the conceptualization of this book was the fact that the world is advancing rapidly; which makes it crucial to document the progress in every field. I am aware that a lot of data is already available, yet, there is a lot more to learn. Hence, I accepted the responsibility of editing this book and contributing my knowledge to the community.

Public health is the combination of all the measures required for the facilitation of health and prevention of disease. It makes an effort to provide complete care through surveillance of cases, health indicators and promotion of healthy habits. This discipline incorporates behavioral health, health economics, public policy, insurance medicine, biostatistics, etc. This book elucidates the concepts and innovative models around prospective developments with respect to public health. It explores all the important aspects of this discipline in the present day scenario. The various studies that are constantly contributing towards advancing technologies and evolution of this field are examined in detail. The extensive content of this book provides the readers with a thorough understanding of the subject. Students, researchers, doctors, public health professionals, experts and all associated with this area will benefit alike from this book.

While editing this book, I had multiple visions for it. Then I finally narrowed down to make every chapter a sole standing text explaining a particular topic, so that they can be used independently. However, the umbrella subject sinews them into a common theme. This makes the book a unique platform of knowledge.

I would like to give the major credit of this book to the experts from every corner of the world, who took the time to share their expertise with us. Also, I owe the completion of this book to the never-ending support of my family, who supported me throughout the project.

Editor

National evaluation of strategies to reduce safety violations for working from heights in construction companies: results from a randomized controlled trial

Henk F. van der Molen[1,2*], Aalt den Herder[2], Jan Warning[2] and Monique H.W. Frings-Dresen[1]

Abstract

Background: The objective of this study is to evaluate the effectiveness of a face-to-face strategy and a direct mail strategy on safety violations while working from heights among construction companies compared to a control condition.

Methods: Construction companies with workers at risk for fall injuries were eligible for this three-armed randomized controlled trial. In total, 27 cities were randomly assigned to intervention groups–where eligible companies were given either a face-to-face guidance strategy or a direct mailing strategy with access to internet facilities–or to a control group. The primary outcomes were the number and type of safety violations recorded by labor inspectors after three months. A process evaluation for both strategies was performed to determine reach, program implementation, satisfaction, knowledge and perceived safety behavior. A cost analysis was performed to establish the financial costs for each intervention strategy. Analyses were done by intention to treat.

Results: In total, 41 % (n = 88) of the companies eligible for the face-to-face intervention participated and 73 % (n = 69) for direct mail. Intervention materials were delivered to 69 % (face-to-face group) and 100 % (direct mail group); completion of intervention activities within companies was low. Satisfaction, increase in knowledge, and safety behavior did not differ between the intervention groups. Costs for personal advice were 28 % higher than for direct mail. Ultimately, nine intervention companies were captured in the 288 worksite measurements performed by the labor inspectorate. No statistical differences in mean number of safety violations (1.8–2.4) or penalties (72 %–100 %) were found between the intervention and control groups based on all worksite inspections.

Conclusions: No conclusions about the effect of face-to-face and direct mail strategies on safety violations could be drawn due to the limited number of intervention companies captured in the primary outcome measurements. The costs for a face-to-face strategy are higher compared with a direct mail strategy. No difference in awareness and attitude for safe working was found between employers and workers between both strategies.

Trial registration: NTR 4298 on 29-nov-2013.

Keywords: Evaluation, Safety hazards, Working from heights, Safety behavior, Construction industry

* Correspondence: h.f.vandermolen@amc.nl
[1]Coronel Institute of Occupational Health, Academic Medical Center, University of Amsterdam, P.O. Box 22660 1100 DD Amsterdam, The Netherlands
[2]Arbouw, P.O. Box 213 3840 AE Harderwijk, The Netherlands

Background

Construction workers are frequently exposed to various types of injury-inducing hazards, especially falling from heights [1–3]. Most fall accidents from scaffolds can be prevented through compliance with regulations [2]. Psychosocial factors can also contribute to occupational accidents. For the construction industry, high time pressure and exposure to violence and harassment by colleagues or supervisors are associated with occupational accidents [4]. Both organizational and project levels are reported as being important for promoting safety performance; leadership and commitment are important at the organization level, while risk assessment and management are important at the project level [5].

More than 80 % of Dutch construction sites violate safety regulations for working from heights (personal communication), while 14 % of the construction workers report that unsafe situations regularly prevail at worksites [6]. Specifically concerning small companies in the construction industry, there seems to be a lack of information on hazard recognition [7]. To increase compliance with safety procedures, employers and workers need to select, implement, and monitor safety measures. To facilitate this behavioral change [8], stimulating knowledge awareness [9] and personalized feedback [10, 11] are behavior change techniques that are frequently advocated. In addition, education and subject matter training could improve occupational safety and health of the small business workforce in the residential construction industry [7]. The involvement of unions, employers' organizations (e.g. [12]) and the labor inspectorate (e.g. [13]) is recommended when executing national programs to improve safety and health at job, company or branch level.

For this study, two behavior change strategies were developed, based on aspects of awareness-raising and personalized feedback. These consisted of: 1) face-to-face contacts with safety consultants; and 2) direct mail with internet links. We hypothesize that both guidance strategies will reduce safety violations with rolling scaffolds, ladders and stairs compared to the control condition of a general announcement of inspection in construction companies. In addition, the face-to-face strategy is thought to be superior to the direct mail strategy due to a higher impact of personalized feedback. The financial costs are expected to be higher in the face-to-face guidance strategy, especially due to hiring safety consultants and their coordinator for worksite visits.

The objective of this study is to evaluate the effectiveness of a face-to-face strategy and a direct mail strategy on safety violations for working from heights among construction companies compared to the control condition of only announcing safety inspections by the labor inspectorate. For both guidance strategies, a process and cost evaluation will be performed.

Methods

Design

A three-armed randomized controlled trial (RCT) was performed to compare the effectiveness of two behavior change strategies: a face-to-face guidance strategy and a direct mailing strategy, with a control condition. For the description of the design of the safety intervention and the two guidance strategies, in compliance with the CONSORT statement, we refer to [14]. No changes to methods or outcomes after trial reporting [14] and commencement occurred. The reporting of this study adheres to the CONSORT guideline for reporting randomized trials.

In addition to the RCT, a process evaluation and a cost evaluation took place for each guidance strategies. In total, 27 large cities were stratified within three regions in the Netherlands (North-East, West, South) and each city was assigned to one of two intervention groups or the control group using nQuery Advisor® Version 7.0. As a result of the inspection procedure of the Dutch Labor Inspectorate, i.e. unannounced worksite inspections in a well-defined area and time period in the Netherlands, the interventions took place at construction companies working in larger cities. The study protocol did not meet the criteria of the "Medical-scientific research with human participants Act", i.e. it was not a study of a medical nature and the subjects do not receive a particular treatment or are asked to behave in a particular way [15]. The ethics committee of the Academic Medical Center in Amsterdam confirmed that the study did not meet the criteria of the 'Medical-scientific research with human participants Act' and therefore no ethics approval was required. For the full description of the design of the safety intervention and the two guidance strategies, we refer to [14].

Subjects

The guidance strategies were given to construction companies. Inclusion criteria of the construction companies were: 1) involved in the painting and maintenance of buildings; and 2) working in one of the 18 pre-randomized bigger cities in the Netherlands during May 2014.

Construction companies willing to participate were contacted in December 2013/January 2014 for further arrangements concerning the proposed interventions, and employers and workers were formally asked for their consent when sending completed questionnaires. The research population included construction sites of the participating companies. With the exception of a general national announcement of inspection in construction companies, no guidance strategies took place in the control group. Allocation occurred on the basis of eligibility, i.e. the companies that were assumed to have construction projects in one of the randomized cities during May

2014 (four to five months after allocation). The researcher (HM) assigned companies to the interventions, while a call center enrolled eligible companies.

Interventions

The safety measures covered by the two guidance strategies were based on the inspection module of the labor inspectorate and the guidelines of the Dutch construction safety and health institute Arbouw. For this study, two behavior change strategies were developed in collaboration with employers' organizations and unions to reduce the number of safety violations during the installation and use of rolling scaffolds, ladders and stairs among painters, in addition to the announcement of safety inspections by the labor inspectorate (interventions are described in detail in [14]). No blinding for the assignment of interventions was possible.

Face-to-face guidance strategy

The face-to-face guidance strategy consisted of personal advice at construction companies with a maximum of three visits during which workers were informed about preventing falling hazards with rolling scaffolds, ladders and stairs. Company visits took place at the company or at worksites on dates and times agreed on with the contact person of each company during a three-month period. Each visit consisted of a one- to two-hour interactive consultancy meeting with the contact person and workers of the construction company. Information was exchanged concerning selection, implementation and monitoring of safety measures with regard to rolling scaffolds, ladders and stairs. The safety consultant wrote a short report of the findings and the advised safety measures. In total, six safety consultants experienced in equipment for working from heights were involved in the face-to-face strategy.

Direct mail guidance strategy

The direct mail guidance strategy consisted of sending direct mail to the construction companies informing workers about the prevention of falling hazards with rolling scaffolds, ladders and stairs. The information consisted of a poster with URLs for the Internet approach (www.schilderenophoogte.nl) to four types of information and instruction materials: brochures and poster, checklists (instructions for safe installation and use of equipment), video, and a toolbox to inform and instruct workers during toolbox meetings.

Measurements

Primary outcome measure

Safety violations were the primary outcome measure and were defined as the number and type of safety violations during the installation and use of equipment for working from heights. The labor inspectorate checked safety violations concerning equipment of rolling scaffolds, ladders and stairs on worksites of painters during a three-week period. The safety violations consist of 0 to 30 safety hazards [14].

Process measures

The following indicators for the implementation of the program were evaluated [16, 17]: reach, dose delivered, dose received. Satisfaction with the intervention (score 0–10), increase in perceived knowledge on safety measures (score 0–10) and perceived effectiveness on safety behavior (score 0–10) were used as indicators for acceptability concerning the interventions [18]. The process outcomes were measured during and after the intervention period by means of logbooks and questionnaires sent to the companies and their workers.

Reach was defined as the attendance rate of the construction companies at the intervention. Attendance rate was defined as the number of construction companies participating in this study relative to the number of eligible construction companies invited through the recruitment strategies. The attendance was assessed by means of a logbook during the recruitment of the construction companies.

Dose delivered referred to the proportion of the intended intervention that was actually delivered to the participating contact persons of the construction companies. For the face-to-face guidance strategy, the number of company visits and company reports including advice delivered by the safety consultants to the contact person of the construction companies was assessed by means of a logbook filled in by the safety consultants. For the direct mailing strategy, dose delivered was assessed by means of the number of direct postal mails and emails sent to the contact person of the construction companies. The dose delivered was rated as sufficient when more than 90 % of the companies received the interventions.

Dose received referred to the proportion of activities in the intervention that were actually performed by the employer and workers of the construction companies. For both intervention strategies, dose received was assessed by questions to the employer and workers after completion of the intervention period.

Satisfaction was measured by asking the employers and workers how they rated their satisfaction with the intervention as a whole and its individual components, on a scale from 0 (not satisfied) to 10 (very satisfied). Increased knowledge about working safely with rolling scaffolds, ladders and stairs was measured by asking the employers and workers to what extent their knowledge increased from (0–10; 0 = not more knowledge, 10 = much more knowledge). The rates were defined as not more knowledge (0), little (≥ 0 and <6), moderate (≥ 6 and <7.5)

or much more knowledge (≥7.5) [14]. Effect on working safely with rolling scaffolds, ladders and stairs was measured by asking the employers and workers to what extent they rated the perceived effect on safety behavior (0–10, 0 = no effect, 10 = large effect). The rates were defined as poor (<6), moderate (≥6 and <7.5) or good (≥7.5).

The costs of the face-to-face strategy were calculated by multiplying the number of company visits by the fixed cost per visit, plus travel costs, coordination costs and the cost of information materials. The cost of the direct mailing strategy was calculated by totaling the coordination costs, the costs of developing information materials and the website, and the costs of direct mailing.

Statistical analyses

At least 64 construction locations involved in painting and maintenance per group had to be captured to detect a reduction in safety violations of 15–25 % with an alpha of 0.05 (two-tailed) and a power of (1-beta) = 0.80. Differences in the mean number of safety violations and proportion of penalties were tested using Kruskal-Wallis one-way analysis of variance and Chi-Square tests respectively. The three process measurements were posttested and differences between the interventions were examined using non-parametric tests. Statistical significance was defined as p < 0.05 for all outcome measures. The costs calculation for each intervention strategy was analyzed descriptively. The statistical analysis occurred after the pre-defined ending of the trial and after ascertainment of the required number of inspected companies (June 2014).

Results

In total, 157 companies were included for participation to the face-to-face intervention or direct mail intervention. Figure 1 shows a flow diagram for the enrollment, allocation, follow-up and analysis of the construction companies for both intervention groups and control group.

In both intervention groups, 37 employers of companies responded to the questionnaire for the process measures dose received and perceived effectiveness (response rates face-to-face and direct mail, respectively 27 % and 19 %). Sixty-nine workers from 24 companies returned questionnaires: 45 workers from 15 companies in the face-to-face group and 24 workers from nine companies in the direct mail group. All process measures are presented below and summarized in Table 1.

Reach

In total, 2188 painting companies were contacted by a call center requesting participation in one of the two interventions. With 666 companies, a structured interview was possible to determine the eligibility of the companies for this study, i.e. working in one of the 18 predetermined cities in the Netherlands during May 2014. With 1522 companies, no structured interview was possible due to the absence of a valid telephone number (729), not answering the telephone, or refusing to participate in the interview (793). Of those with completed interviews, 202 companies expected to work during the measurement period in the nine cities assigned to the face-to-face intervention; 94 companies expected to work during the measurement period in the nine cities assigned to the direct mail intervention.

In total, 41 % (83/202) of the eligible companies for the face-to-face intervention and 73 % (69/94) of the eligible companies for direct mail participated. Spontaneously, five companies were included in the group of personal advice after a request placed in a newsletter of the branch's organizations (see Table 1). Reported reasons for not participating were: already sufficiently informed, safety sufficiently settled, no external advice, own professional workers, no time, no necessity.

Interventions delivered and received

In the face-to-face group, 69 % (61/88) of the companies were visited by a safety consultant while 57 % (81/142) of the intended number of visits and 60 % (53/88) of the company reports were achieved. In the direct mail group, 100 % (69/69) received documentation (postal and email) while 52 % (36/69) visited the internet site and 13 % (9/69) did the safety test. In three companies, workers were allowed to be emailed directly (n = 10).

The majority of the employers reported that they provided feedback to their workers about safe working and had undertaken safety actions; in the face-to-face group, this proportion was higher than in the direct mailing group (91 % and 88 % vs. 78 % and 62 %). Additionally, the majority of the responding workers reported that they had been informed and had taken action.

Satisfaction, perceived effectiveness and costs

Employers and workers were satisfied with the delivered intervention activities (means ranging from 7.4 to 7.9). Perceived increase in knowledge and safe work was rated between 5.7 to 7.5. No statistical differences between the interventions were found.

Costs for intervention activities for face-to-face intervention were €32,026 (safety consultants: 63 %; documentation materials 4 %; coordination: 33 %) and for direct mail intervention €25,000 (documentation materials and mailing: 49 %; website: 32 %; coordination: 20 %).

National evaluation of strategies to reduce safety violations for working...

5

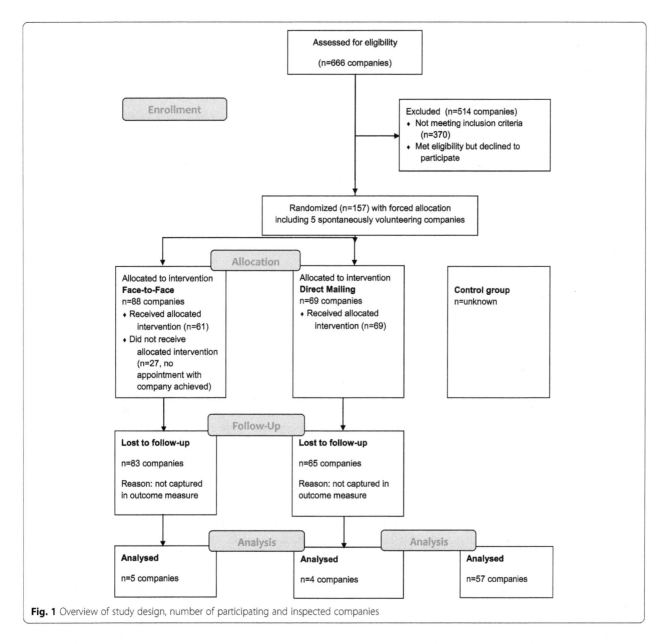

Fig. 1 Overview of study design, number of participating and inspected companies

Safety violations

Ultimately, nine intervention worksites of nine companies and 60 control worksites of 57 companies were captured in the 288 inspected worksites of painting companies. No statistical differences in mean number of safety violations and penalties were found between the intervention and control groups (see Table 2). The mean number of recorded violations and proportion of penalties varied between 1.8–2.4, respectively 72–100 %.

Discussion

The present randomized controlled intervention study evaluated two frequently advocated strategies to reduce safety violations in the construction industry and gain insight into their effect, implementation and acceptability.

No conclusions about the effect of face-to-face and direct mail strategies on safety violations could be drawn due to the limited number of intervention companies captured in the primary outcome measurements. Perceived increase in knowledge and safe work did not differ between the intervention strategies. Financial costs for the face-to-face strategy were 28 % higher than the direct mail strategy.

Methodological considerations

A strength of this national evaluation study was the double blinding in the assessment of the primary outcome measures. However, this advantage turned out to also be the major limitation of this study in terms of the low capture of intervention companies in the outcome measurements. Although the intended inspection sites

Table 1 Overview of process evaluation measures on company level (reach and dose delivered), individual level among employers and workers (dose received, satisfaction, knowledge and safe work) and intervention level (costs)

		Face-to-face	Direct mail
Reach	Participating companies (%)	83/202 (41 %)	69/94 (73 %)
	Spontaneously volunteering companies	5	-
Dose delivered	Intervention activities delivered	61/88 (69 %)	69/69 (100 %)
Dose received	Employers shared information with workers	91 % (n = 21)	78 % (n = 9)
	Employers took action	88 % (n = 24)	62 % (n = 13)
	Workers received information	75 % (n = 44)	88 % (n = 24)
	Workers took action	62 % (n = 45)	58 % (n = 24)
Satisfaction (0–10)	Employers (mean, sd)	7.9 (1.27) (n = 22)	7.4 (0.88) (n = 9)
	Workers (mean, sd)	7.7 (1.07) (n = 34)	7.5 (0.98) (n = 21)
Increase in knowledge (0–10)	Employers (mean, sd)	5.7 (2.95) (n = 22)	6.6 (2.56) (n = 9)
	Workers (mean, sd)	7.5 (1.12) (n = 33)	6.8 (2.23) (n = 21)
Increase in safe work (0–10)	Employers (mean, sd)	6.8 (2.80) (n = 21)	6.8 (0.97) (n = 9)
	Workers (mean, sd)	7.5 (1.40) (n = 33)	6.9 (1.84) (n = 21)
Costs		€ 32,026	€ 25,000

by the labor inspectorate–based on power analyses and expected loss to follow-up and inspection of non-painting construction sites–were achieved (in total 288 worksites: 122 worksites in cities assigned to face-to-face intervention group, 106 worksites in cities assigned to direct mailing intervention group and 60 worksites assigned to cities in control group), only nine intervention companies were captured in the outcome measurements by the labor inspectorate. Due to ethical reasons, i.e. introducing unequal risk of incurring financial penalties when safety violations were established by the labor inspectorate, all construction sites in the 27 cities were able to be the subject of inspection and the researchers could not reveal the names of the 18 intervention cities nor the names of the participating painting companies. Intervention research in the construction industry remains a challenge because of the many workplace factors prevalent in the construction setting that may need to be accounted for in research design [19]. Among others, a jobsite moves from place to place, and most construction employees work on

several jobsites each year, while placing bids for work often do not include specification requirements for health and safety equipment and procedures [19].

Furthermore, the program implementation in terms of dose delivered and dose received was insufficient. It was difficult to make appointments with the construction companies for worksite visits in the group of companies with the face-to-face strategy. Although in the companies with the email strategy dose delivered in terms of sending information was guaranteed, the uptake of information was low in terms of consulting the internet or testing the knowledge.

The practice base has been incorporated to the maximum in both interventions [14]. For both guidance strategies, the content and approach has been developed by the Dutch institute on safety and health in the construction industry. The safety consultants were experienced in safety in construction work and the information materials were adapted to the context of painters. In addition, construction companies were free to choose how they wanted

Table 2 Mean number of safety violations and proportion of penalties in intervention groups and control group

		Face-to-face	Direct mail	Control	P-value
Number inspected companies (worksites) by labor inspectorate		5 (5)	4 (4)	57 (60)[a]	
Penalty for companies		4 (80 %)	4 (100 %)	43 (72 %)	0.435
of which	...urging	-	1 (25 %)	4 (9 %)	
	...warning	4 (100 %)	2 (50 %)	24 (56 %)	
	...paying	-	1 (25 %)	7 (16 %)	
	...shutting down	2 (50 %)	1 (25 %)	17 (40 %)	
Mean number (SD) violations		2.4 (2.70)	1.8 (1.71)	1.9 (2.05)	0.847
Range number violations		0–7	0–4	0–8	

[a]In control group at three companies two independent worksites

to control the safety hazards when working with rolling scaffolds, ladders and stairs. Possibly, this practice base in combination with the recruitment strategy with structured telephone interviews [14] contributed to the high recruitment rates for the face-to-face interventions and the direct mail strategy with much higher rates than reported in other intervention studies in the construction industry [20, 21], and especially for small construction companies in voluntary safety programs or safety research [22]. Possibly due to the fact that there was no need to make further appointments in the direct mail strategy compared with the face-to-face intervention, the direct mail intervention achieved the highest recruitment rate of over 70 %.

A strength in this design was the process measurements that gave insight into the acceptance and perceived increase in knowledge and safe work among employers and workers. However, due to *a priori* agreed restrictions in approaching the companies for research goals, process measures could not be evaluated in more detail, e.g. performed safety measures and involved number of workers. Many reviews on intervention studies stipulate the importance of process evaluations alongside the effect evaluations [23].

Practice implications

In both interventions, three important implementation measures were assessed: knowledge in safe working (awareness); satisfaction and perceived safety (attitude); and safety violations (behavior). Both among employers and workers, increase in knowledge was rated as moderate for the direct mail strategy; for the face-to-face strategy, increase in knowledge was rated as low among employers and high among workers. This lower rate among employers for the face-to-face strategy could be due to higher expectations regarding personal knowledge transfer. Since attitude in terms of perceived increase in safe work and satisfaction were moderate to high in both strategies among employers and workers, both strategies are acceptable for stimulation of safety behavior.

Possibly, additional strategies for the stimulation of personal feedback could be built in for internal organized feedback in both the face-to-face strategy and direct mail approach. An example could be the coaching of construction site foremen to include safety in their daily verbal exchanges with workers that showed a positive and lasting effect on the level of safety [24].

The effect on actual safety behavior in terms of safety violations did not differ between intervention and control groups, but—as stated in the methodological considerations—this result is biased due to the low number of intervention companies in the outcome measurements. However, the mean number of violations and penalties did not differ between the nine captured intervention companies and the other 279 inspected companies. Consequently, there are no indications of any effect of the interventions on safety violations. The high prevalence of penalties at inspected construction sites underlines the need to counteract unsafe working with rolling scaffolds, ladders and stairs.

Finally, the costs for the face-to-face strategy are 28 % higher compared with the direct mail strategy. Taking into account the difference in actual delivered implementation, this difference increases from €250 to €525 per company.

Lessons learned

From a methodological point of view, two lessons can be learned, namely the efficient and successful procedure of recruitment of companies and the lack of data triangulation of the primary outcome measure. Firstly, many eligible companies were identified through a call center, and an adequate number of companies were willing to participate. In many studies, especially in the construction industry, the recruitment phase takes a long time. Secondly, allowing researchers extra effort in visiting the intervention companies to assess the primary outcome measure—besides the measurements by the labor inspectorate—would have resulted in a sufficient number of analyzed companies, thereby making it possible to answer the first research question. Unfortunately, a limited number of intervention companies were actually working in the assigned cities during the follow-up measurement period specified by the labor inspectorate, probably due to the short and alternating duration of many construction projects. Therefore, choosing inspector assessment as outcome measure alone resulted in too few assessments of intervention companies. This might be overcome by another study design, e.g. more qualitative and explorative designs alongside a thorough process evaluation. For example, in-depth interviews with employers and workers during the intervention could provide insight into barriers and facilitators for increasing the intervention uptake. Also, more participatory approaches with active involvement of researchers could increase insight into the intervention process.

From a practical point of view, one main lesson has been learned, namely the low intensity of the delivered and received interventions due to variable work settings at construction sites. Since behavioral change requires continuous attention and feedback to tackle barriers at organizational and worksite level, e.g. appointments with suppliers of rolling scaffolds or using instructions when setting up and using climbing materials.

Conclusions

No conclusions about the effect of face-to-face and direct mail strategies on safety violations could be drawn due to the limited number of intervention companies captured in the primary outcome measurements. The costs for a face-to-face strategy are higher compared with a direct mail strategy. No difference in awareness and attitude for safe working was found among employers and workers between both strategies.

Competing interests

The authors declare that they have no competing interests.

Authors' contributions

HM conceived and designed the study and drafted the manuscript. MFD participated in the design of the study and the manuscript preparation. JW and AH participated in all phases of this study and manuscript preparation. All authors read and approved the final manuscript.

Acknowledgments

We would like to thank the Dutch Labor Inspectorate, Annemarie Arensen and participating construction companies for data collection, coordination and participation. This study has been funded by Arbouw.

References

1. Hsiao H, Stout N. Occupational injury prevention research. Saf Health Work. 2010;1:107–11.
2. Ohdo K, Hino Y, Takahashi H. Research on fall prevention and protection from heights in Japan. Ind Health. 2014;52:399–406.
3. Schoenfisch A, Lipscomb H, Cameron W, Adams D, Silverstein B. Rates of and circumstances surrounding work-related falls from height among union drywall carpenters in Washington State, 1989–2008. J Safety Res. 2014;51:117–24.
4. van der Klauw M, Oude Hengel K, Bakhuys Roozeboom M, Koppes L, Venema A. Occupational accidents in the Netherlands: incidence, mental harm, and their relationship with psychosocial factors at work incidence. Int J Inj Contr Saf Promot. 2014. doi:10.1080/17457300.2014.966119.
5. Mahmoudi S, Ghasemi F, Mohammadfam I, Soleimani E. Framework for continuous assessment and improvement of occupational health and safety issues in construction companies. Saf Health Work. 2014;5:125–30.
6. Arbouw. Atlas of workers health surveillance data in construction industry of 2012. (http://www.arbouw.nl/werkgever/tools/bedrijfstakatlas-2012/ [Accessed on 10th March 2014].
7. Choi SD, Carlson K. Occupational safety issues in residential construction surveyed in Wisconsin, United States. Ind Health. 2014;52:541–7.
8. Prochaska JO, Velicer WF. The transtheoretical model of health behavior change. Am J Health Promot. 1997;12:38–48.
9. Leeman J, Baernholdt M, Sandelowski M. Developing a theory-based taxonomy of methods for implementing change in practice. J Adv Nurs. 2007;58:191–200.
10. Diclemente CC, Marinilli AS, Singh M, Bellino LE. The role of feedback in the process of health behavior change. Am J Health Behav. 2001;25:217–27.
11. Choudhry RM. Behavior-based safety on construction sites: a case study. Accid Anal Prev. 2014;70:14–23.
12. Jensen LK, Friche C. Effects of training to implement new tools and working methods to reduce knee load in floorlayers. Appl Ergon. 2007;38:655–65.
13. Laitinen H, Päivärinta K. A new-generation safety contest in the construction industry-a long-term evaluation of a real-life intervention. Safety Sci. 2010; 48:680–6.
14. Van der Molen HF, Frings-Dresen MHW. Strategies to reduce safety violations for working from heights in construction companies: study protocol for a randomized controlled trial. BMC Public Health. 2014;14:541. doi:10.1186/1471-2458-14-541.
15. CCMO (Central Committee on Research Involving Human Subjects). Your research: does it fall under the Medical Research Involving Human Subjects Act (WMO). http://www.ccmo.nl/en/your-research-does-it-fall-under-the-wmo [Accessed on 10th March 2014].
16. Linnan L, Steckler A. Process evaluation for public health interventions and research. San Francisco, California: Jossey-Bass; 2002.
17. Murta SG, Sanderson K, Oldenburg B. Process evaluation in occupational stress management programs: a systemic review. Am J Health Promot. 2007;21:248–54.
18. Bowen DJ, Kreuter M, Spring B, Cofta-Woerpel L, Linnan L, Weiner D, et al. How we design feasibility studies. Am J Prev Med. 2009;36:452–7.
19. Wolford R. Intervention research in construction: a hypothetical case study of painters. Am J Ind Med. 1996;29:431–4.
20. Oude Hengel KM, Blatter BM, van der Molen HF, Joling CI, Proper KI, Bongers PM, et al. Meeting the challenges of implementing an intervention to promote work ability and health-related quality of life at construction worksites: a process evaluation. J Occup Environ Med. 2011;53:1483–91.
21. Boschman JS, van der Molen HF, Sluiter JK, Frings-Dresen MHW. Improving occupational health care for construction workers: a process evaluation. BMC Public Health. 2013;13:218.
22. Kidd P, Parshall M, Wojcik S, Struttmann T. Overcoming recruitment challenges in construction safety intervention research. Am J Ind Med. 2004; 45:297–304.
23. Robson LS, Shannon HS, Goldenhar LM, Hale AR. Guide to evaluating the effectiveness of strategies for preventing work injuries: how to show whether a safety intervention really works. Department of Health and Human Services, NIOSH. NIOSH: Cincinnati, OH; 2001.
24. Kines P, Andersen LPS, Spangenberg S, Mikkelsen KL, Dyreborg J, Zohar D. Improving construction site safety through leader-based verbal safety communication. J Safety Res. 2010;41:399–406.

Crude incidence in two-phase designs in the presence of competing risks

Paola Rebora[1]* , Laura Antolini[1], David V. Glidden[2] and Maria Grazia Valsecchi[1]

Abstract

Background: In many studies, some information might not be available for the whole cohort, some covariates, or even the outcome, might be ascertained in selected subsamples. These studies are part of a broad category termed two-phase studies. Common examples include the nested case-control and the case-cohort designs. For two-phase studies, appropriate weighted survival estimates have been derived; however, no estimator of cumulative incidence accounting for competing events has been proposed. This is relevant in the presence of multiple types of events, where estimation of event type specific quantities are needed for evaluating outcome.

Methods: We develop a non parametric estimator of the cumulative incidence function of events accounting for possible competing events. It handles a general sampling design by weights derived from the sampling probabilities. The variance is derived from the influence function of the subdistribution hazard.

Results: The proposed method shows good performance in simulations. It is applied to estimate the crude incidence of relapse in childhood acute lymphoblastic leukemia in groups defined by a genotype not available for everyone in a cohort of nearly 2000 patients, where death due to toxicity acted as a competing event. In a second example the aim was to estimate engagement in care of a cohort of HIV patients in resource limited setting, where for some patients the outcome itself was missing due to lost to follow-up. A sampling based approach was used to identify outcome in a subsample of lost patients and to obtain a valid estimate of connection to care.

Conclusions: A valid estimator for cumulative incidence of events accounting for competing risks under a general sampling design from an infinite target population is derived.

Keywords: Two-phase design, Competing risks, Crude incidence, Case-control, Case-cohort, Missing data, Subdistribution hazard

Background

In many longitudinal studies, some information might not be measured/available for the whole cohort, in fact biomarkers/additional covariates, or even outcome, might be ascertained only in selected subsamples. These studies are part of a broad category termed two-phase studies [1], in fact they imply two sampling phases: the first one being usually a random sample from the target population, ending up in the entire cohort (phase I sample), and the second one applying some kind of sampling (e.g. efficient or of convenience) to collect additional information or the selection of subjects with no missing data

(phase II sample). Common examples of efficient second phase sampling include the nested case-control and the case-cohort designs [2–5]. In other situations the outcome itself is collected only for a subsample [6]. Two-phase sampling, or more generally, multiphase sampling, is a general design that includes any valid probability sample of the data, in which each subsampling can depend on all the currently observed data at each step [7]. The actual sampling probabilities will depend on the specific design. The acknowledgement of these sampling phases, even in the commonly applied designs, can be very useful to improve efficiency and to allow flexibility in the analysis (e.g. different time-scales or different models can be applied) by using information available for the whole cohort [8].

Efficient designs are particularly useful to identify new biomarkers when the combination between large cohorts

*Correspondence: paola.rebora@unimib.it
[1] Center of Biostatistics for Clinical Epidemiology, School of Medicine and Surgery, University of Milano-Bicocca, via Cadore 48, 20900 Monza, Italy
Full list of author information is available at the end of the article

and expensive new technologies make it infeasible to measure the biomarkers on the entire cohort. The Women's Health Initiative program, for example, stored serum and plasma from participants and used them for specialized studies [9]. Also the Cardiovascular Health Study collected DNA from most participants to study different genetic factors underlying cardiovascular or other diseases and only subsets of the cohort have been genotyped in different projects [10].

In our first motivating clinical example, the aim was to evaluate the role of different genetic polymorphisms on treatment failure due to relapse in childhood acute lymphoblastic leukemia (ALL) using clinical information and biological samples available from a clinical trial that enrolled nearly 2000 patients. In this situation, a parsimonious use of these specimens motivated the choice of an efficient/optimal two-phase sampling design [11]. We present also a further application where the aim was to estimate engagement to care of HIV patients in resource limited settings. Here the outcome itself was missing in a group of patients due to possibly informative loss to follow-up. The outcome was tracked in a random sample of those lost to follow-up to obtain a valid estimate of engagement to care [12].

For two-phase studies, appropriate weighted survival estimates have been derived, both in the presence of additional covariates measured in the second phase [7, 13, 14], as well as in cohorts where the outcome/follow-up is not available for everyone [15]. A Cox model adapted for two-phase designs has also been derived [14]. However no estimator of cumulative incidence accounting for competing events in the general framework of two-phase designs has been proposed, while it has been developed for specific designs, such as nested case-control studies [16, 17]. This is relevant in the presence of multiple types of events, such as relapse and (toxic) death in cancer patients, as in the motivating examples presented here, where estimation of event type specific quantities are needed for evaluating outcome.

The aim of this paper is to develop a non parametric estimator of the crude incidence of events accounting for possible competing events in the general framework of two-phase designs, where subgroups of analysis might be defined according to explanatory variables ascertained in the phase II sample, or the outcome itself assessed only in the second phase sample.

In the Methods section we propose a weighted crude incidence estimator for application in two-phase designs. The theoretical properties of the proposed method are derived in appendix and investigated through simulations under different scenarios, which results are reported in Results section. In this section we also report the examples on childhood ALL and HIV patients. Conclusions is dedicated to the discussion.

Methods

Notation and basics

Let T be the failure time variable and suppose there are K possible causes of failure denoted by $\varepsilon = 1, 2, \ldots K$. Let the cause-specific hazard function of the kth event be:

$$\lambda_k(t) = \lim_{dt \to 0} \frac{1}{dt} P(t \leq T < t + dt; \varepsilon = k | T \geq t)$$

and $\Lambda_k(t) = \int_0^t \lambda_k(s) ds$. Define

$$F_k(t) = P(T \leq t; \varepsilon = k) \tag{1}$$

as the probability that a failure due to cause k occurs by time t, that is the quantity that we aim to estimate. Define also $S(t) = P(T > t) = 1 - \sum_k F_k(t)$ as the probability of surviving from any cause of failure.

A convenient representation of the crude incidence function (1) as product limit estimator naturally arises starting from the subdistribution hazard introduced by Gray [18] and defined as:

$$\begin{aligned} \lambda_k^*(t) &= \lim_{dt \to 0} \frac{1}{dt} P\{t \leq T < t + dt; \varepsilon \\ &= k | T \geq t \cup (T < t; \varepsilon \neq k)\} \end{aligned} \tag{2}$$

This hazard has been shown to be very useful to compare the crude cumulative hazard functions in different groups, since it restores a one-to-one relationship between the hazard and the cumulative probability of a particular failure type: $F_k(t) = 1 - \exp\{-\Lambda_k^*(t)\} = 1 - \prod_{s \leq t}[1 - \Lambda_k^*(ds)]$, with $\Lambda_k^*(t) = \int_0^t \lambda_k^*(s) ds$ and where the product integral notation $\prod$ is used to suggest a limit of finite products $\prod$ [18, 19]. Of note, the one-to-one relationship between the hazard and the cumulative probability is not satisfied from the cause-specific hazard in the presence of competing events [20]. The subdistribution hazard can be thought as the hazard of an artificial variable $T_k^* = T \cdot I\{\varepsilon = k\} + \infty \cdot I\{\varepsilon \neq k\}$ that extends to infinity the time to event k when another competing event is observed. In fact, for any finite t, $T_k^* \leq t$ is equivalent to $T \leq t$ and $\varepsilon = k$; thus, given definition (1), $P(T_k^* \leq t) = F_k(t)$. The definition of T_k^* is consistent with the argument that when an event other than k occurs as first, the latter will never be observed as first and thus the corresponding time is infinity.

Let $(T_i, \varepsilon_i, C_i, Z_i)$, with $i = 1 \ldots N$, be N independent replicates of (T, ε, C, Z), where C is the censoring time and Z a vector of covariates. We will refer to these N subjects as the phase I sample. Define $X = \min(T, C)$ and $\Delta = I(T \leq C)$. We will assume that failure and censoring times are conditionally independent, $T \perp C | Z$. Let $Y_i(t) = I(X_i \geq t)$, $N_{ik}(t) = I(X_i \leq t, \Delta_i \varepsilon_i = k)$ and $N_{i\cdot}(t) = \sum_{k=1}^K N_{ik}(t)$, where $I(\cdot)$ is the indicator function. Define $G(t) = P(C > t)$ as the probability to remaining uncensored up to t.

Suppose that complete information on $(X_i, \Delta_i \varepsilon_i, Z_i)$ is available only for a subset $n < N$ of subjects drawn based on a possibly complex sampling design and let ξ_i indicate whether subject i is selected into this sample. We will refer to the $n = \sum_i \xi_i$ subjects as the phase II sample, even if multiple phases of sampling could actually be involved to obtain the final complete sample [7]. Let $\pi_i = P(\xi_i = 1 | X_i, \Delta_i \varepsilon_i, Z_i)$ being the inclusion probability of subject i for the phase II sample, conditional on being selected at the first phase. In a random sample this probability is equal for every subject. However sampling is often stratified on some variables to increase efficiency; in this case, the probability to be selected for the phase II sample is common for all subjects in the same stratum and differs between strata. In particular, it is usually higher for the more informative strata (e.g. strata including subjects with the event of interest as in case-control studies). For nested case-control designs the sampling probability of cases will be 1, while the one of controls might be derived as the probability that individual i is ever selected as control, following Samuelsen [4]. We denote the pairwise sampling probability for any two subjects $(i, j$, with $i \neq j)$ by $\pi_{ij} = P(\xi_i = 1, \xi_j = 1 | X_i, \Delta_i \varepsilon_i, Z_i, X_j, \Delta_j \varepsilon_j, Z_j)$. As commonly assumed in survey theory, the sampling method should have the following properties: the sampling probabilities π_i and π_{ij} must be non zero for all i, j in the population and must be known for each i, j in the sample [7].

Incidence estimation in the presence of competing risks
Overall survival/incidence estimate
Under a two-phase design it is common to be interested in estimating survival in subgroups related to variables ascertained only in phase II sample (i.e. biomarkers). Another possible situation is that, instead of covariates, the outcome itself is not available for the whole cohort. Thus, in both cases an estimate of the incidence of event using only the phase II sample is very useful. The total number of events of type k up to t and the total number of persons at risk at time t for the entire phase I sample can be estimated from the phase II sample (accounting for the sample design) by $\hat{N}_{.k}(t) = \sum_{i=1}^{N} [\xi_i N_{ik}(t)/\pi_i]$ and $\hat{Y}_.(t) = \sum_{i=1}^{N} [\xi_i Y_i(t)/\pi_i]$, respectively. Note that these estimates are valid under general sampling designs, where π_i and π_{ij}, the so-called 'design weights', are known for the observations actually sampled [21].

The estimate of the overall survival has been shown by several authors in different contexts of complex sampling [13–15]:

$$\hat{S}(t) = \prod_{s \leq t} \left[1 - \hat{\Lambda}(ds) \right] \tag{3}$$

where the overall hazard can be obtained by $\hat{\Lambda}(t) = \sum_{k=1}^{K} \hat{\Lambda}_k(t)$ and $\hat{\Lambda}_k(t) = \int_0^t \hat{N}_{.k}(ds)/\hat{Y}_.(s)$ [22]. It has

been shown that $\sqrt{N}[\hat{\Lambda}(t) - \Lambda(t)]$ converges weakly to a zero-mean Gaussian process [14, 15].

Competing risk
The goal is to estimate the crude incidence of a given cause k, $F_k(t) = 1 - \prod_{s \leq t} [1 - \Lambda_k^*(ds)]$, using the phase II sample, which is also called subdistribution function and is the probability that a failure due to cause k occurs within t [23, 24]. The estimate of $\Lambda_k^*(t)$ is based on the count of events due to cause k and the count of subjects at risk for T_k^*, denoted by $\hat{Y}_{.k}^*(s)$ (see Appendix A.1):

$$\hat{Y}_{.k}^*(s) = \sum_{i=1}^{N} \frac{\xi_i}{\pi_i} Y_i(s) + \sum_{i=1}^{N} \frac{\xi_i}{\pi_i} \left[\sum_{l \neq k} N_{il}(s^-) \cdot \hat{G}(s^- | X_i^-) \right] \tag{4}$$

The estimate of the cumulative subdistribution hazard in (2) can now be estimated, using only the phase II sample, by:

$$\hat{\Lambda}_k^*(t) = \int_0^t \frac{\hat{N}_{.k}(ds)}{\hat{Y}_{.k}^*(s)}. \tag{5}$$

Note the complement of $F_k(t)$ can be thought as the survival probability of T_k^* [18, 20, 25], thus a product limit type estimator can be directly derived as:

$$\hat{F}_k(t) = 1 - \prod_{s \leq t} \left[1 - \hat{\Lambda}_k^*(ds) \right] = 1 - \prod_{s \leq t} \left[1 - \frac{\hat{N}_{.k}(ds)}{\hat{Y}_{.k}^*(s)} \right] \tag{6}$$

Interestingly, this estimator is algebraically equivalent to the Aalen-Johansen type estimator, shown by [18] for random sampling, and in the Appendix A.2 for general sampling:

$$\hat{F}_k(t) = 1 - \prod_{s \leq t} \left[1 - \hat{\Lambda}_k^*(ds) \right] = \int_0^t \hat{S}(s^-) \hat{\Lambda}_k(ds) \tag{7}$$

It is easy to see that in the absence of competing events, $\hat{Y}_{.k}^*(s)$ in (4) degenerates to the usual risk set $\hat{Y}_.(s)$, thus $\hat{\Lambda}_k^*(t) = \hat{\Lambda}(t)$ and $\hat{F}_k(t)$ equals the complement of 1 of the weighted Kaplan-Meier estimator for two-phase studies [13]. Under no censoring, the weight $\hat{G}(s^- | X_i)$ becomes 1 and the risk set $Y_{.k}^*$ is eroded in time only by events of type k, therefore $\hat{F}_k(t)$ degenerates into the proportion of events of type k estimated by the phase II sample (weighted number of events of type k out of the estimated total size of the cohort, phase I). If every subject in phase I is sampled ($\xi_i = 1 \forall i$), then (5) becomes the standard subdistribution cumulative hazard [19, 20] and (6) the standard estimator of the crude incidence.

For simplicity of notation, in (6) we estimated the overall incidence regardless of covariates, but the estimator can also be applied on subgroups defined by Z. The censoring probability $G(t)$ should also be estimated in subgroups defined by Z. The overall estimator is reasonable when we make the more restrictive assumption $T \perp C$, otherwise separate estimators conditional on Z would be more appropriate (and eventually an average, weighted on the frequencies of Z, between the conditional estimates).

Variance and confidence intervals

Following Breslow and Wellner [26], we can express
$$\sqrt{N}\left[\hat{\Lambda}_k^*(t) - \Lambda_k^*(t)\right] = \sqrt{N}\left[\tilde{\Lambda}_k^*(t) - \Lambda_k^*(t)\right] + \sqrt{N}\left[\hat{\Lambda}_k^*(t) - \tilde{\Lambda}_k^*(t)\right]$$ where $\tilde{\Lambda}_k^*(t)$ represents the crude cumulative incidence estimator that we would have obtained if complete information $(X_i, \Delta_i\varepsilon_i, Z_i)$ was known for all the subjects in phase I sample $(i = 1\dots N)$ [18]. The two terms are asymptotically independent [14, 26]. The first term converges weakly to a zero-mean Gaussian process [19] with covariance that we denote as $\sigma_{kI}^2(t)$. By the arguments in Appendix A.3, the second term converges weakly to a zero-mean Gaussian process with covariance $\sigma_{kII}^2(t)$. Hence, $\sqrt{N}\left[\hat{\Lambda}_k^*(t) - \Lambda_k^*(t)\right]$ converges weakly to a zero-mean Gaussian process with covariance being the sum of the contribution of each sampling phase: $\sigma_k^2(t) = \sigma_{kI}^2(t) + \sigma_{kII}^2(t)$. The first one represents the irreducible minimum uncertainty that would remain if everyone in phase I would be sampled and the second one accounts for the fact that complete information is available only in the phase II sample [13, 14, 26].

Each contribution to the variance can be estimated by the influence function approach [27]. The influence function of an estimator describes how the estimator changes when single observations are added or removed from the data and has the property that the difference between the estimate and the population quantity can be expressed as the sum of influence functions over all the subjects in the sample. By denoting with $z_{ik}^*(t)$ the influence function of subject i on $\hat{\Lambda}_k^*(t)$ we have that [28]:

$$\hat{\Lambda}_k^*(t) - \Lambda_k^*(t) = \sum_{i=1}^{N} z_{ik}^*(t) + o(1/\sqrt{N}) \qquad (8)$$

The influence function of subject i on $\hat{\Lambda}_k^*(t)$ has been derived in Appendix A.4.

By using the Horvitz-Thompson variance [29] on the weighted influence function, the contribution of the variance of phase II will be:

$$\hat{\sigma}_{kII}^2(t) = v\hat{a}r\left[\sum_{i=1}^{N} \frac{\xi_i}{\pi_i} z_{ik}^*(t)\right] = \\ = \sum_{i=1}^{n}\sum_{j=1}^{n}\left[\frac{z_{ik}^*(t) \cdot z_{jk}^*(t)}{\pi_i \cdot \pi_j} - \frac{z_{ik}^*(t) \cdot z_{jk}^*(t)}{\pi_{ij}}\right] \qquad (9)$$

For phase I, the variance $\hat{\sigma}_{kI}^2(t)$ can also be estimated using (9) by setting sampling probabilities to 1 [13].

Given the one-to-one relationship between $F_k(t)$ and $\Lambda_k^*(t)$, the variance of the crude cumulative incidence (6) can now be estimated as:

$$v\hat{a}r\left[\hat{F}_k(t)\right] = \left[1 - \hat{F}_k(t)\right]^2 \cdot \hat{\sigma}_k^2(t) \qquad (10)$$

In analogy with the survival estimate for two-phase designs, we derived confidence intervals for (6) on the logarithm scale by:

$$\exp\left\{\log[\hat{F}_k(t)] \pm q_{\alpha/2}\frac{1 - \hat{F}_k(t)}{\hat{F}_k(t)}\hat{\sigma}_k(t)\right\} \qquad (11)$$

where $q_{\alpha/2}$ denotes the $\alpha/2$ quantile of the standard Gaussian distribution.

Software

By using suitable weights for both study design and censoring, any software allowing for time dependent weights can be used to derive the modified risk set and to estimate the crude cumulative incidence function (6). These weights have been implemented in R in function `crprep` in the `mstate` package [30] and in STATA in the `stcrprep` function. However, any software can be used to derive the ingredients for the modified risk set in (4) and these can be used to estimate (6) and its variance by the Horvitz-Thompson approach.

The complete code to compute this estimate has been developed in R software [31] using the `survey` package [32] and is available at [33]. An example of the application of this function is given in the subsection Genotype ascertained on a subset of a clinical trial cohort.

Results
Simulations
Simulations protocol

We considered two competing events with independent latent times T_1 and T_2 and constant marginal hazard of 0.1, the crude incidences are then $F_1(t) = F_2(t) = \frac{1}{2}(1 - e^{-0.1t})$. We focused on the crude incidence of event 1 up to $t = 2$ units of time (i.e. years). This implies a fraction of 82 % with no events at $t = 2$ (administrative censoring) and a crude incidence of about 9 %. The independence between the latent times T_1 and T_2 is not restrictive given the non identifiability issue [34]. The censoring time followed an uniform distribution on ranges (0.5,30.5) and (0.5,10.5), leading to around 5 % and 15 % censored before $t = 2$, respectively.

We drew $B = 1000$ random first-phase samples of size $N = 1000$, from which we sampled a phase II sample according to different study designs:

1. random sample, with $n = 50, 100$ units;
2. case-control sampling: we randomly sampled $n/2$ individuals among those who experienced event 1

(cases) up to time 2 and $n/2$ individuals among the others (controls), with $n = 50, 100$ units;

3. stratified sampling: we considered the phase I sample divided into 4 strata defined by the variable $Z = \{0, 1\}$ (with frequencies 70 % and 30 % for $Z = 0$ and $Z = 1$, respectively) and the occurrence or not of event 1 up to time 2. The hazard rates were assumed to be 0.08 and 0.2 with $Z = 0$ and with $Z = 1$, respectively. An equal number of subjects ($n/4$) were sampled for each strata (balanced sampling), with $n = 50, 100$ units.

4. nested case-control design: we selected all cases and m controls for each case with no events at the time of event of the case, fixing $m = 1, 2$. Under this design we cannot fix a total sample size a priori, but we expect around 90 events and $90 \cdot m$ controls. Sampling probabilities for each included subject were derived according to Samuelsen [4].

$B = 1000$ was chosen in order to get a ± 5 % level of accuracy in the estimate of the crude incidence ($F_1(t), t > 0.3$) in about 95 % of the samples. For each sample, $\hat{F}_1(t)$ has been computed by (6), with $\hat{\Lambda}_1^*(dt)$ estimated by (5), and it has been compared with $F_1(t)$ in order to assess bias in each sample: $\hat{F}_{1b}(t) - F_1(t), b = 1 \ldots B$. Bias has been computed and reported for 20 different time points $t = 0.1, 0.2, \ldots, 2$. For each simulation, we also computed standard error of $\hat{F}_1(t)$ according to (10) and the 95 % confidence interval (CI) of $\hat{F}_1(t)$ on the logarithm scale (11) to evaluate coverage and length.

Simulations results

Figure 1 compares the average of the estimated standard error of $\hat{F}_1(t)$ in each simulation with the empirical standard error at the 20 different times of observation in the four different scenarios with random censoring of 15 %. They were found to be very close in all scenarios, as expected.

Figure 2 reports the distribution of bias in each one of the 1000 simulated samples under random (panel a), case-control (panel b), stratified (panel c) and nested case-control sampling ($m = 1$, panel d). Bias fluctuates around 0 in each scenario, but it has more variability in the random sampling compared to other scenarios, resulting also in a higher mean value of absolute bias over the B simulations (still always lower than 0.2 %). The lower performance of the estimator in the first scenario is due to the fact that random sampling is not a convenient design in the simulated setting. In fact, in phase I cohort we expect around 90 events of type 1 (incidence of 9 % and sample size of 1000), thus if we randomly sample 100 subjects from the phase I cohort, we expect to observe only 9 events (in phase II sample). With such a small number of events, unbiasedness is in fact not sufficient to ensure a reasonable behaviour and to get enough information

on event incidence. To address this issue, the other study designs (scenarios 2, 3, and 4) are indeed thought to guarantee to sample more events of type 1. Thus we recommend adopting efficient designs accounting for the event of interest. Relative and standardized biases were always lower than 6 % (data not shown). The mean square error, not shown, slightly increases with time, in fact variability is increasing in time (as confirmed by the empirical standard error of $\hat{F}_1(t)$ and by Fig. 2). The average length of the confidence interval was consistently increasing with time, ranging between 7 % and 12 % in the random sampling and between 2 % and 4 % in the case-control, stratified and nested case-control sampling (data not shown). This comparison underscores the advantages of a careful selection of the subsample.

Figure 3 reports results on coverage for the random, case-control, stratified and nested case-control sampling. The coverage was very close to the nominal value of 95 %, ranging mostly within a minimum of 94 % and a maximum of 97 %, except for very early times in the random setting.

In the same setting, we also considered a longer follow-up time, t = 50, with around 500 events of type 1 expected in phase I sample (under no censoring), and confirmed the performance of our estimator in a scenario with higher variability, with similar results for the different sampling schemes (data not shown).

Motivating examples
Genotype ascertained on a subset of a clinical trial cohort
A study on childhood ALL evaluated the role of a genetic polymorphism (glutathione S-transferase-θ, GST-T1) on treatment failure due to relapse (in different sites), in the presence of a competing event (toxic death). GST-T1 is a common genetic polymorphism in Caucasians, with 13–26 % of individuals displaying a homozygous deletion of the gene (null genotype). Subjects carrying the null variants fail to express the GST-T1 enzyme, that is involved in drug metabolism. Clinical information were available for a cohort of 1999 consecutive patients (mainly European Caucasians, aged between 1 and 17 years, median age: 5 years) newly diagnosed with ALL in the Italian Associazione Italiana di Ematologia Pediatrica centers between September 2000 and July 2006. Biological samples stored at diagnosis were available, but genotype was ascertained only in a subgroup (phase II sample) for an efficient use of specimens [11, 13]. The interest was to evaluate incidence at different relapse sites by GST-T1, that can only be estimated using phase II data. In order to select the subgroup to be genotyped we adopted an optimal strategy that is carefully described in [11, 13]. Briefly, sampling was done after classifying patients into 6 strata according to the event of interest (relapse/no relapse) and to 3 groups, defined by prognostic features in the treatment protocol, that modulate the intensity of treatment, we will call them

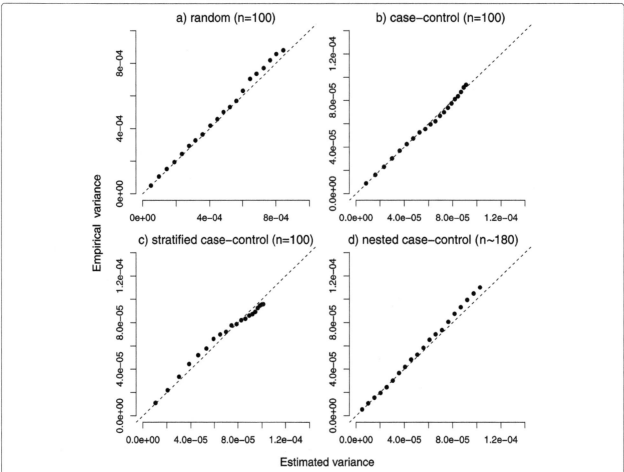

Fig. 1 Estimated and empirical variances. Comparison between estimated and empirical variance under random (panel **a**), case-control (panel **b**), stratified (panel **c**) and nested case-control sampling ($m = 1$, panel **d**). For the first three scenarios a sample size of 100 was used, while in the nested case-control sampling a mean of 180 subjects was considered. Data were subject to a random censoring of 15 % (plus administrative censoring). Dashed lines represent the main bisector corresponding to the equality between estimated and empirical reference

treatment protocols (Table 1). Strata were not defined based on the competing event death due to toxicity- 58 events - for efficiency reasons given that the event of interest was relapse. Patients were sampled at random without replacement from the 6 strata, with the sampling from each stratum conducted independently (stratified sampling) and with higher probability in the more informative strata according to an optimal design [13]. The full cohort of 1999 patients represents the phase I sample, for which clinical information are available, while genotype is ascertained in the phase II sample only ($n = 601$).

Relapses were classified according to the site, in particular we distinguished relapses involving bone-marrow (BM) from the others (extramedullary). We estimated the crude incidence of BM relapse by GST-T1 deletion using (6) and (10) and found higher relapse incidence for patients with GST-T1 deletion, with 5-year crude incidence of 19.3 % (95 % CI: 13.4 − 27.7 %) versus 12.4 % (95 % CI: 10.7 − 14.4 % for non deleted patients, Fig. 4 panel a).

This was derived accounting for the competing risk of other sites of relapse as well as for death due to toxicity.

We report here the R code used to compute these estimates:

```
library(survey)
d.std<-twophase(id=list(~upn,~upn),
subset=~!is.na(GST_T),strata=list
(NULL,~interaction(rel,elfin)),data=dat)
GSTse<-svycr(Surv(time,event>0)~GST_T,
etype="BMrelapse",d.std,se=TRUE)
```

The `twophase` function in the `survey` package describes the design and produces a survey object [32]. The `svycr` function, available at [33], performs the estimate of crude incidence by the influence approach and uses 3 variables: `time` is the time of event, `event` the censoring indicator (1 if an event of any type is observed and 0 otherwise) and `BMrelapse` indicates whether a BM relapse is observed or not. Details on the `survey` package can be found in [7, 32].

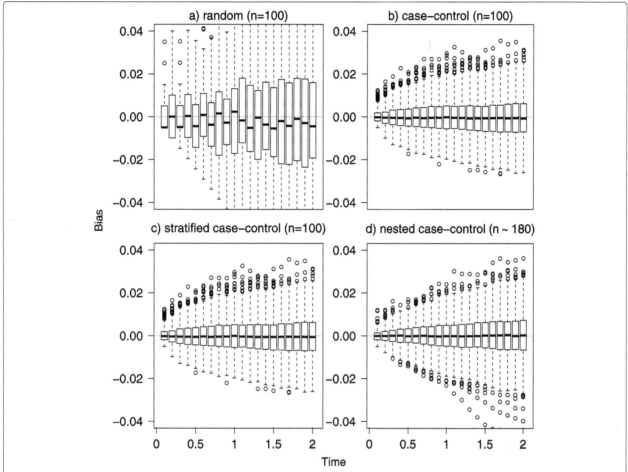

Fig. 2 Bias distribution. Distribution of bias in the 1000 simulated samples under random (panel **a**), case-control (panel **b**), stratified (panel **c**) and nested case control sampling ($m = 1$, panel **d**). For the first three scenarios a sample size of 100 was used, while in the nested case-control sampling a mean of 180 subjects was considered. Data were subject to a random censoring of 15 % (over administrative censoring). The box represent the first and third quartile, the black line the median and the empty dots represent outliers defined as bias more than 1.5 times the interquartile range above the third quartile (or more than 1.5 times the interquartile range below the first quartile). Dotted lines represent the reference for bias (bias equal to 0)

The right panel of Fig. 4 represents the incidence of extramedullary relapses by GST-T1 showing that the difference in relapse incidence between GST-T1 deleted and other patients is mainly due to relapse involving the BM, that represents the most relevant type of relapse in childhood ALL. A Cox model adapted for two-phase design [14], when applied to the cause specific hazard of BM relapse, gives an hazard ratio (HR) of 1.53 (95 % CI 0.98–2.37) for GST-T1 deleted patients versus non deleted; after adjusting for relevant factors (treatment protocol, gender, age), the HR dropped to 1.38 (95 % CI 0.90–2.13). For extramedullary relapses the HR was 1.22 (95 % CI 0.60–2.49). Of note, in order to compare patients with and without deletion of the GST-T1 gene, we used a cause-specific model, thus we actually compared the cause-specific hazard of relapse. In fact, a subdistribution model accounting for the two-phase design is not available. This would be useful to compare the actual incidences of relapse in the two groups, however the cause-specific model is still very useful to address the impact of the genotype on relapse by an aetiological point of view.

Outcome ascertained on a subset of patients lost to follow-up
In the evaluation of the effectiveness of the global effort to provide antiretroviral therapy (ART) for HIV-infected patients in resource limited settings, the estimate of the number of patients who continue to access care after starting ART is essential. This estimate is hampered, however, by the fact that some patients die shortly after their last visit to clinic - a group of individuals who cannot be considered as "stopping care" nor censored for the event of stopping care. In addition, the number of patients who are starting care is large and a high fraction have unknown outcomes (i.e., are lost to follow-up), generating informative censoring. Given that lost patients could reasonably be not in care, but they could also have changed clinic or

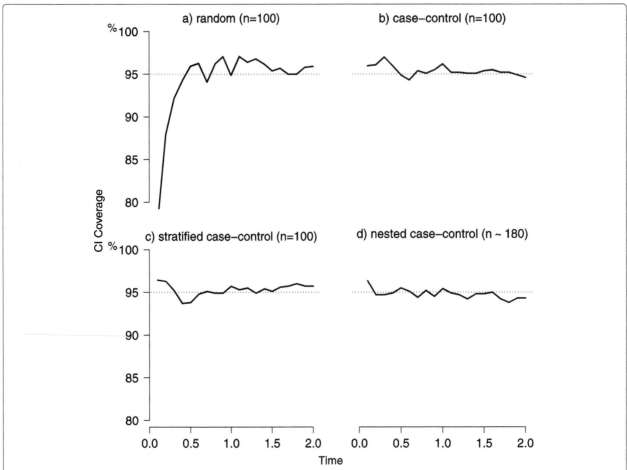

Fig. 3 Coverage of confidence intervals. Simulation results for the coverage of confidence intervals (CI) under random (panel **a**), case-control (panel **b**), stratified (panel **c**) and nested case-control sampling ($m = 1$, panel **d**). For the first three scenarios a sample size of 100 was used, while in the nested case control sampling a mean of 180 subjects was considered. Data were subject to a random censoring of 15 % (over administrative censoring). Dotted lines represent the reference for CI coverage (nominal 95 %)

be dead, one approach to obtain outcomes estimates has been to identify a numerically small, but random, sample of those who are lost [15], intensively seeking their outcomes, and using them to correct outcomes among the lost.

Table 1 Distribution of phase I (N_s) and II (n_s) samples in the 6 strata and sampling fractions expressed as percentages in parenthesis for Phase II

	Treatment protocol			
	Standard	Medium	High	
		n_s/N_s (%)		Total
No relapse	54/487 (11.1)	193/987 (19.6)	109/219 (49.8)	356/1693
Relapse	21/28 (75.0)	147/186 (79.0)	77/92 (83.7)	245/306
Total	75/515	340/1173	186/311	601/1999

To illustrate, a cohort of 13,321 HIV-infected adult patients, who initiated ART treatment, were followed from ART initiation to either death, disengagement or administrative database closure (see Fig. 5). Among them, 2451 patients were lost to follow-up [35], defined as not being seen at the clinic for at least 90 days (after the last return visit). A tracker went into the community to determine the outcome of a random subsample of 428 among the 2451 lost patients and got information on 306 patients (110 patient were found to be in care in other clinics, 80 died while in care and 116 were found to be not treated/disengaged) [12]. The 10,870 patients no lost to follow-up and the 306 tracked patients can been considered as the second phase sample of the whole cohort, stratified on lost to follow-up.

We used the methods developed in the Methods section to estimate crude cumulative incidence, where the 306 tracked patients represented the 2451 lost patients by the

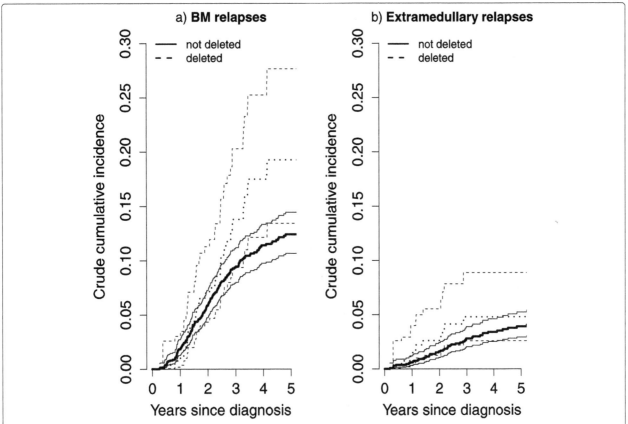

Fig. 4 Crude cumulative incidence of relapse in ALL data. Panel **a** reports the crude cumulative incidence estimate of relapse involving the bone marrow in patients with normal (estimate and confidence limits reported with solid lines) and deleted (dashed lines) GST-T1 gene. Panel **b** reports the crude cumulative incidence estimate of relapse in extramedullary sites in patients with normal (solid lines) and deleted (dashed lines) GST-T1 gene

sampling probability 306/2451, while the other 10,870 had sampling weight one. The crude incidence estimate of disengagement is reported in Fig. 6, the curve starts to rise after 90 days from ART start, that is the earliest possible time of disengagement, by definition. At 1 year, disengagement resulted 6.8 % (CI 95 % 5.7–8.2 %). This was subject to a strong influence of the competing event death in care that resulted 7.7 % (CI 95 % 6.8–8.9 %) at 1 year. A naïve (but less expensive) approach to deal with informative censoring would be to treat all lost patients as events or, contrarily, as censored observations. We plotted the two corresponding curves in Fig. 6, obtaining estimates of crude incidence at 1 year since ART treatment of 18.5 % and 0.2 %, respectively. We can consider that the true incidence will lie between these two estimates (that are however quite far in this context), as in fact it does

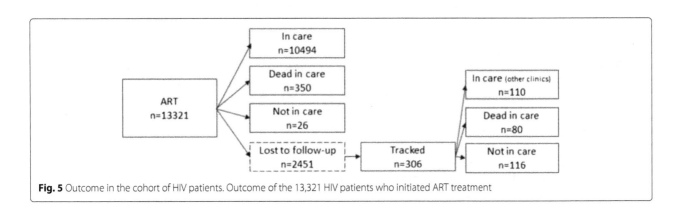

Fig. 5 Outcome in the cohort of HIV patients. Outcome of the 13,321 HIV patients who initiated ART treatment

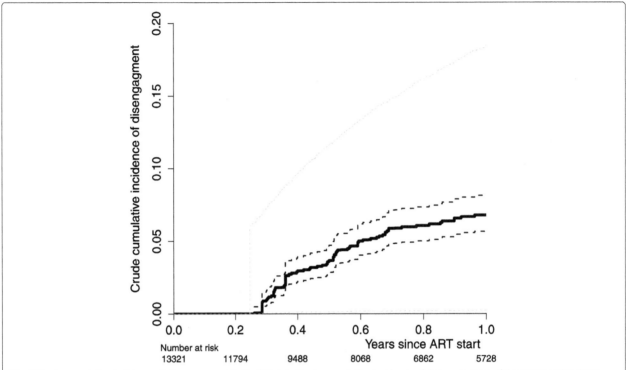

Fig. 6 Crude cumulative incidence of disengagement in the HIV data. Crude cumulative incidence of disengagement of the 13,321 HIV patients who initiated ART treatment (black line) with confidence intervals (dashed lines). In the bottom part of the plot the number of patients at risk in time is reported (weighed to represent the whole cohort of 13,321). The dashed grey lines report the crude cumulative incidence of disengagement computed by treating all lost patients as event or censored observation, respectively

the estimate we got by tracking a random sample of lost patients and using the proposed estimator.

Availability of supporting data

The R code to compute the proposed estimate of crude cumulative incidence is available at [33]. The results of simulations presented in the Simulations section and the related code are also available at [33].

Conclusions

We have derived an estimator for cumulative incidence of events based on the subdistribution hazard accounting for competing risks under a general sampling design from an infinite target population. The estimator shows good performance in simulations under different scenarios and the variance, derived by the influence function of the subdistribution hazard and the Horvitz-Thompson theory, was very close to the empirical variance, therefore we expect it to be very close to the one obtainable by replicate weights (e.g. bootstrap) [7]. Confidence intervals, derived on the log scale, provided good coverage in simulations, but alternative confidence intervals might also be considered such as the complementary log-log transformation [36]. The proposed estimator was used to estimate incidence of relapse by genotype in a cohort of childhood ALL patients,

where the genotype was ascertained only on a subsample of the cohort chosen by an optimal sampling approach based on relapse as the event of interest. Interestingly, we can also analyze the incidence of the competing event (toxic death) or of the combined endpoint (relapse or toxic death), but the efficiency could be lower unless the sub-sampling is adapted to this new endpoint by including a further strata on toxic death in the sampling process. This is particularly important since toxic death is a rare event in this context. We should also remember to avoid random sampling when the event of interest is rare, as discussed in the Simulations section.

In the second case, we dealt with a missing data problem, in which the outcome itself was not available for everybody, since some patients were lost to follow-up. A subsample of lost patients had been tracked to ascertain the outcome, but if this tracking was not possible, a more basic/naïve approach to deal with this informative censoring could have been to identify the variables affecting missingness, post-stratify the sample in homogeneous strata and use the missing probabilities for each strata as sort of sampling weights to adjust the incidence estimate. This approach would make an important assumption of missing at random that might be not appropriate and cannot be tested [7, 15, 21, 37]. However this underlines how the proposed estimator could be applied also in the presence of missing data.

The code to compute this estimate has been developed in R software [31] under the `survey` package [32] and is available at [33]. The survey package is a flexible package for complex surveys including also two-phase studies. It provides flexible functions to describe the design of the study and to derive sampling fraction accordingly. The package includes functions to estimate survival and to perform a weighted Cox model with standard error properly adjusted for the design and with the possibility to use general weights, as calibrated weights. Our function takes advantage of the facilities of the package (see an example of use in Genotype ascertained on a subset of a clinical trial cohort).

In order to recover the representativeness of the sub-cohort (phase II) for the entire cohort, we used weights related to the inverse of the probability to be sampled, similarly to the weights of Barlow for case-cohort studies [38]. More general weights can be used, such as calibration weights [7, 39, 40]. The use of calibration weights is advantageous when there is availability of phase I variables that are strongly related to the additional variables ascertained in phase II. This would provide results more representative of phase I data and increase precision. When phase II variables are common genetic polymorphisms, as in our first example, it is unlikely to find any strong relation between phase I and II variables, therefore no big advantage would be expected by calibration.

The estimator can also be extended to a situation where an individual may move among a finite number of states to estimate the Aalen-Johansen probabilities of transition among each state in a multistate framework [41] in the presence of general sampling design.

In order to derive a model-based estimate of incidence (adjusted for possible covariates) two main approaches have been followed in the context of competing risk, the first one based on the cause-specific hazard inspired by Benichou and Gail [16, 42, 43] and the other one based on the subdistribution hazard [19, 44]. The crude cumulative estimator developed by Kovalchik and Pfeiffer [45] for two-phase studies for finite population follows the first approach, and the Cox model for two-phase designs [14] could be used to extend it for infinite population. Under this model we can estimate the effect of a covariate on the cause-specific hazard to address its impact on the event by an aetiological point of view. However it is well known that this does not reflect the impact of the variable on the crude cumulative incidence. The latter effect, even if affected by the incidence of the other competing events, could still be of interest for a public health prospective. Future work will concern the development of a regression model to assess the effect of a covariate on the crude cumulative incidence. The Fine and Gray regression model [19] could be extended to complex sampling by weighting the estimating function of the parameter of interest and working out their influence function.

A   Appendix

A.1   Derivation of the risk set for T_k^*

The risk set for the usual survival time T at s is commonly obtained in standard analysis by counting the observed times greater then s. It can be also written as:

$$\hat{Y}.(s) = \hat{P}(T > s^-)\hat{P}(C > s^-) = \hat{Y}.(0)\hat{S}(s^-)\hat{G}(s^-) \quad (12)$$

where $\hat{G}(s)$ is the probability to be free of censoring up to s and is estimated considering censored observations as events and viceversa according to (3). This can proved also in the case of a two-phase design by the following:

$$\hat{Y}.(0)\hat{S}(s^-) \cdot \hat{G}(s^-) = \hat{Y}.(0) \prod_{u<s}\left[1 - \frac{\hat{N}..(du)}{\hat{Y}.(u)}\right] \cdot$$

$$\prod_{u<s}\left[1 - \frac{\hat{N}^c(du)}{\hat{Y}.(u) - \hat{N}..(du)}\right] =$$

$$= \hat{Y}.(0) \prod_{u<s}\left[\frac{\hat{Y}.(u) - [\hat{N}..(du) + \hat{N}^c(du)]}{\hat{Y}.(u)}\right] =$$

$$= \hat{Y}.(0) \prod_{u<s}\frac{\hat{Y}.(u^+)}{\hat{Y}.(u)} = \frac{\hat{Y}.(0)\hat{Y}.(s)}{\hat{Y}.(0)} =$$

$$= \sum_{i=1}^{N}[\xi_i Y_i(s)/\pi_i]$$

$$(13)$$

where $\hat{N}^c(t) = \sum_{i=1}^{N}[\xi_i I(X_i \le t, \Delta_i = 0)/\pi_i]$ denotes the number of censoring up to time t and $\hat{N}..(t) = \sum_{i=1}^{n}\hat{N}_i.(t)$ the total count of events observed up to time t.

The derivation of the risk set for T_k^* at s can be obtained by:

$$\hat{Y}^*_{.k}(s) = \hat{P}\left(T_k^* > s^-\right)\hat{P}(C > s^-) = \hat{Y}.(0) \cdot \left[1 - \hat{F}_k(s^-)\right]\hat{G}(s^-) =$$

$$= \hat{Y}.(0) \cdot \left[\hat{S}(s^-) + \sum_{l \ne k}\hat{F}_l(s^-)\right] \cdot \hat{G}(s^-) =$$

$$= \hat{Y}.(s) + \hat{Y}.(0) \cdot \sum_{l \ne k}\hat{F}_l(s^-) \cdot \hat{G}(s^-)$$

$$(14)$$

By writing $\hat{F}_l(s^-)$ as empirical cumulative distribution function $\hat{F}_l(s^-) = \frac{1}{\hat{Y}.(0)}\sum_{i=1}^{N}\frac{\xi_i}{\pi_i}\frac{I(X_i \le s^-; \varepsilon_i = l)}{\hat{G}(X_i^- \wedge s^-)}$ [25, 46], the risk set becomes:

$$\hat{Y}_{.k}^*(s) = \hat{Y}_{.}(s) + \sum_{l \neq k} \sum_{i=1}^{N} \frac{\xi_i}{\pi_i} I(X_i \leq s^-; \varepsilon_i = l) \frac{\hat{G}(s^-)}{\hat{G}(X_i^- \wedge s^-)}$$

$$(15)$$

that can be simplified to

$$\sum_{i=1}^{N} \frac{\xi_i}{\pi_i} Y_i(s) + \sum_{i=1}^{N} \frac{\xi_i}{\pi_i} \left[\sum_{l \neq k} N_{il}(s^-) \cdot \hat{G}\left(s^- | X_i^-\right) \right] \quad (16)$$

that is equivalent to (4).

The first summation estimates the usual total number of subjects at risk at s, where the condition $X_i = \min(T_i, C_i) \geq s$ is satisfied. This in fact implies $\min(T_{ki}^*, C_i) \geq s$, i.e. being at risk for T implies being also at risk for T_k^*. The second summation estimates the number of subjects who had other events before s, satisfying the condition $X_i = \min(T_i, C_i) < s$, $\Delta_i = 1$ and $\varepsilon_i \neq k$ which implies $T_{ki}^* = \infty > s$ and completes the number at risk at s for T_k^*. While the first part is exposed to censoring, the contribute of each subject observed to fail of cause $l \neq k$, $\sum_{l \neq k} N_{il}(s^-)$, would remain equal to 1 up to ∞, thus ignoring possible censoring, given that C_i is (usually) not observable if $T_i < C_i$. A possible way to deal with this inconsistency is to mimic the presence of random censoring acting on the infinite times, by weighting the unitary contributions $\sum_{l \neq k} N_{il}(s^-)$ by the estimate $\hat{G}(s^- | X_i^-)$ of $P(C > s^- | C > X_i^-) = G(s^- | X_i)$, where $G(t) = P(C > t)$ is estimated by $\hat{G}(t) = \prod_{s \leq t} \left[1 - \frac{\sum_{i=1}^{N} \xi_i N_i^c(ds)/\pi_i}{\sum_{i=1}^{N} \xi_i Y_i(s)/\pi_i} \right]$, with $N_i^c(s) = I(X_i \leq s, \Delta_i = 0)$. This weight assumes value 1 before X_i and decreases afterword according to the censoring distribution.

Of note, an alternative expression for $\hat{Y}_{.k}^*(s)$ derives substituting $\hat{Y}_{.}(0)\hat{G}(s^-) = \frac{\hat{Y}_{.}(s)}{\hat{S}(s^-)}$ from (12) in (14):

$$\hat{Y}_{.k}^*(s) = \hat{Y}_{.}(0)\hat{G}(s^-) \cdot \left[1 - \hat{F}_k(s^-) \right] = \hat{Y}_{.}(s) \frac{\left[1 - \hat{F}_k(s^-) \right]}{\hat{S}(s^-)}$$

$$(17)$$

This shows as $\hat{Y}_{.}(s)$ is upweighted by a multiplier that gets greater as the action of competing events gets larger, accounting for the fact that subjects that experienced events of type $l \neq k$ will never experience event k as first.

A.2   Proof of equivalence (7)

The equality between the cumulative incidence of the artificial variable T^* in (6) and the Aalen-Johansen type estimator (that for the purpose of this proof will be denoted as $\hat{F}_k^{AJ}(t)$) holds true if and only if, $\forall t$:

$$\hat{F}_k^{AJ}(t) = \int_0^t \hat{S}(s^-)\hat{\Lambda}_k(ds) = 1 - \prod_{s \leq t} \left[1 - \hat{\Lambda}_k^*(ds) \right] = \hat{F}_k(t)$$

$$(18)$$

which can be proved by induction. Both quantities are step functions, changing value at each occurrence of type k events. At the time t where the first event of type k is observed, $\hat{\Lambda}_k(dt) = \hat{\Lambda}_k^*(dt)$ being from (4) $\hat{Y}_{.}(t) = \hat{Y}_{.k}^*(t)$. If this was the first event overall, then $\hat{S}(0) = 1$ and Eq. 18 is satisfied, otherwise $\hat{F}_k^{AJ}(t) = [1 - 1/\hat{Y}_{.}(0)] \cdot 1/[\hat{Y}_{.}(0) - 1] = 1/\hat{Y}_{.}(0) = 1 - [1 - 1/\hat{Y}_{.}(0)] = \hat{F}_k(t)$.

Now, assuming that (18) holds true for a given t^-, this implies $\hat{F}_k^{AJ}(t) = \hat{F}_k(t)$ if and only if, from (18):

$$\hat{F}_k^{AJ}(t^-) + \hat{S}(t^-)\hat{\Lambda}_k(dt) = 1 - (1 - \hat{F}_k(t^-)) \left(1 - \hat{\Lambda}_k^*(dt) \right)$$

and using the equality at t^-:

$$\hat{F}_k(t^-) + \hat{S}(t^-)\hat{\Lambda}_k(dt) = \hat{F}_k(t^-) + \left[1 - \hat{F}_k(t^-) \right] \hat{\Lambda}_k^*(dt)$$

$$\hat{S}(t^-)\hat{\Lambda}_k(dt) = \left[1 - \hat{F}_k(t^-) \right] \hat{\Lambda}_k^*(dt)$$

$$\hat{\Lambda}_k(dt) = \frac{1 - \hat{F}_k(t^-)}{\hat{S}(t^-)} \hat{\Lambda}_k^*(dt)$$

$$\frac{\hat{N}_k(dt)}{\hat{Y}_{.}(t)} = \frac{1 - \hat{F}_k(t^-)}{\hat{S}(t^-)} \frac{\hat{N}_k(dt)}{\hat{Y}_{.k}^*(t)}$$

$$\hat{Y}_{.k}^*(t) = \hat{Y}_{.}(t) \cdot \frac{1 - \hat{F}_k(t^-)}{\hat{S}(t^-)}$$

That is proved by (17).

A.3   Weak convergence of $\hat{\Lambda}_k^*(t)$

Lin showed that the normalised Horvitz-Thompson estimators of the number of events $\sqrt{N}\left[\hat{N}_{.}(t) - N_{.}(t) \right]$, number at risk $\sqrt{N}\left[\hat{Y}_{.}(t) - Y_{.}(t) \right]$, cumulative hazard $\sqrt{N}[\hat{\Lambda}(t) - \Lambda(t)]$ and survival function $\sqrt{N}\left[\hat{S}(t) - S(t) \right]$ (and analogously $\sqrt{N}\left[\hat{G}(t) - G(t) \right]$) are asymptotically multivariate zero-mean normal [14]. Firstly, we concentrate on the normalised Horvitz-Thompson estimators of the modified at risk process: $\sqrt{N}\left[\hat{Y}_{.k}^*(t) - Y_{.k}^*(t) \right] = \sqrt{N} \sum_{i=1}^{N} \frac{\xi_i - \pi_i}{\pi_i} Y_{.k}^*(t) = \sqrt{N} \sum_{i=1}^{N} \frac{\xi_i - \pi_i}{\pi_i} Y_{.k}(t) + \sqrt{N} \sum_{i=1}^{N} \frac{\xi_i - \pi_i}{\pi_i} \sum_{l \neq k} N_{il}(t^-)\hat{G}(t^- | X_i)$. The first term represents the estimator of the number at risk, that Lin showed to be asymptotically multivariate zero-mean normal [14]. We concentrate now on the second term:

$$\sqrt{N} \sum_{i=1}^{N} \left[\frac{\xi_i}{\pi_i} \cdot \sum_{l \neq k} N_{il}(t^-) \hat{G}(t^-|X_i) - \sum_{l \neq k} N_{il}(t^-) \hat{G}(t^-|X_i) \right] =$$

$$= \sqrt{N} \sum_{i=1}^{N} \left[\hat{G}(t^-|X_i) \left\{ \frac{\xi_i}{\pi_i} \sum_{l \neq k} N_{il}(t^-) - \sum_{l \neq k} N_{il}(t^-) \right\} \right] =$$

$$= \sqrt{N} \left[\hat{G}(t^-|X_i) \left\{ \sum_{l \neq k} \hat{N}_{\cdot l}(t^-) - \sum_{l \neq k} \sum_{i=1}^{N} N_{il}(t^-) \right\} \right] =$$

$$= \sqrt{N} \int_0^{t^-} \hat{G}(s^-|X_i) \left\{ \sum_{l \neq k} \hat{N}_{\cdot l}(ds-) - \sum_{l \neq k} \sum_{i=1}^{N} N_{il}(ds^-) \right\} =$$

$$= \sqrt{N} \int_0^{t^-} G(t^-|X_i) \left\{ \sum_{l \neq k} \hat{N}_{\cdot l}(ds-) - \sum_{l \neq k} \sum_{i=1}^{N} N_{il}(ds^-) \right\} +$$

$$+ o_p(1)$$

that using Lemma 1 in [14] also converges to a zero-mean Gaussian process.

We want to prove that also $\sqrt{N} \left[\hat{\Lambda}_k^*(t) - \Lambda_k^*(t) \right] = \sqrt{N} \left[\tilde{\Lambda}_k^*(t) - \Lambda_k^*(t) \right] + \sqrt{N} \left[\hat{\Lambda}_k^*(t) - \tilde{\Lambda}_k^*(t) \right]$ converges to a zero-mean normal, where $\tilde{\Lambda}_k^*(t)$ represents the crude cumulative incidence estimator that we would have obtained if complete information $(X_i, \Delta_i \varepsilon_i, Z_i)$ was known for all the subjects in phase I sample $(i = 1 \ldots N)$ [18]. Fine and Gray proved that the first term converges weakly to a zero-mean Gaussian process [19].

The second term results:

$$\sqrt{N} \left[\hat{\Lambda}_k^*(t) - \tilde{\Lambda}_k^*(t) \right] = \sqrt{N} \left[\int_0^t \frac{\hat{N}_k(ds)}{\hat{Y}_{\cdot k}^*(s)} - \int_0^t \frac{N_k(ds)}{Y_{\cdot k}^*(s)} \right] =$$

$$= \sqrt{N} \left[\int_0^t \frac{\hat{N}_k(ds)}{\hat{Y}_{\cdot k}^*(s)} - \int_0^t \frac{N_k(ds)}{Y_{\cdot k}^*(s)} + \int_0^t \frac{N_k(ds)}{\hat{Y}_{\cdot k}^*(s)} - \int_0^t \frac{N_k(ds)}{\hat{Y}_{\cdot k}^*(s)} \right] =$$

$$= \sqrt{N} \left[\int_0^t \frac{\hat{N}_k(ds) - N_k(ds)}{\hat{Y}_{\cdot k}^*(s)} - \int_0^t \frac{N_k(ds) \left[\hat{Y}_{\cdot k}^*(s) - Y_{\cdot k}^*(s) \right]}{\hat{Y}_{\cdot k}^*(s) Y_{\cdot k}^*(s)} \right].$$

It then follows that also $\sqrt{N} \left[\hat{\Lambda}_k^*(t) - \tilde{\Lambda}_k^*(t) \right]$ converges weakly to a zero-mean Gaussian process.

A.4 Influence function for $\hat{\Lambda}_k^*(t)$

The estimator $\hat{\Lambda}_k^*(t)$ can be expressed as a differentiable function g of the estimated total number of events of type k and total number at risk for T^* up to t:

$$\hat{\Lambda}_k^*(t) = g(\hat{N}_{\cdot k}(dt), \hat{Y}_{\cdot k}^*(t)) = \int_0^t \frac{\hat{N}_{\cdot k}(ds)}{\hat{Y}_{\cdot k}^*(s)} =$$

$$= \int_0^t \frac{\sum_{i=1}^N \xi_i \cdot N_{ik}(ds) w_i}{\sum_{i=1}^N \xi_i \cdot Y_{ik}^*(s) w_i} \tag{19}$$

where $w_i = 1/\pi_i$ and ξ_i indicates whether subject i is withdrawn in the phase II sample.

The difference between the true and estimated cumulative hazard can be expressed as a sum of influence functions: $\hat{\Lambda}_k^*(t) - \Lambda_k^*(t) = \sum_{i=1}^N z_{ik}^* + o(1/\sqrt{N})$, where z_{ik}^* is the influence function of the ith subject. Demnati and Rao [27] proved that we can express the influence function of subject i as $z_{ik}^*(t) = \frac{\partial g\left(\hat{N}_{\cdot k}(dt), \hat{Y}_{\cdot k}^*(t) \right)}{\partial w_i}$. The influence function of $\hat{\Lambda}_k^*(t)$ of the ith subject can thus be derived as:

$$z_{ik}^*(t) = \int_0^t \frac{N_{ik}(ds) \hat{Y}_{\cdot k}^*(s) - \frac{\partial \hat{Y}_{\cdot k}^*(s)}{\partial w_i} \hat{N}_{\cdot k}(ds)}{\hat{Y}_{\cdot k}^*(s)^2} \tag{20}$$

Being $\hat{Y}_{\cdot k}^*(s) = \sum_{i=1}^N \xi_i w_i \cdot \left[Y_i(s) + \frac{I(X_i \leq s^-; \varepsilon_i \neq k) \hat{G}(s^-)}{\hat{G}(X_i^- \wedge s^-)} \right]$ and being $\hat{G}(s) = \prod_{u \leq s} \left[1 - \frac{\sum_{i=1}^N \xi_i N_i^c(du)/\pi_i}{\sum_{i=1}^N \xi_i Y_i(u)/\pi_i} \right]$, the derivative of $\hat{Y}_{\cdot k}^*(s)$ with respect to w_i results:

$$\frac{\partial \hat{Y}_{\cdot k}^*(s)}{\partial w_i} = \frac{\partial \left\{ \xi_i w_i \cdot \left[Y_i(s) + \frac{I(X_i \leq s^-; \varepsilon_i \neq k) \hat{G}(s^-)}{\hat{G}(X_i^- \wedge s^-)} \right] + \sum_{j \neq i} \xi_j w_j \cdot \left[Y_j(s) + \frac{I(X_j \leq s^-; \varepsilon_j \neq k) \hat{G}(s^-)}{\hat{G}(X_j^- \wedge s^-)} \right] \right\}}{\partial w_i} =$$

$$= \xi_i Y_i(s) + \xi_i \frac{\partial \left[w_i \frac{I(X_i \leq s^-; \varepsilon_i \neq k) \hat{G}(s^-)}{\hat{G}(X_i^- \wedge s^-)} \right]}{\partial w_i} + \frac{\partial \left[\sum_{j \neq i} \frac{\xi_j w_j I(X_j \leq s^-; \varepsilon_j \neq k) \hat{G}(s^-)}{\hat{G}(X_j^- \wedge s^-)} \right]}{\partial w_i} = \tag{21}$$

$$= \xi_i Y_i(s) + \xi_i \frac{I(X_i \leq s^-; \varepsilon_i \neq k) \hat{G}(s^-)}{\hat{G}(X_i^- \wedge s^-)} + \sum_{j=1}^N \xi_j w_j I(X_j \leq s^-; \varepsilon_j \neq k) \frac{\partial}{\partial w_i} \left[\frac{\hat{G}(s^-)}{\hat{G}(X_j^- \wedge s^-)} \right].$$

Please note that the last addendum accounts for the fact that $\hat{G}(t)$ is estimated using information of subject i. For $v \leq u$:

$$\frac{\partial}{\partial w_i}\left[\frac{\hat{G}(u)}{\hat{G}(v)}\right] = \frac{\hat{G}(u)\int_0^u \frac{dN_i^c(s)-\hat{\lambda}^c(s)Y_i(s)}{\hat{Y}_\cdot(s)}\hat{G}(v) - \hat{G}(v)\int_0^v \frac{dN_i^c(s)-\hat{\lambda}^c(s)Y_i(s)}{\hat{Y}_\cdot(s)}\hat{G}(u)}{\hat{G}(v)^2} =$$

$$= \frac{\hat{G}(u)\hat{G}(v)\int_{v+}^u \frac{dN_i^c(s)-\hat{\lambda}^c(s)Y_i(s)}{\hat{Y}_\cdot(s)}}{\hat{G}(v)^2} = \frac{\hat{G}(u)\int_{v+}^u \frac{dN_i^c(s)-\hat{\lambda}^c(s)Y_i(s)}{\hat{Y}_\cdot(s)}}{\hat{G}(v)}$$

(22)

where the superscript c indicates the quantities related to the censoring process, i.e. $N_i^c(u) = I(X_i \leq u, \Delta_i = 0)$ is the indicator of censoring for subject i up to time u and $\hat{\lambda}^c(u) = \hat{N}_\cdot^c(du)/\hat{Y}_\cdot(u)$ the instantaneous hazard of censoring. The derivative of $\hat{Y}_{\cdot k}^*(u)$ becomes:

$$\frac{\partial \hat{Y}_{\cdot k}^*(s)}{\partial w_i} =$$

$$Y_i(s) + I(X_i \leq s^-; \varepsilon_i \neq k) \cdot \frac{\hat{G}(s^-)}{\hat{G}\left(X_i^- \wedge s^-\right)} + \sum_{j=1}^N \xi_j w_j I(X_j \leq s^-; \varepsilon_j \neq k)\frac{\hat{G}(s^-)}{\hat{G}\left(X_j^- \wedge s^-\right)}\left[\int_{X_j}^{s^-} \frac{N_i^c(du)-\hat{\lambda}^c(u)Y_i(u)}{\hat{Y}_\cdot(u)}\right]$$

(23)

Thus, the influence function of $\hat{\Lambda}_k^*(t)$ of the ith subject results:

$$z_{ik}^*(t) = \int_0^t \frac{N_{ik}(ds)\hat{Y}_{\cdot k}^*(s) - \hat{N}_{\cdot k}(ds)\left[Y_i(s) + \frac{I(X_i \leq s^-;\varepsilon_i \neq k)\hat{G}(s^-)}{\hat{G}(X_i^- \wedge s^-)} + \sum_{j=1}^N \frac{\xi_j w_j I(X_j \leq s^-;\varepsilon_j \neq k)\hat{G}(s^-)}{\hat{G}(X_j^- \wedge s^-)}\int_{X_j}^{s^-}\frac{N_i^c(du)-\hat{\lambda}^c(u)Y_i(u)}{\hat{Y}_\cdot(s)}\right]}{\hat{Y}_{\cdot k}^*(s)^2} =$$

$$= \int_0^t \frac{N_{ik}(ds) - \hat{\Lambda}_k^*(ds)\left[Y_i(s) + \frac{I(X_i \leq s^-;\varepsilon_i \neq k)\hat{G}(s^-)}{\hat{G}(X_i^- \wedge s^-)} + \sum_{j=1}^N \frac{\xi_j I(X_j \leq s^-;\varepsilon_j \neq k)\hat{G}(s^-)}{\pi_j \hat{G}(X_j^- \wedge s^-)}\int_{X_j}^{s^-}\frac{N_i^c(du)-\hat{\lambda}^c(u)Y_i(u)}{\hat{Y}_\cdot(u)}\right]}{\hat{Y}_{\cdot k}^*(s)}$$

(24)

where $w_j = 1/\pi_j$. By defining $M_i^c(s,t) = \int_s^t \frac{N_i^c(du)-\hat{\lambda}^c(u)Y_i(u)}{\hat{Y}_\cdot(u)}$ as the influence function of subject i on censoring, $v_j = \frac{\xi_j}{\pi_j}\sum_{l \neq k} N_{jl}(s^-)\hat{G}(s^-|X_j^-)$, and $M_{ik}(s) = \left[N_{ik}(s) - \hat{\Lambda}_k^*(s)Y_{ik}^*(s)\right]/\hat{Y}_{\cdot k}^*(s)$.
Thus it can be reduced as:

$$z_{ik}^*(t) = \int_0^t \frac{N_{ik}(ds) - \hat{\Lambda}_k^*(ds)Y_{ik}^*(s) - \hat{\Lambda}_k^*(ds)\left[\sum_{j=1}^N \frac{\xi_j}{\pi_j}\sum_{l \neq k} N_{jl}(s^-)\hat{G}\left(s^-|X_j^-\right)M_i^c\left(X_j,s^-\right)\right]}{\hat{Y}_{\cdot k}^*(s)} =$$

$$= \int_0^t M_{ik}(ds) - \frac{\hat{\Lambda}_k^*(ds)\left[\sum_{j=1}^N v_j M_i^c\left(X_j,s^-\right)\right]}{\hat{Y}_{\cdot k}^*(s)}$$

Abbreviations

ALL: Acute lymphoblastic leukemia; ART: Antiretroviral therapy; BM: Bone-marrow; CI: Confidence interval; GST-T1: Glutathione S-transferase-θ; HR: Hazard ratio.

Competing interests

The authors declare that they have no competing interests.

Authors' contributions

PR performed the theoretical derivation, analyses and simulation studies and drafted the manuscript. LA, DVG, MGV contributed to the analyses and to the manuscript. All authors read and approved the final manuscript.

Acknowledgements

The authors thank Thomas Lumley for useful comments, Raffaella Franca and Marco Rabusin for the ALL data and Jeff Martin and Elvin Geng for the HIV data. PR was supported by the grant SIR RBSI14LOVD of the Italian Ministry of Education, University and Research. This research was partially supported by AIRC (2013-14634, MGV) and by NIH (U01 AI069911).

Author details

[1]Center of Biostatistics for Clinical Epidemiology, School of Medicine and Surgery, University of Milano-Bicocca, via Cadore 48, 20900 Monza, Italy. [2]Department of Epidemiology and Biostatistics, University of California, San Francisco, California.

References

1. Neyman J. Contribution to the theory of sampling human populations. J Am Stat Assoc. 1938;33(201):101–16.
2. Borgan Ø, Samuelsen SO. A review of cohort sampling designs for Cox's regression model: Potentials in epidemiology. Norsk Epidemiol. 2003;13: 239–48.
3. Prentice RL. A case-cohort design for epidemiologic cohort studies and disease prevention trials. Biometrika. 1986;73(1):1–11.
4. Samuelsen SO. A psudolikelihood approach to analysis of nested case-control studies. Biometrika. 1997;84(2):379–94.
5. Langholz B, Borgan Ø. Counter-matching: a stratified nested case-control sampling method. Biometrika. 1995;82(1):69–79.
6. Rudolph KE, Gary SW, Stuart EA, Glass TA, Marques AH, Duncko R, et al. The association between cortisol and neighborhood disadvantage in a US population-based sample of adolescents. Health Place. 2014;25:68–77.
7. Lumley TS. Complex Surveys: A Guide to Analysis Using R. 1st ed. Inc JWS, editor. Wiley Series in Survey Methodology. Hoboken, New Jersey: John Wiley & Sons; 2010.
8. Breslow N, Lumley T, Ballantyne C, Chambless L, Kulich M. Using the Whole Cohort in the Analysis of Case-Cohort Data. Am J Epidemiol. 2009;169(11):1398–405.
9. Anderson GL, Manson J, Wallace R, Lund B, Hall D, Davis S, et al. Implementation of the women's health Initiative study design. Ann Epidemiol. 2003;13(9, Supplement):S5–17.
10. Fried LP, Borhani NO, Enright P, Furberg CD, Gardin JM, Kronmal RA, et al. The Cardiovascular Health Study: design and rationale. Ann Epidemiol. 1991;1(3):263–76.
11. Franca R, Rebora P, Basso G, Biondi A, Cazzaniga G, Crovella S, et al. Glutathione S-transferase homozygous deletions and relapse in childhood acute lymphoblastic leukemia: a novel study design in a large Italian AIEOP cohort. Pharmacogenomics. 2012;13(16):1905–16.
12. Geng E, Emenyonu N, Bwana M, Glidden D, Martin J. Sampling-based approach to determining outcomes of patients lost to follow-up in antiretroviral therapy scale-up programs in Africa. JAMA. 2008;300(5): 506–7. Available from: http://dx.doi.org/10.1001/jama.300.5.506.
13. Rebora P, Valsecchi MG. Survival estimation in two-phase cohort studies with application to biomarkers evaluation. Stat Methods Med Res. 2014. in press. doi:10.1177/0962280214534411.
14. Lin DY. On fitting Cox's proportional hazards models to survey data. Biometrika. 2000;87(1):37–47.
15. Frangakis CE, Rubin DB. Addressing an idiosyncrasy in estimating survival curves using double sampling in the presence of self-selected right censoring. Biometrics. 2001;57(2):333–42.
16. Borgan Ø. Estimation of covariate-dependent Markov transition probabilities from nested case-control data. Stat Methods Med Res. 2002;11(2):183–202.
17. Aalen OO, Borgan Ø, Fekjær H. Covariate adjustment of event histories estimated from Markov chains: the additive approach. Biometrics. 2001;57(4):993–1001.
18. Gray RJ. A class of K-sample tests for comparing the cumulative incidence of a competing risk. The Annals of Statistics. 1988;16(3):1141–54.
19. Fine JP, Gray RJ. A proportional hazards model for the subdistribution of a competing risk. J Am Stat Assoc. 1999;94(446):496–509.
20. Antolini L, Biganzoli EM, Boracchi P. Crude cumulative incidence in the form of a Horvitz-Thompson like and Kaplan-Meier like estimator. COBRA Preprint Series. 2006. 10 http://biostats.bepress.com/cobra/art10.
21. Särndal C, Swensson B. A general view of estimation for two phases of selection with applications to two-phase sampling and nonresponse. Int Stat Rev. 1987;55(3):279–94.
22. Kang S, Cai J. Marginal hazards model for case-cohort studies with multiple disease outcomes. Biometrika. 2009;96(4):887–901.
23. Marubini E, Valsecchi MG. Analysing survival data from clinical trials and observational studies. Chichester, England: Wiley-Interscience; 2004.
24. Bernasconi D, Antolini L. Description of survival data extended to the case of competing risks: a teaching approach based on frequency tables. Epidemiol Biostat Public Heal. 2013;11(1):. e8874–1:e8874–10.
25. Satten GA, Datta S. The Kaplan-Meier estimator as an inverse-probability-of-censoring weighted average. Am Stat. 2001;55(3): 207–10.
26. Breslow NE, Wellner JA. Weighted likelihood for semiparametric models and two-phase stratified samples, with application to cox regression. Scand J Stat. 2007;34(1):86–102.
27. Demnati A, Rao JNK. Linearization variance estimators for model parameters from complex survey data. Surv Methodol. 2010;36:193–201.
28. Breslow NE, Lumley T, Ballantyne CM, Chambless LE, Kulich M. Improved Horvitz–Thompson estimation of model parameters from two-phase stratified samples: applications in epidemiology. Stat Biosci. 2009;1(1):32–49.
29. Horvitz DG, Thompson DJ. A generalization of sampling without replacement from a finite universe. J Am Stat Assoc. 1952;47(260):663–85.
30. de Wreede LC, Fiocco M, Putter H. mstate: An R Package for the Analysis of Competing Risks and Multi-State Models. J Stat Softw. 2011;38(7):1–30. Available from: http://www.jstatsoft.org/v38/i07/.
31. R Core Team. R: A Language and Environment for Statistical Computing. Vienna, Austria: R Foundation for Statistical Computing; 2014. Available from: http://www.R-project.org.
32. Lumley T. Analysis of complex survey samples. J Stat Softw. 2004;9(8):1–19.
33. Rebora P. R code to estimate crude incidence in two-phase designs. 2015. Accessed: 2015-10-27. http://dx.doi.org/10.6070/H4F18WRG.
34. Tsiatis AA. A nonidentifiability aspect of the problem of competing risks. Proc Natl Acad Sci U S A. 1975;72(1):20–2.
35. Geng EH, Glidden DV, Bwana MB, Musinguzi N, Emenyonu N, Muyindike W, et al. Retention in care and connection to care among HIV-infected patients on antiretroviral therapy in Africa: estimation via a sampling-based approach. PLoS One. 2011;e21797:7.
36. Glidden DV. Robust inference for event probabilities with Non-Markov event data. Biometrics. 2002;58(2):361–68.
37. Lin DY, Ying Z. Cox regression with incomplete covariate measurements. J Am Stat Assoc. 1993;88:1341–9.
38. Barlow W, Ichikawa L, Rosner D, Izum iS. Analysis of case-cohort designs. J Clin Epidemiol. 1999;52(12):1165–72.
39. Scott AJ, Wild CJ. Fitting regression models with response-biased samples. Can J Stat. 2011;39(3):519–36.
40. Rudolph KE, Diaz I, Rosenblum M, Stuart EA. Estimating population treatment effects from a survey sub-sample. Am J Epidemiol. 2014;180: 737–48.
41. Aalen OO, Johansen S. An empirical transition matrix for non-homogeneous Markov chains based on censored observations. Scand J Stat. 1978;5(3):141–50. Available from: http://www.jstor.org/stable/4615704.

42. Benichou J, Gail MH. Estimates of absolute cause-specific risk in cohort studies. Biometrics. 1990;46(3):813–26. Available from: http://www.jstor.org/stable/2532098.

43. Langholz B, Borgan Ø. Estimation of absolute risk from nested case-control data. Biometrics. 1997;53(2):767–74.

44. Wolkewitz M, Cooper BS, Palomar-Martinez M, Olaechea-Astigarraga P, Alvarez-Lerma F, Schumacher M. Nested case-control studies in cohorts with competing events. Epidemiology. 2014;25(1):122–5.

45. Kovalchik S, Pfeiffer R. Population-based absolute risk estimation with survey data. Lifetime Data Anal. 2014;20(2):252–75.

46. Jewell NP, Lei X, Ghani AC, Donnelly CA, Leung GM, Ho LM, et al. Non-parametric estimation of the case fatality ratio with competing risks data: an application to Severe Acute Respiratory Syndrome (SARS). Stat Med. 2007;26(9):1982–98.

Post cardiac arrest care and follow-up in Sweden – a national web-survey

Johan Israelsson[1,2,3*], Gisela Lilja[4,5], Anders Bremer[6,7], Jean Stevenson-Ågren[8,9] and Kristofer Årestedt[10,2]

Abstract

Background: Recent decades have shown major improvements in survival rates after cardiac arrest. However, few interventions have been tested in order to improve the care for survivors and their family members. In many countries, including Sweden, national guidelines for post cardiac arrest care and follow-up programs are not available and current practice has not previously been investigated. The aim of this survey was therefore to describe current post cardiac arrest care and follow-up in Sweden.

Methods: An internet based questionnaire was sent to the resuscitation coordinators at all Swedish emergency hospitals ($n = 74$) and 59 answers were received. Quantitative data were analysed with descriptive statistics and free text responses were analysed using manifest content analysis.

Results: Almost half of the hospitals in Sweden ($n = 27$, 46 %) have local guidelines for post cardiac arrest care and follow-up. However, 39 % of them reported that these guidelines were not always applied. The most common routine is a follow-up visit at a cardiac reception unit. If the need for neurological or psychological support are discovered the routines are not explicit. In addition, family members are not always included in the follow-up.

Conclusions: Although efforts are already made to improve post cardiac arrest care and follow-up, many hospitals need to focus more on this part of cardiac arrest treatment. In addition, evidence-based national guidelines will have to be developed and implemented in order to achieve a more uniform care and follow-up for survivors and their family members. This national survey highlights this need, and might be helpful in the implementation of such guidelines.

Keywords: Heart arrest, Survivors, Family members, Follow-up, Quality of life, Guidelines

Background

Every year, approximately 275 000 persons in Europe suffer from an out-of-hospital cardiac arrest (OHCA) [1] whereas the number of in-hospital cardiac arrest (IHCA) is not known. Recent decades have shown major improvements in survival rates and in Sweden more than 1 000 persons survive cardiac arrest (CA) annually [2]. Most CAs are caused by a cardiovascular disease [2] and survivors are at risk of suffering cardiac complications [3]. Survival may also be associated with neurological impairments due to the lack of oxygen to the brain at the time of the arrest. Severe brain injuries in survivors are uncommon but mild to moderate cognitive impairments, e.g., memory problems have been reported in as many as 30–50 % of the survivors [4, 5]. Additionally, psychological impairments may be present [6]. Surviving a life-threatening event such as CA will affect the lives of both survivors and their family members [7, 8]. Following a near death experience, survivors may become more aware of their vulnerability. Family members can be forced to confront feelings of unreality, uncertainty, hopelessness and, in addition, they can experience feelings of inadequacy and an overwhelming responsibility in the situation [7]. Moreover, patients and family members are at risk of psychological stress due to the critical illness *per se*. It is well-known that patients recovering from critical illness and intensive care are at risk for psychological problems such as anxiety, depression and post-traumatic stress disorders [9], which may affect the patient's ability to perform activities in everyday life and participate in society.

* Correspondence: johani@ltkalmar.se

[1]Department of Internal Medicine, Division of Cardiology, Kalmar County Hospital, SE-39185 Kalmar, Sweden

[2]Department of Medical and Health Sciences, Division of Nursing Science, Linköping University, SE-58185 Linköping, Sweden

Full list of author information is available at the end of the article

Psychological problems, cognitive dysfunction and difficulties in performing activities of daily life have been associated with decreased health among CA survivors [10]. A review article concludes that health and quality of life (QoL) among survivors appears to be acceptable or good, but also reports major variations between different studies and within study populations [11]. Some studies report that suffering a CA has negative effects on QoL, and that survivors have poorer QoL compared to a normal population [10, 12, 13]. Other studies have not been able to show any differences [14–16].

In order to address problems caused by CA and to support health among survivors and their family members, structured post CA care is needed. Today, national guidelines for post CA care and follow-up programs are not available in Sweden. The Swedish Resuscitation Council (SRC) has recommended an information package for survivors and their family members since 2011 [17]. This material contains information about CA in general and stories of experiencing CA, told by survivors and their family members, in particular. However, the success of the implementation is unknown. Patients suffering CA are often admitted to intensive care units (ICU) [2]. In Sweden, patients with critical illness in general participate in follow-ups performed by intensive care nurses post ICU discharge. However, these follow-ups have been described as varying extensively in design and not being available for all [18]. The goal of the ICU follow-up is to promote the patients' recovery by focusing on three domains: the past, the present and the future. The past aims to support patients' understanding, the present includes actual physical, cognitive and psychological status, and the future includes rehabilitation or other interventions to promote health. The last step has been the weakest point so far in Scandinavia [18], where other countries promote more structured guidelines for rehabilitation, as in the UK with the National Institute for Health and Clinical Excellence (NICE) guidelines [19]. Whether these ICU follow-ups include the majority of CA survivors is unknown.

Since cardiac etiology is common [2], CA survivors are likely to receive cardiovascular follow-up, primarily focused on physiological secondary prevention [20]. However, because they are at risk of also suffering neurological and emotional complications [5, 6], which might affect their QoL [10], specific care and follow-up is necessary [6, 21–23]. Previous research describing specific post CA care and follow-up is sparse [24–27]. In many countries, including Sweden, national guidelines for post CA care and follow-up programs are not available, and current practice has, to our knowledge, not previously been investigated. The aim of this survey was therefore to describe current post CA care and follow-up in Sweden.

Methods

Design

This national survey had a descriptive cross-sectional design. The overall theoretical rationale for this study was based on a perspective of health as a multidimensional concept. Health can be enhanced over time, through a process supported by health care, especially regarding the development of coping strategies and learning within the family. Nursing is viewed as a science of health-promoting interactions: to actively promote patient and family strengths, to help them cope with a life-changing event, and to achieve life goals [28]. The study was designed and conducted in accordance with the World Medical Association Declarations of Helsinki [29] and Swedish Ethics Legislation concerning informed consent and confidentiality [30]. Formal ethical approval was not required, according to ethics legislation in Sweden (SFS 2003:460), since no sensitive personal information was collected and the participants answered in their role as health care professionals. Participation was voluntary and confidential, and participants were assured that hospitals and individuals would be impossible to trace in the published material. Informed consent was presumed if the participant chose to complete the questionnaire.

Data collection

A study specific questionnaire was developed for this survey (Additional file1, English translation). The development was guided by a conceptual framework of health care quality, a comprehensive literature review, and the authors' own experience. The framework of health care quality, described by Donabedian [31], comprises three components; structure, process and outcome. These three components cover: 1) contextual factors in which care is provided such as physical equipment, facilities, environments, human resources and organizational characteristics, 2) health care actions taken by professionals, patients and family members, and 3) effects of health care on patients, family members or populations. In developing the tool, all three components were included.

The initial version of the questionnaire included 11 closed-ended questions covering six topics: local guidelines (3 questions), routines for follow-up visits (3 questions), content of the follow-up visits (1 question), family involvement (1 question), patient reported outcome measures (PROMs) and information material (2 questions), and quality registry (1 question). To ensure content validity [32], an expert group including researchers, members of the SRC, health care professionals and a psychometrician evaluated the questionnaire. The expert group critically reviewed the questionnaire, which was then revised, guided by their comments. In addition to minor refinements, an open-ended question was added.

Thus, the final questionnaire had a total of 12 questions. Six questions were constructed as statements, e.g., "At my hospital we have explicit guidelines for post CA care", answered by a Likert type scale with four response options: "Agree", "Partly agree", Disagree" or "Don't know". Four questions included possible content of post CA care and follow-up, and were constructed to be answered with "Yes", "No" or "Don't know". One multiple choice question was posed to elucidate the timing of follow-up visits.

The final question had an open-ended format where respondents were given the opportunity to write their own comments, thoughts and/or proposals in relation to the previous questions and answers. This question aimed to provide supplementary information for a better understanding of the quantitative findings.

With assistance from the SRC, a web-based version of the questionnaire was sent out to the resuscitation coordinators at all Swedish emergency hospitals ($n = 74$) in January 2013. After 2 reminders, 59 answers (80 %) were received.

Data analysis

Quantitative data were analysed with descriptive statistics, using STATA 13.1 for Mac (StataCorp LP, College Station, TX, USA). The qualitative free text responses (open-ended question) were independently analysed (by AB and JI) using manifest content analysis [33], aiming to describe and compare the respondents' answers to the six topics in the questionnaire, to identify responses with similar content. The data were then read several times to become familiar with the content. The qualitative data were deductively grouped according to the topics, followed by inductive categorization and abstraction of the data. Finally, the findings were discussed between all researchers until agreement was reached.

Results

Quantitative and qualitative results are reported together in connection with each topic. The categories and sub-categories, identified by manifest content analysis, are presented in Table 1.

Local guidelines for post CA care – lack of guidelines

Almost half of the hospitals in Sweden ($n = 27$, 46 %) reported having local guidelines for post CA care. However, 39 % of these hospitals reported that guidelines were not always applied. More than half of the hospitals did not have local guidelines.

Open-ended responses revealed that a few participants ($n = 2$) were aware of this deficiency:

"Unfortunately we do not have any guidelines."

Table 1 Categories and sub-categories based on manifest content analysis of answers to the open-ended question; "Do you have any other considerations or suggestions related to post cardiac arrest care and follow-up?"

Sub-category	Category
No follow up structure	Lack of guidelines
Instructions are missing	
Planning for care programs	
Varying time intervals	Varying routines
Different professionals involved	
Follow up based on needs	
Routines are missing	
Diagnosis guide follow up	Inexplicable differences
Cause of the CA guide follow up	
Type of hospital ward guide follow up	
Insufficient family follow up	Invited or forgotten
Lack of time	

One participant seemed to have become aware of the problem while answering the survey:

"Here it seems like we need help to improve post cardiac arrest care. This survey made this very clear."

Routines for follow-up visits – varying routines

The most common routine was a follow-up visit at a cardiac reception unit to meet with a cardiologist ($n = 42$, 70 %) and/or a cardiac nurse ($n = 36$, 61 %) (Fig. 1). In general, the follow-up visits took place within one month ($n = 23$, 39 %) and/or within 3 months ($n = 22$, 37 %). However, 42 % ($n = 25$) did not know the time for the follow-up visits (Fig. 2). A minority of the hospitals reported to have routines for follow-up visits to other occupational categories; intensive care nurse ($n = 5$, 9 %), neurologist ($n = 2$, 3 %), counselor ($n = 7$, 12 %), occupational therapist ($n = 4$, 7 %) and physiotherapist ($n = 14$, 24 %) (Fig. 1).

Respondents' comments in the open-ended question showed how the follow-up was organized regarding professionals involved ($n = 4$), and time intervals ($n = 3$):

"At the cardiology section follow-up for cardiac arrest patients is always performed by a cardiologist eight weeks after discharge."

Sometimes respondents ($n = 5$) indicated that there was a need for follow-up involving other professionals with various expertise:

"It would be good to have routine follow-up visits to e.g.: Neurologist, Occupational therapist, Counselor, Psychologist."

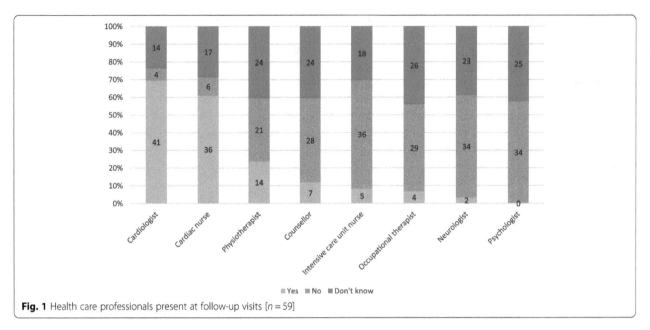

Fig. 1 Health care professionals present at follow-up visits [*n* = 59]

If the need for neurological or psychological support is discovered the routines are not explicit. One respondent indicated that this situation is not optimal:

"There is a lot we could do for the survivors and their family members. For example, a follow-up visit to me. Unfortunately, there is not enough time. All the time is needed to make things work at the hospital with all the education."

Content of the follow-up visits – inexplicable differences
The most common standardized content at the follow-up visits were; tiredness and fitness (*n* = 35, 59 %), physical symptoms (*n* = 36, 61 %), general health (*n* = 32,

54 %) and return to daily activities (*n* = 36, 61 %). In 48 % (*n* = 28) cognitive function and in 39 % (*n* = 23) psychological problems were followed up. The questions about the content of post CA care were frequently answered with "don't know" (36–54 %) (Fig. 3).

In the open-ended question, respondents (*n* = 3) commented that the content of post CA care was dependent on care settings:

"The post cardiac arrest care looks different depending on what ward the patients are admitted to."

According to a few respondents (*n* = 2), the content could also be dependent on aetiology:

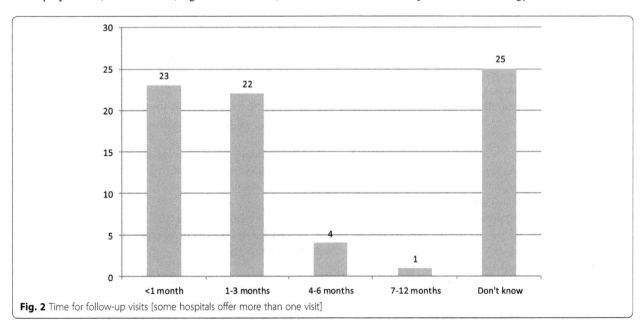

Fig. 2 Time for follow-up visits [some hospitals offer more than one visit]

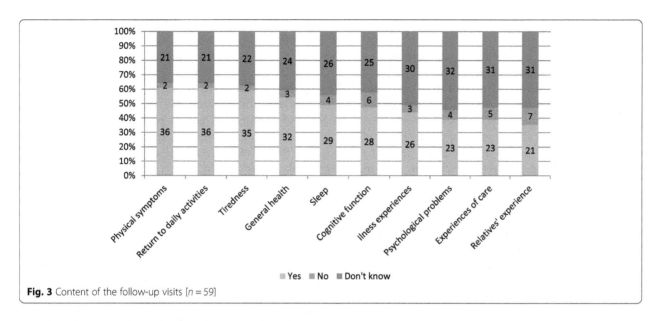

Fig. 3 Content of the follow-up visits [n = 59]

"The follow-up is dependent on the cause of cardiac arrest and may therefore vary quite a lot."

Family involvement in post CA care – invited or forgotten

In total, 44 % (n = 26) of the hospitals had as a routine to involve family members by inviting them to participate in post cardiac arrest care and follow-up. Further, 17 % (n = 10) of the hospitals invited family members occasionally, but not as a routine. The rest of the hospitals had no such routine or did not know, 3 % (n = 2) and 36 % (n = 21) respectively.

In the open-ended question, one respondent emphasised the importance of routines for involving family members in post CA care and follow-up:

"The patients and their family members meet our cardiac rehabilitation nurse two weeks after discharge. Also a follow-up visit to a cardiologist one month after discharge."

Patient reported outcome measures and information material

A minority (n = 12, 20 %) of the hospitals used PROMs to detect problems experienced by the patients themselves, e.g., EuroQol-5 Dimensions, Short Form-36 and Visual Analogue Scale for well-being. The majority of the hospitals (n = 44, 75 %) in some way used the national information material from the SRC as a routine to support survivors and their family members.

Quality registry in post CA care

In order to follow and evaluate CA care and follow-up, a majority of Swedish hospitals (n = 51, 86 %) report data to the Swedish registry for cardiopulmonary resuscitation. The registry is internet based and data are collected

on three occasions: CA event, hospital discharge and 30 days post arrest [2].

Discussion

Despite the need for structured post CA care for survivors and family members, few studies have described these aspects [24–27]. Overall, this survey showed that guidelines are not available at many hospitals in Sweden, and consist mainly of traditional cardiac rehabilitation with follow-up visits at cardiac reception units. Resuscitation coordinators in general lack knowledge about how post CA care is organized. Answers to the open-ended question confirm these findings. This raises the question of whether the hospitals meet post CA care needs, among survivors and family members, in order for health to be restored and improved over time.

Since cardiac follow-up does not include all CA patients and ICU follow-ups seem to be uncommon, there is no clear pathway for CA survivors and their family members. According to answers from the open-ended question, differences could depend on diagnosis, cause of CA and type of hospital ward. In addition, our results imply great variability in care between hospitals. In contrast to national intentions, striving for equal care [34], our findings showed that quality of post CA care and follow-up seems to depend on where the patient lives. This is not unique to Sweden and corresponds to the results of a Canadian study by Keenan, et al. [35]. In their study, regional differences in ICU care after CA were also described. However, the results entail the importance of local, national and international guidelines. Encouragingly, written information material with the aim to support patients' and family members' recovery seemed to be implemented as an element of post CA care at the majority of the Swedish hospitals, and therefore in some ways can help to create uniformity. Further, processes that promote families' ability to cope with the life-threatening event might be strengthened by learning from the experiences of others [28].

As in previous investigations of post ICU care and follow-up [18], the content of the visits in our survey mainly included the present status of the patients (e.g. assessing current physical function, daily activities and health). The lack of routines on how to handle problems identified, shows low focus on rehabilitation in order to support and promote health and recovery over time. A randomized controlled follow-up intervention especially designed for CA survivors has been tested in the Netherlands [36]. This [37] is one of few health-promoting interventions intended for CA survivors and their caregivers, which have been described in detail. This individualized, semi-structured psychosocial intervention, 'Stand still..., and move on', is designed for early detection of emotional and cognitive problems, and for providing information and support. It also aims to promote self-management as well as an early referral to specialized care if needed. The intervention consists of one to six consultations conducted by specially trained nurses [36]. The recently published results showed that the intervention improved QoL and decreased anxiety among CA survivors at one-year post CA. However, it did not improve outcome for caregivers. These results are very likely to contribute to improvements in post CA care and follow-up [25].

Less than half of the hospitals reported that they had as a routine to invite family members to participate in post CA care. However, it remains unclear how and if concerns among family members are detected. Maybe they are invited to participate in follow-up, or maybe they are forgotten. Since mild cognitive dysfunction appears to be common among OHCA survivors [4, 5], and cognitive dysfunction among survivors has been shown to be associated with strain among family members [38], it is important for family members to be included in post CA care. In addition, stress, anxiety and decreased QoL among relatives have been reported [23]. As previous dyad studies show that patients and spouses affect each other's health [39, 40], survivors and their family members will likely affect each other in the same way. There is also reason to assume that the function of the family is affected by, as well as affects, health and QoL among both patients and family members [41]. Family members might play an important part in the post CA care. Therefore, nursing should actively promote strengths and health among both survivors and their family members [28].

A minority of the hospitals used PROMs to detect problems among survivors. After this study was conducted, the Swedish registry for cardiopulmonary resuscitation began including PROMs in the follow-up, for example, health-related quality of life among survivors using questionnaires and telephone interviews. PROM data will contribute to better knowledge of the life situation among survivors, since the number of patients available for research will increase. This knowledge could constitute a starting point for the testing of screening methods and health promoting interventions as well as the creating of national guidelines. In addition, PROMs play a key role for person centred care, by influencing the care based on patient specific information [42]. In a recently published editorial, Smith and Bernard [16] highlight the need for more research to determine what outcome measures accurately describe obstacles important to patient- and family health after a CA event. They argue that good measurements, with the ability to capture predictors for poor health, could aim to target and evaluate interventions. Consensus has not been reached concerning what assessments to use to evaluate outcome after a CA. However, one of the most descriptive guidelines can be found in the recommendations of the American Heart Association from 2011 [43]. In a recently published study of 249 OHCA survivors [38] it was concluded that questionnaires and telephone interviews to assess cognitive function and QoL can be recommended for CA research.

In the present study, most of the follow-up visits took place within the first three months after the CA. However, a few open-ended responses indicated that follow up visits were sometimes based on patients' needs. This might indicate a growing awareness of health as multidimensional [28], making the patient perspective essential. Further, there is a lack of knowledge and guidance about optimal timing and intervals for evaluating the patient's QoL after a CA. The UK NICE guidelines for follow-up after a general critical illness suggest a structured pathway for assessments: at ICU stay (during the stay and before discharge), at ward-based care (during and before discharge), and at a follow-up visit 2–3 months after discharge [19]. A structured pathway for rehabilitation of present findings has further been suggested by Jones [9]. However, these guidelines are not designed especially for a CA group and most of the interventions still lack sufficient evidence. In addition, many survivors, especially those suffering IHCA, may not be admitted to an ICU at all.

Nurses, in particular those working at cardiac- and intensive care reception units, should be aware that CA patients and relatives could be at risk of not receiving optimal post CA care. Therefore, they should pay special attention to individual needs and possible health-problems. In order to improve post CA care and follow-up, future research should focus on the needs of CA survivors and their family members and on the testing of health promoting interventions. Such knowledge will be helpful for improving hospital care and developing guidelines.

Limitations

Cross-sectional surveys with descriptive designs are beneficial approaches for health care researchers, particularly in new area of inquiry. However, they have some drawbacks that need to be considered [44]. The questionnaire was developed specifically for this study and had not undergone any extensive validation. However, the tool development was guided by a well-used conceptual framework about health care quality [31, 45]. Although the questions cover all three components, i.e. structure, process and outcome, not all aspects of these were included. This choice was made to make the questionnaire short and easy to complete. The open-ended question allowed respondents to provide supplementary answers to the closed-ended questions, as well as to express other aspects of post CA care. In addition, content validity was determined by a researcher with extensive experience in instrument development and psychometrics. The response rate was high, which indicated that the questions were easy to understand and complete. This also indicated an interest for the study. In addition to a high response rate, the respondents were well spread geographically and there were different types of cities, and small and large hospitals. Despite the high response rate, the findings should be interpreted and generalized with some caution.

Another limitation was sparse qualitative data from the open-ended question, reported by 15 of the respondents. For this reason, qualitative data were deductively grouped according to the six established topics, followed by inductive categorization and abstraction of the data. With more extensive material, it would have been preferable to start the analysis by coding the data. Despite this limitation, the qualitative data contributed to a better understanding of the quantitative findings.

In this study, we sent the questionnaire to resuscitation coordinators, since they were most likely to know the routines at the hospitals. However, in order to get more comprehensive results, answers from other groups, e.g., cardiac rehabilitation nurses or nurses responsible for post ICU care and follow-up, might also have been of interest. Another weakness is that we cannot say anything about which hospitals completed the questionnaire and which did not, since the answers were given anonymously. Still our results imply the need for improvements in post CA care, e.g., by finding structured pathways for referral and including other specialities, in order to increase the chances of promoting all aspects of health and QoL among survivors and their families, especially emotional and cognitive aspects.

Conclusions

Although efforts have already been made to improve post CA care and follow-up, many hospitals need to focus more on this part of CA treatment. In addition, evidence-based national guidelines will have to be developed and implemented in order to achieve more uniform care and follow-up for survivors and their family members. This national survey highlights this need and might be helpful in the implementation of such guidelines.

Abbreviations
CA: Cardiac arrest; IHCA: In-hospital cardiac arrest; ICU: Intensive care unit; NICE: National Institute for Health and Clinical Excellence; OHCA: Out-of-hospital cardiac arrest; PROMs: Patient reported outcome measures; SRC: Swedish Resuscitation Council; QoL: Quality of life.

Competing interests
The authors declare that they have no competing interests.

Authors' contributions
JI, GL and KÅ participated in designing the study, analysing and making interpretation of the data, and drafting the manuscript. AB and JSÅ participated in analysing and making interpretation of the data, and revised the manuscript. All authors read and approved the final manuscript.

Acknowledgements
We would like to thank Elisabeth Sevborn at Kalmar County Hospital and Solveig Aune at Sahlgrenska University Hospital for their assistance with the data collection. The Medical Research Council of Southeast Sweden and the Swedish Heart and Lung Association funded this study.

Author details
[1]Department of Internal Medicine, Division of Cardiology, Kalmar County Hospital, SE-39185 Kalmar, Sweden. [2]Department of Medical and Health Sciences, Division of Nursing Science, Linköping University, SE-58185 Linköping, Sweden. [3]Kalmar Maritime Academy, Linnaeus University, SE-39182 Kalmar, Sweden. [4]Department of Clinical Science, Division of Neurology, Lund University, Lund, Sweden. [5]Department of Neurology and Rehabilitation Medicine, Skane University Hospital, SE-22185 Lund, Sweden. [6]Faculty of Caring Science, Work Life and Social Welfare and the Centre for Prehospital Research, University of Borås, SE-50190 Borås, Sweden. [7]Division of Emergency Medical Services, Kalmar County Hospital, SE-39185 Kalmar, Sweden. [8]Information School, University of Sheffield, Regent Court, 211 Portobello Street, Sheffield S1 4DP, England. [9]eHealth Institute, Linnaeus University, SE-39182 Kalmar, Sweden. [10]Center for Collaborative Palliative Care, Linnaeus University, SE-39182 Kalmar, Sweden.

References
1. Atwood C, Eisenberg MS, Herlitz J, Rea TD. Incidence of EMS-treated out-of-hospital cardiac arrest in Europe. Resuscitation. 2005;67:75–80.
2. Herlitz J. The Swedish national registry for cardiopulmonary resuscitation - Annual report 2014. Gothenburg: The Swedish national registry for cardiopulmonary resuscitation; 2014. Swedish.
3. Bunch TJ, White RD, Gersh BJ, Meverden RA, Hodge DO, Ballman KV, et al. Long-term outcomes of out-of-hospital cardiac arrest after successful early defibrillation. N Engl J Med. 2003;348:2626–33.

4.   Cronberg T, Lilja G, Rundgren M, Friberg H, Widner H. Long-term neurological outcome after cardiac arrest and therapeutic hypothermia. Resuscitation. 2009;80:1119–23.

5.   Moulaert VR, Verbunt JA, van Heugten CM, Wade DT. Cognitive impairments in survivors of out-of-hospital cardiac arrest: a systematic review. Resuscitation. 2009;80:297–305.

6.   Wilder Schaaf KP, Artman LK, Peberdy MA, Walker WC, Ornato JP, Gossip MR, et al. Anxiety, depression, and PTSD following cardiac arrest: a systematic review of the literature. Resuscitation. 2013;84:873–7.

7.   Bremer A, Dahlberg K, Sandman L. Experiencing out-of-hospital cardiac arrest: significant others' lifeworld perspective. Qual Health Res. 2009;19:1407–20.

8.   Bremer A, Dahlberg K, Sandman L. To survive out-of-hospital cardiac arrest: a search for meaning and coherence. Qual Health Res. 2009;19:323–38.

9.   Jones C. What's new on the post-ICU burden for patients and relatives? Intensive Care Med. 2013;39:1832–5.

10. Moulaert VR, Wachelder EM, Verbunt JA, Wade DT, van Heugten CM. Determinants of quality of life in survivors of cardiac arrest. J Rehabil Med. 2010;42:553–8.

11. Elliott VJ, Rodgers DL, Brett SJ. Systematic review of quality of life and other patient-centred outcomes after cardiac arrest survival. Resuscitation. 2011;82:247–56.

12. Graf J, Muhlhoff C, Doig GS, Reinartz S, Bode K, Dujardin R, et al. Health care costs, long-term survival, and quality of life following intensive care unit admission after cardiac arrest. Crit Care. 2008;12:R92.

13. Nichol G, Stiell IG, Hebert P, Wells GA, Vandemheen K, Laupacis A. What is the quality of life for survivors of cardiac arrest? A prospective study. Acad Emerg Med. 1999;6:95–102.

14. Harve H, Tiainen M, Poutiainen E, Maunu M, Kajaste S, Roine RO, et al. The functional status and perceived quality of life in long-term survivors of out-of-hospital cardiac arrest. Acta Anaesthesiol Scand. 2007;51:206–9.

15. Torgersen J, Strand K, Bjelland TW, Klepstad P, Kvale R, Soreide E, et al. Cognitive dysfunction and health-related quality of life after a cardiac arrest and therapeutic hypothermia. Acta Anaesthesiol Scand. 2010;54:721–8.

16. Smith K, Bernard S. Quality of life after cardiac arrest: how and when to assess outcomes after hospital discharge? Resuscitation. 2014;85:1127–8.

17. Andersson B, Marklund E, Bervall M-J, Lilja G. Cardiac arrest – stories of survivors and relatives. Stockholm: Swedish Resuscitation Council; 2011. Swedish.

18. Egerod I, Risom SS, Thomsen T, Storli SL, Eskerud RS, Holme AN, et al. ICU-recovery in Scandinavia: a comparative study of intensive care follow-up in Denmark, Norway and Sweden. Intensive Crit Care Nurs. 2013;29:103–11.

19. Plowright C. National Institute for Health and Clinical Excellence announces guideline on critical illness rehabilitation. Nurs Crit Care. 2009;14:159–61.

20. Piepoli MF, Corrà U, Benzer W, Bjarnason-Wehrens B, Dendale P, Gaita D, et al. Secondary prevention through cardiac rehabilitation: from knowledge to implementation. A position paper from the Cardiac Rehabilitation Section of the European Association of Cardiovascular Prevention and Rehabilitation. Eur J Cardiovasc Prev Rehabil. 2010;17:1–17.

21. Cronberg T, Lilja G. Cognitive decline after cardiac arrest – It is more to the picture than hypoxic brain injury. Resuscitation. 2015;91:A3–4.

22. Goossens PH, Moulaert VR. Cognitive impairments after cardiac arrest: implications for clinical daily practice. Resuscitation. 2014;85:A3–4.

23. Wachelder EM, Moulaert VR, van Heughten C, Verbunt JA, Bekkers SC, Wade DT. Life after survival: long-term daily functioning and quality of life after an out-of-hospital cardiac arrest. Resuscitation. 2009;80:517–22.

24. Dougherty CM, Thompson EA, Levis FM. Long-term outcomes of a telephone intervention after an ICD. Pacing Clin Electrophysiol. 2005;28:1157–67.

25. Moulaert VR, van Heughten CM, Winkens B, Bakx WG, de Krom MC, Gorgels TP, et al. Early neurologically-focused follow-up after cardiac arrest improves quality of life at one year: A randomised controlled trial. Int J Cardiol. 2015;193:8–16.

26. Kim C, Jung H, Choi HE, Kang SH. Cardiac rehabilitation after acute myocardial infarction resuscitated from cardiac arrest. Ann Rehabil Med. 2014;38:799–804.

27. Takahashi H, Sasanuma N, Itani Y, Tanaka T, Domen K, Masuyama T, et al. Impact of early interventions by a cardiac rehabilitation team on the social rehabilitation of patients resuscitated from cardiogenic out-of-hospital cardiopulmonary arrest. Intern Med. 2015;54:133–9.

28. Allen FM, Warner M. A developmental model of health and nursing. J Fam Issues. 2002;8:96–135.

29. World Medical Association. Declaration of Helsinki: ethical principles for medical research involving human subjects (Doc. 17.c). Adopted by the 59th WMA General Assembly. Seoul: 2008.

30. SFS 2003:460. (Swedish Ethics Legislation). Stockholm: 2003. Swedish.

31. Donabedian A. Evaluating the quality of medical care. Milbank Q. 2005;83:691–729.

32. Streiner DL, Norman GR. Health measurement scales: a practical guide to their development and use. 4th ed. Oxford: Oxford University Press; 2008.

33. Elo S, Kyngäs H. The qualitative content analysis process. J Adv Nurs. 2008;62:107–11.

34. SOU 2013:44. (Official report of the Swedish government). Stockholm: 2013. Swedish.

35. Keenan SP, Dodek P, Martin C, Priestap F, Norena M, Wong H. Variation in length of intensive care unit stay after cardiac arrest: where you are is as important as who you are. Crit Care Med. 2007;35:836–41.

36. Moulaert VR, Verbunt JA, van Heugten CM, Bakx WG, Gorgels AP, Bekkers SC, et al. Activity and Life After Survival of a Cardiac Arrest (ALASCA) and the effectiveness of an early intervention service: design of a randomised controlled trial. BMC Cardiovasc Disord. 2007;7:26.

37. Moulaert VR, Verbunt JA, Bakx WG, Gorgels AP, de Krom MC, Heuts PH, et al. 'Stand still …, move on', a new early intervention service for cardiac arrest survivors and their caregivers: rationale and description of the intervention. Clin Rehabil. 2011;25:867–79.

38. Beesems SG, Wittebrood KM, de Haan RJ, Koster RW. Cognitive function and quality of life after successful resuscitation from cardiac arrest. Resuscitation. 2014;85:1269–74.

39. Chung ML, Moser DK, Lennie TA, Rayens MK. The effects of depressive symptoms and anxiety on quality of life in patients with heart failure and their spouses: testing dyadic dynamics using Actor-Partner Interdependence Model. J Psychosom Res. 2009;67:29–35.

40. Rayens MK, Svavarsdottir EK. A new methodological approach in nursing research: an actor, partner, and interaction effect model for family outcomes. Res Nurs Health. 2003;26:409–19.

41. Miller IW, McDermut W, Gordon KC, Keitner GI, Ryan CE, Norman W. Personality and family functioning in families of depressed patients. J Abnorm Psychol. 2000;109:539–45.

42. Jayadevappa R, Chhatre S. Patient centered care - a conceptual model and review of the state of the art. The Open Health Services and Policy Journal. 2011;4:15–25.

43. Holmes Jr DR, Becker JA, Granger CB, Limacher MC, Page 2nd RL, Sila C. ACCF/AHA 2011 health policy statement on therapeutic interchange and substitution: a report of the American College of Cardiology Foundation Clinical Quality Committee. Circulation. 2011;124:1290–310.

44. Grimes DA, Schulz KF. Descriptive studies: what they can and cannot do. Lancet. 2002;359:145–9.

45. Stelfox HT, Straus SE. Measuring quality of care: considering measurement frameworks and needs assessment to guide quality indicator development. J Clin Epidemiol. 2013;60:1320–7.

4

Pattern of acute poisoning at two urban referral hospitals in Lusaka, Zambia

Jessy Z'gambo[1,2*], Yorum Siulapwa[2] and Charles Michelo[1]

Abstract

Background: Poisoning remains an important public health problem contributing significantly to the global burden of disease. Evidence on the exact burden and pattern of acute poisoning in Zambia is limited. We aimed to characterise acute poisoning with regard to demographic and epidemiologic factors of cases reported at the University Teaching Hospital and Levy Mwanawasa General Hospital; two large referral hospitals in Lusaka, Zambia.

Methods: This was a cross-sectional study involving retrospective collection of data on all poisoning cases recorded in hospital records from 1 January to 31 December 2012. A pretested data collection form was used to extract demographic and other data such as poisonous agents used, circumstance of poisoning, route and outcome of poisoning. All analyses were performed in STATA (StataCorp. 2013. Stata Statistical Software: Release 13. College Station, TX: StataCorp LP).

Results: A total of 873 poisoning cases were reviewed with almost similar proportions of males (52 %) and females (49 %). Poisoning cases were highest in the 0-12 years age category (36 %) followed by the 20-30 years age category (31 %). Accidental poisoning characterised most (65 %) cases in children aged < 13 years. The common route of exposure to poisonous agents was ingestion. Overall, the mortality rate was 2.6 per 100 cases, the majority of deaths were observed in men (78 %). Poisonous agents associated with most cases were pesticides (57 %) and pharmaceuticals (13 %).

Conclusions: The high risk of accidental poisoning observed in children calls for special health education on chemical safety, tailored for mothers and caregivers to prevent chemical exposure in this important age group whose access to toxic agents is mainly in homes or their immediate environment. The results also call for additional regulatory controls on pesticides and pharmaceuticals, which were the most common toxic agents.

Keywords: Acute, Poisoning, Chemical, Hospital, Toxic agent, Lusaka, Zambia

Background

Poisoning remains a significant public health problem associated with over 340 000 unintentional poisoning deaths and an estimated global loss of over 7.4 million years of healthy life (disability adjusted life years, DALYs). Furthermore, there are almost one million suicides each year and a significant number of these deaths are related to chemicals [1, 2]. Low and middle-income countries suffer the highest burden of unintentional and suicidal poisoning – a phenomenon exacerbated by crippled chemicals management structures and health care delivery systems [2].

In Southern Africa, acute poisoning has been identified as a significant cause of both morbidity and mortality with hospital prevalence ranging from 1 to 17 % [3].

As has been reported, more than 25 % of the global burden of disease is linked to environmental factors including exposures to and inappropriate use of toxic chemicals [4]. Current trends show an increase in use of chemicals in the global economy and daily modern life which may be linked to increased human exposure [5, 6]. Limiting the availability of and access to highly toxic chemicals such as pesticides has been shown to reduce the number of deaths due to poisoning. For instance, the withdrawal of all World Health Organisation (WHO) class I pesticides as well as endosulfan through a number of targeted legislative initiatives in Sri Lanka resulted in a 50 % drop in

* Correspondence: jessyzgambo88@yahoo.co.uk
[1]Department of Public Health, Epidemiology & Biostatistics Unit, School of Medicine, University of Zambia, Lusaka, Zambia
[2]Department of Public Health, Environmental Health Unit, School of Medicine, University of Zambia, Lusaka, Zambia

suicides and even greater reduction in fatal poisonings [7, 8]. A call has been made to modify the WHO classification based on new evidence on human lethality from acute poisoning of certain pesticides [7, 8].

Though much is known and documented on acute poisoning globally, the opposite is true for Zambia. The lack of up-to-date information can be attributed to the unavailability of published data in accessible databases, an absence of poison centres and national surveillance systems, including the non-mandatory notification of poisoning cases. Similar challenges have been observed in other countries such as China, Botswana and South Africa [3, 9, 10].

This dearth of information on circumstances, substances and populations at risk is a barrier to effective poisoning prevention and targeted intervention programmes. Therefore, the need for a current review of poisoning patterns in Zambia is imperative.

This study sought to characterise acute poisoning with regard to demographic factors (i.e. age, sex and residence), common toxic agents used and their case fatality rates as well as the overall mortality rate of acute poisoning.

Methods

Study area

The study was conducted in Lusaka district, the capital and largest city of Zambia. Lusaka district has a total land area of 375 km^2 and a total population of 1.7 million inhabitants with almost equal proportions of males and females (i.e. 49 % and 51 % respectively) [11, 12]. The city is Zambia's most densely populated city with a population density close to 5000 persons per square kilometre. Over 70 % of people in Lusaka district reside in peri urban areas which are characterised by squatter settlements and regularised informal settlements known as Improved Areas [12]. The majority of low income social groups reside in the peri urban areas of Lusaka.

The central location of Lusaka district makes it easily accessible to most parts of the country and provides a ready market for goods and services. The main economic activities in the district are manufacturing, transport, wholesale and retail trading. In addition, despite Lusaka being a built-up urban area and as more productive agricultural land continues to be taken for urban processes, urban agriculture is also an important economic activity consisting of crop cultivation and animal husbandry [12].

Lusaka district is well covered with regard to health care delivery services. The district has 3 third level (i.e. tertiary) hospitals, 1 second level (i.e. secondary) hospital, 9 first level (i.e. primary) hospitals, 170 urban health centres and 11 health post. Of these health facilities, 44 are run by the government while the rest are of private ownership [13]. The University Teaching Hospital (UTH) is a third level

referral hospital which caters for a catchment population of approximately over 800 000. Levy Mwanawasa General Hospital (LMGH) is a second level referral hospital intended to cater for a catchment area of between 200 000 and 800 000 people. Both UTH and LMGH receive referral cases from health facilities within Lusaka district as well as from other parts of the country [13]. The first point of contact with the health care service system for the patients presenting with poisoning is at health centres and primary level hospitals. Depending on the level of care required, complicated cases are moved up the chain of care to the secondary (i.e. LMGH) and tertiary hospital (i.e. UTH). However, some patients go straight to the secondary and tertiary level hospitals.

Population and sampling procedures

The study was cross-sectional and made use of retrospective extraction of data on acute poisoning cases from records at Levy Mwanawasa General Hospital (LMGH) and the University Teaching Hospital (UTH). Filter clinic and the department of paediatrics at UTH provided the adult and children populations respectively. Filter clinic is a medical emergency unit that attends to all medical emergencies in adults including poisoning cases. The department of paediatrics handles all paediatric emergencies including poisoning cases. The department of casualty at LMGH provided both adult and children populations.

Data collection and extraction

All cases of poisoning recorded in hospital out-patient registers, patient case files and death registers covering a period of one year from 1st January to 31st December 2012 were listed and included in the study. Demographic (i.e. sex, age and residence) and epidemiologic data such as toxic agents used, route of exposure, circumstance (i.e. accidental, deliberate self-harm and recreational) and outcome (i.e. recovery, injury or death) of poisoning were collected using a pretested data collection form. Data collection was done by trained research assistants. The first point of extraction was from out-patient registers which list all patients passing through the selected hospital departments. Serial numbers from out-patient registers were used to locate patient case files containing detailed information about each case. Death registers provided data on all deaths as a result of acute poisoning. Data on route of exposure and circumstance of poisoning were collected as recorded in patient case files. Poisonous agents were described and grouped based on their use, chemical properties and groupings used in other studies.

Statistical analysis

For quality assurance, data collection forms were checked daily for accuracy, consistency and completeness. Analyses were done in STATA (StataCorp. 2013. Stata Statistical Software: Release 13. College Station, TX: StataCorp LP). Chi Square test was used to examine associations of variables. P ≤ 0.05 was used to determine significance.

Ethical consideration

Permission was obtained from the hospital administration to access hospital records that contain private information about patients. Patients were only identified by serial numbers as recorded in the hospital registers and all the information was kept confidential. In addition, approval to conduct research was sought from the Excellence in Research Ethics and Science (ERES) Institutional Review Board (IRB) (I.R.B. No. 00005948).

Results

Participation and socio-demographic distribution

A total of 1 061 cases were reviewed, 188 of these cases were found to be with incomplete data and were excluded resulting in 873 poisoning cases. The age of patients ranged from 0 to 76 years with a mean age of 22 years (±22 years). Poisoning cases were highest in the 0-12 years age category (36 %) followed by the 20-30 years age category (31 %). Overall, there were almost similar proportions of poisoning cases in males (52 %) and females (49 %) (Table 1). Females had the largest proportion (75 %) of poisoning cases in the 13-19 years age category (Table 2). The majority (64 %) of cases reported were from peri urban areas, others were from urban (27 %) and rural (7 %) residential areas of Lusaka (Table 1). The residence was not known in 1 % of the cases.

Circumstance of poisoning and route of exposure

Most poisoning cases were due to accidental circumstances (52 %, Table 1), only 2 of these cases were linked to occupational chemical exposures. Sixty five percent of accidental poisoning cases were in children aged 0-12 years (Table 3). Deliberate self-harm was associated with 39 % (Table 1) of the poisoning cases and more than half (52 %, Table 3) of these cases were in adults between the ages of 20 and 30 years. Pesticides were the common toxic agents used in deliberate self-harm for most of the cases (43 %, Table 3). Of the cases reviewed, 91 % were exposed to toxins orally while others were exposed by inhalation (2 %), dermal absorption (0.1 %) as well as through animal/insect bites (7 %) (Table 1).

Acute poisoning mortality

Of all the cases reviewed, 23 had died representing a mortality rate of 2.6 per 100 cases. There were 3 injuries recorded and these were predominantly oesophageal injuries which were a result of damage caused by corrosive chemicals ingested by the patients. Death in men was as high as 78 % while only 22 % of the deaths were

Table 1 Baseline characteristics of poisoning cases reviewed from all data collection sites, from January to December 2012 (n = 873)

Patient Characteristics	Frequency	Proportion
Sex		
Male	450	51.6
Female	423	48.5
Age		
0 to 12 years	300	36.3
13 to 19 years	149	18.0
20 to 30 years	253	30.6
Over 30 years	125	15.1
Mean age (SD)	22 years (22 years)	
Residence		
Urban	239	27.4
Peri-urban	562	64.4
Rural	60	6.9
Circumstance of poisoning		
Accidental	453	51.9
Deliberate self-harm	336	38.5
Recreational	3	0.3
Outcome of poisoning		
Recovery	847	97.0
Injury	3	0.3
Death	23	2.6
Route of poisoning		
Ingestion	793	90.8
Inhalation	14	1.6
Absorption (Dermal)	1	0.1
Animal/Insect bites	60	6.9
Toxic agent involved		
Household chemicals	44	5.0
Pharmaceutical	123	14.1
Animal/insect venom	60	6.9
Pesticides	187	21.4
Food Poisoning	115	13.2
Narcotics	3	0.3
Traditional medicine	7	0.8
Plants	19	2.2
Unspecified agents	173	19.8
Other agents	142	16.3

• Marital status and occupation were not included in the table because the variables were found to be missing in the hospital records for most cases
• Pharmaceuticals were predominantly oral but difficult to disaggregate
• The circumstance of poisoning for the cases was based on details of information recorded in the case files
• The category 'other agents' included chemicals that could not fit into the categories created prior to data collection. The specific agents have been tabulated in Table 5

Table 2 Distribution of poisoning cases according to age categories

Patient characteristics	Frequency [Number (%)]			
	0 - 12 years (n = 300)	13 - 19 years (n = 149)	20 - 30 years (n = 253)	> 30 years (n = 125))
Sex				
Male	177 (59.0)	37 (24.8)	121 (47.8)	84 (67.2)
Female	123 (41.0)	112 (75.2)	132 (52.2)	41 (32.8)
Residence				
Urban	72 (24.7)	46 (30.1)	72 (28.8)	41 (32.8)
Peri urban and rural	220 (75.3)	103 (69.1)	178 (71.2)	84 (67.2)
Route of poisoning				
Ingestion	286 (95.3)	135 (90.6)	226 (89.3)	106 (84.8)
Inhalation	0	4 (2.7)	5 (2)	2 (1.6)
Absorption	1 (0.3)	0	0	0
Animal/insect bites	13 (4.3)	10 (6.7)	19 (7.5)	17 (13.6)
Circumstance of poisoning				
Accidental	288 (98.0)	43 (31.2)	63 (27.8)	49 (49.0)
Deliberate self-harm	6 (2.0)	95 (68.8)	164 (72.3)	51 (51.0)
Outcome of poisoning				
Recovered	300 (100)	148 (99.3)	245 (96.8)	118 (94.4)
Died	0	1 (0.6)	8 (3.16)	7 (5.6)
Toxic agent involved				
Pharmaceutics and narcotics	25 (10.4)	30 (25.0)	51 (24.5)	11 (11.3)
Pesticides	39 (16.3)	32 (26.7)	73 (35.1)	29 (29.9)
Domestic and industrial	98 (40.8)	29 (24.2)	37 (17.8)	15 (15.5)
Plant, animal and food poisoning	78 (32.5)	29 (24.2)	47 (22.6)	42 (43.3)

Category for unknown information not shown for all variables

observed in females (p = 0.009) (Table 4). There were no deaths observed in children during the period reviewed and none of those who were accidentally poisoned had died. Most of the deaths were observed in patients of the age categories 20-30 years (50 %) and over 30 years (44 %) (p < 0.001, Table 4). The most common route of exposure to toxic chemicals for patients who had died was ingestion (74 %). The majority (73 %) of those who died resided in peri urban and rural areas of Lusaka (Table 4).

Toxic agents and their case fatality rates
Overall, pesticides (57 %) and pharmaceuticals (13 %) were associated with a larger proportion of deaths, representing case fatalities of 7 % and 2 % respectively. Narcotics were responsible for 4 % of the poisoning cases with a lone fatality (33 % case fatality). Poisoning by pesticides was more prevalent in men (n = 102, 55 %) compared to females (n = 85, 45 %) (Fig. 1). On the contrary, poisoning by pharmaceuticals was more prevalent in females (59 %) particularly among young adults (51 %) and teenagers (34 %) (Table 2). Of the industrial chemicals identified, kerosene (49 %) was more predominant and the majority

of cases (86 %) were in children in the age category of 0-12 years (results not shown). The toxic agent involved in poisoning could not be identified in a significant proportion of cases (20 %). The primary toxicant of interest was recorded in 25 cases were the patients ingested more than one agent. In 17 of these cases, alcohol (unspecified) was ingested with pesticides (n = 13) and pharmaceuticals (n = 4). All the toxic agents involved (with an exception of alcohol) in such cases were listed and included in Table 5 which outlines all the specific toxic agents involved in poisoning.

Discussion
In the present study, it was observed that the majority of poisoning cases were in children involving accidental circumstances. Literature shows that although accidental poisoning can occur at any age, it is most common in children with peak age around two years [10, 14–16]. Hand to mouth behaviour of inquisitive children as they explore the world around them, coupled with the lack of knowledge of consequences puts the children at a higher risk of poisoning [2, 17]. Overall, non sex differentiation was observed in the distribution of poisoning cases

Table 3 Factors associated with circumstance of poisoning

Patient characteristics	Circumstance of poisoning [Number (%)]		
	Accidental	DSH[a]	P-Value*
Sex			0.002
Male	254 (56.1)	158 (45.1)	
Female	199 (43.9)	186 (54.9)	
Age			< 0.001
0 to 12 years	288 (65.0)	6 (1.9)	
13 to 19 years	43 (9.7)	95 (30.1)	
20 to 30 years	63 (14.2)	164 (51.9)	
Over 30 years	49 (11.1)	51 (16.1)	
Route of poisoning			< 0.001
Ingestion	382 (84.3)	338 (99.7)	
All other routes combined[b]	71 (15.6)	1 (0.21)	
Residence			0.006
Urban	140 (31.4)	76 (22.6)	
Peri urban; rural	306 (68.6)	261 (77.5)	
Outcome of poisoning			< 0.001
Recovered	453 (100)	322 (95.0)	
Died	0	17 (5.0)	
Toxic agent involved			
Pharmaceutics and narcotics	27 (7.0)	93 (33.6)	< 0.001
Pesticides	61 (15.8)	120 (43.3)	
Domestic and industrial	126 (32.7)	55 (19.9)	
Plant, animal and food poisoning	171 (44.4)	9 (3.3)	

*P-values were derived using chi square
[a]DSH = Deliberate Self-Harm
[b]Comprised of inhalation, bites/stings and dermal routes

Table 4 Factors associated with outcome of poisoning

Patient characteristics	Outcome of poisoning [Number (%)]		
	Recovery	Death	P-Value*
Sex			0.009
Male	432 (50.8)	18 (78.3)	
Female	418 (49.2)	5 (21.7)	
Age			< 0.001
0 to 12 years	300 (37.0)	0	
13 to 19 years	148 (18.3)	1 (6.25)	
20 to 30 years	245 (30.2)	8 (50.0)	
Over 30 years	118 (14.6)	7 (43.8)	
Route of poisoning			0.004
Ingestion	776 (91.3)	17 (73.9)	
All other routes combined[a]	74 (8.7)	6 (26.1)	
Residence			0.959
Urban	233 (27.8)	6 (27.3)	
Peri urban; Rural	606 (73.2)	16 (72.7)	
Circumstance of poisoning			< 0.001
Accidental	453 (58.5)	0	
Deliberate self-harm	322 (41.6)	17 (100)	
Toxic agent involved			< 0.001
Pharmaceutics and narcotics	122 (17.9)	4 (22.2)	
Pesticides	174 (25.5)	13 (72.2)	
Domestic and industrial	185 (27.1)	1 (5.6)	
Plant, animal and food poisoning	201 (29.5)	0	

*P - values were derived using chi square
[a]Comprised of inhalation, bites/stings and dermal routes

reviewed in this study. Age and sex distribution of poisoning burden vary in different geographic regions and time periods due to the interaction and influence of socioeconomic, cultural and behavioural factors in the general population [17–19].

The mortality rate of 2.6 per 100 cases noted in this study was similar to findings in a study conducted in South Africa [3]. A male predominance in deaths was observed in the poisoning cases reviewed in this study. This pattern has been observed by others and has been attributed to the male tendency to choose more violent and successful means of self-harm than women [16, 19]. Furthermore, high case fatality rates were associated with pesticide poisoning. This observation can be attributed to the high toxicity of these agents. However, other toxicological factors - such as potency of toxic agent and amount exposed to - also need to be put into consideration with regard to survival of the victims. While mortality is usually high in patients of deliberate self-harm, a study in rural Sri Lanka found that the choice of poison was based on availability and not toxicity of the poison [20].

The finding that the most prevalent chemical agents involved in poisoning were pesticides and pharmaceuticals was not surprising because these tend to be the most predominant chemicals in poor resource settings. Existing literature shows that toxic agents associated with morbidity and mortality are influenced by various factors such as location, time periods, availability and use of chemicals or poisoning agents, as well as changes in lifestyles, beliefs and traditions of people [21, 22]. To this effect, we observed similarities and differences in findings from our study and those found by others. For instance, a Zimbabwean study revealed that pesticides and pharmaceuticals were the most common toxic agents responsible for hospital admissions [16]. In Francistown and Gaborone, Botswana, household chemicals and pharmaceuticals were the predominant cause of acute poisoning [3]. In Kampala, Uganda, agrochemicals, household chemicals and carbon monoxide were more prevalent among the cases [23]. A study conducted in Hong Kong found sleeping pills and analgesics to be the most common poisons [9]. In Khuzestan region, South Western Iran, envenomation by scorpions, spiders and snakes was the major cause of poisoning [24].

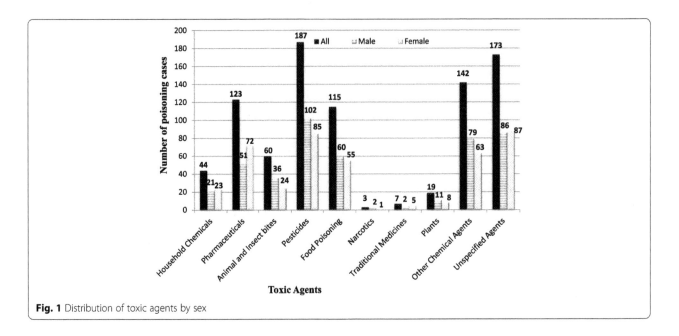

Fig. 1 Distribution of toxic agents by sex

Though only a few cases with narcotic poisoning were recorded in the present study, this observation is of particular importance since Zambia has in recent years become a consumer of hard drugs as evidenced by the increasing number of drug-dependent persons attended to by the Drug Enforcement Commission [25]. This increase in the rate of drug abuse observed poses a threat to public health in the near future. In addition, our study showed that children recorded more cases of poisoning with kerosene. This finding is in support of evidence in the literature that kerosene and paraffin oils are often kept in unsafe non-child-proof containers, resulting in accidental ingestion of the chemicals by children [17].

The number of snake envenomation cases recorded in this study was in accordance with those recorded in studies within countries such as Zimbabwe, Uganda and South Africa where more than 10 % were affected [16, 23]. As noted by the WHO, snake bites are an important public health issue in rural areas of sub-Saharan African countries - like Zambia - where the burden of snakebites is also high [26].

Background factors such as residence and socioeconomic status have been associated with acute poisoning elsewhere [27, 28]. Residential areas in urban Lusaka are classified as high, medium and low-cost housing areas based on the infrastructure and social services available. Studies and surveys have shown distinct differences in socioeconomic characteristics among these classes such as level of education, income and employment status [29]. A gradient in number of cases was observed with regard to area of residence. Most of the cases were from low cost, densely populated residential areas suggesting

an influence of socioeconomic status and living conditions on acute poisoning.

Limitations

The use of secondary data in the study limited control over the quality of data that were collected due to unsatisfactory record-taking and record-keeping. Pages from registers were torn out and some patient files were missing. In the files that were available, certain information such as marital status and occupation was not entered, though provision was made for the collection of such data in the registers. A good number of toxic agents were not specified in the records, making their classification difficult. Also, for most toxic agents identified, only the generic name was indicated which made the classification difficult. Furthermore, this being a hospital-based study we acknowledge that the results may not be representative of the general population. Data from the coroner's reports was not included in the study which may result in omission of some of the deaths which may have been due to poisoning.

Considering that the likelihood of being referred to higher level hospitals increases with clinical complexity and severity of poisoning cases, we acknowledge that some cases could have been missed as not all cases were referred to the study hospitals. This has further implications in that, deaths could be over represented in the study hospitals because they are more likely to receive severe cases. Also, due to their sensitive and delicate nature, children stand a higher chance of being referred as compared to adults and could therefore be over represented in the study hospitals. However, this does not undermine the findings in this study as referral hospitals

Table 5 Specific description of agents involved in poisoning cases reviewed

Toxic agent	Frequency n (%)
Narcotic drugs (n = 3)	
Amphetamines	2 (66.7)
Glue[a]	1 (33.3)
Plants (n = 19)	
Unspecified plants	14 (93.7)
Elephant ear plant[b]	5 (26.3)
Household chemicals (n = 44)	
Disinfectants	19 (43.2)
Cleaning agents	15 (34.1)
Personal care products	8 (18.2)
Food additives	2 (4.6)
Animal/Insect bites (n = 60)	
Snake	53 (88.3)
Bee	4 (6.7)
Wasp	2 (3.3)
Scorpion	1 (1.7)
Pharmaceuticals (n = 128[c])	
Analgesics	56 (43.8)
Antibiotics	20 (15.6)
Unspecified drugs	18 (14.6)
Antipsychotics	7 (5.5)
Nutrition supplements	6 (4.7)
Anticonvulsants	6 (4.7)
Antimalarial drugs	6 (4.7)
Anti-retroviral drugs	4 (3.1)
Antihistamines	2 (1.6)
Family planning pills	1 (0.8)
Antihypertensive drugs	1 (0.8)
Anti-Tuberculosis (TB) drugs	1 (0.8)
Pesticides (n = 187)	
Unspecified organophosphates	97 (51.9)
Insecticides	76 (40.6)
Rodenticides	14 (7.5)
Other agents (n = 142)	
Kerosene	69 (48.6)
Carbon monoxide	26 (18.3)
Acids	23 (16.2)
Construction chemicals	11 (7.8)
Spirit of salt	6 (4.3)
Formalin	3 (2.1)
Diesel	1 (0.7)
Car radiator cooler	1 (0.7)

Table 5 Specific description of agents involved in poisoning cases reviewed *(Continued)*

Brake fluid	1 (0.7)
Silica gel	1 (0.7)

[a]A volatile solvent/inhalant
[b]A plant of the genus *Colocasia*
[c]Counts for both single and combination drug overdose cases

have been shown to be good surrogates for monitoring poisoning in a wider population base [30]. Hence, the information provided is still valuable in describing the pattern of acute chemical poisoning in Lusaka.

Conclusions

It can be concluded that children, whose circumstance of poisoning is mainly unintentional, are at a high risk of poisoning. The study also revealed that although deliberate self-harm was common in young adult females, mortality was higher in males. Most poisoning cases were from the social demographically disadvantaged peri urban areas of Lusaka district. The findings of this study identify the need for health education in the general public on chemical safety, particularly with regard to pesticides and pharmaceuticals to prevent morbidity and mortality due to this problem. Special health education on chemical safety may be tailored for mothers and caregivers to prevent chemical exposure in children whose access to toxic agents is known to be mainly in homes or their immediate environment. In addition, information on the prevention of snake bites may be incorporated in public health messages, especially during the rainy season when most snake bites generally occur. Health education may be supported by strengthening and enforcing regulations addressing the control of pharmaceuticals, pesticides and other chemicals to prevent unnecessary access and exposure.

Further prospective studies are required to explore the pattern of poisoning in other geographical locations of the country and for longer time periods. This may aid in creation of models for predicting poisoning in the different regions which may provide for effective diagnosis, management and prevention of poisoning in Zambia.

Abbreviations
DALY's: Disability Adjusted Life Years; ERES: Excellence in Research Ethics and Science; IRB: Institutional Review Board; LMGH: Levy Mwanawasa General Hospital; UTH: University Teaching Hospital; WHO: World Health Organisation.

Competing interests
The authors have no competing interests to disclose.

Authors' contributions
JZ contributed in conception of the research idea, development and write up of the proposal, as well as in data collection, analysis and interpretation of data. JZ was also involved in drafting of the manuscript. CM played a key role in the consolidation of the research idea, design, analysis and interpretation of results. CM was also involved in critical review of the manuscript. YS assisted in development of data collection tools, analysis and interpretation of results. All authors agree to be accountable for all aspects of the work.

Authors' information
Authors' Academic Qualifications
JZ: Bachelor of Science in Environmental Health 2012, University of Zambia; Master of Science in Epidemiology 2014, University of Zambia; Master of Philosophy in International Health 2015 (Occupational Health), University of Bergen, Norway.
YS: BSc Honours in Occupational Hygiene 1984, Polytechnic of South Bank, London; Master of Public Health 2005, University of Zambia; Post-PhD Master of Science in Biostatistics and Epidemiology 2010, University of the Witwatersrand, Johannesburg, South Africa.
CM: Bachelor of Science in Human Biology 1984, University of Zambia; Bachelor of Medicine and Bachelor of Surgery (MBChB) 1988, University of Zambia; Master of Public Health (MPH) 1999, University of Zambia; MBA 2009, Edith Cowan University, Perth, Australia; PhD (Epidemiology) 2007, University of Bergen, Norway.

Acknowledgements
This study is part of the MSc Epidemiology program supported by Norad's Programme for Master Studies (NOMA, ref No.2010/12841) that provided financial support for developing and running Master's degree programmes in Zambia. We would also like to thank the management for the University Teaching Hospital and Levy Mwanawasa General Hospital providing access to the data that was used in this research. We further acknowledge the support provided by the Research Support Centre at the University of Zambia, School of Medicine (UNZA-SoM) through the Southern African Consortium for Research Excellence (SACORE), which is part of the African Institutions Initiative Grant of the Welcome Trust (company no. 2711000), a charity (no. 210183) registered in England; The National Institutes of Health (NIH) through the Medical Education Partnership Initiative (MEPI) programmatic award No. 1R24TW008873 entitled "Expanding Innovative Multidisciplinary Medical Education in Zambia" at UNZA-SoM; for arranging analytical support.

References

1. World Health Organization WHO. Global Burden of Disease: 2004 update. World Health Organisation: Switzerland; 2008.
2. World Health Organisation WHO. Poisons information, prevention and management. http://www.who.int/ipcs/poisons/en/ (2014). Accessed 05 Jun 2014.
3. Malangu N. Characteristics of acute poisoning at two referral hospitals in Francistown and Gaborone. SA Fam Pract. 2008;50(3):67.
4. World Health Organisation WHO. Manual for the Public Health Management of Chemical Incidents. Geneva, Switzerland: WHO Documentation Production Services; 2009.
5. Chemicals Abstract Services CAS. Content at a Glance. http://www.cas.org/content/at-a-glance (2014). Accessed 16 Jun 2014.
6. Organisation for Economic Co-operation and Development OECD. Environmental Outlook for the Chemicals Industry. http://www.oecd.org/dataoecd/7/45/2375538.pdf (2001). Accessed 15 Jun 2014.
7. Dawson AH, Eddleston M, Senarathna L, Mohamed F, Gawarammana I, Bowe SJ, et al. Acute human lethal toxicity of agricultural pesticides: a prospective cohort study. Plos Med. 2010;7(10), e1000357. doi:10.1371/journal.pmed.1000357.
8. Miller M, Bhalla K. An urgent need to restrict access to pesticides based on human lethality. Plos Med. 2010;7(10), e1000358.
9. Chan YC, Fung HT, Lee CK, Tsui SH, Ngan HK, Sy MY, et al. A prospective epidemiological study of acute poisoning in Hong Kong. Hong Kong J emerg med. 2005;12:156–61.
10. Veale DJ, Wium CA, Muller GJ. Toxicovigilance. I: A survey of acute poisonings in South Africa based on Tygerberg Poison Information Centre data. S Afr Med J. 2013;103(5):293–7. doi:10.7196/SAMJ.6647.
11. Central Statistics Office (CSO). Zambia 2010 Census of Population and Housing: Preliminary Population Figures. 2011. http://unstats.un.org/unsd/demographic/sources/census/2010_PHC/Zambia/PreliminaryReport.pdf. Accessed 15 Jun 2014.
12. United Nations Human Settlements Programme (UN-HABITAT). Zambia: Lusaka Urban Profile. Nairobi: UNON, Publishing Services Section; 2007.
13. Republic of Zambia. The 2012 List of Health Facilities in Zambia: Preliminary Report (Version No. 15). http://www.moh.gov.zm/docs/facilities.pdf (2013). Accessed 20 October 2015.
14. Jepsen F, Ryan M. Poisoning in Children. Current Paediatrics. 2005;15:563–8.
15. Malangu N, Ogunbanjo GA. A profile of acute poisoning at selected hospitals in South Africa. South African Journal of Epidemiology Infection. 2009;24(2):14–6.
16. Tagwireyi D, Ball DE, Nhachi CF. Poisoning in Zimbabwe: a survey of eight major referral hospitals. J Appl Toxicol. 2002;22(2):99–105.
17. Eddleston M. Pattern and problems of deliberate self-poisoning in the developing world. QJ Med. 2000;93:715–31.
18. Hawton K, Fagg J. Trends in deliberate self poisoning and self injury in Oxford, 1976-90. BMJ. 1992;304(6839):1409–11.
19. Camidge DR, Wood RJ, Bateman DN. The epidemiology of self-poisoning in the UK. British Journal of Clinical Pharmacology. 2003;56(6):613–9. doi:10.1046/j.1365-2125.2003.01910.x.
20. Eddleston M, Karunaratne A, Weerakoon M, Kumarasinghe S, Rajapakshe M, Sheriff MH, et al. Choice of poison for intentional self-poisoning in rural Sri Lanka. Clin Toxicol (Phila). 2006;44(3):283–6.
21. Joint WHO/IPCS/CEC Meeting, Kulling P., La Ferla F. Prevention of Acute Chemical Poisoning: High-Risk Circumstances: Munster, 8-12 December 1986. Copenhagen, Europe ROf;1986.
22. Thundiyil JG, Stober J, Besbelli N, Pronczuk J. Acute pesticide poisoning: a proposed classification tool. Bull World Health Organ. 2008;86(3):205–9.
23. Malangu N. Acute poisoning at two hospitals in Kampala-Uganda. Journal of Forensic and Legal Medicine. 2008;15:489–92.
24. Jalali A, Savari M, Dehdardargahi S, Azarpanah A. The pattern of poisoning in southwestern region of Iran: envenoming as the major cause. Jundishapur J Nat Pharm Prod. 2012;7(3):100–5.
25. Drug Enforcement Commission (DEC). Drug Enforcement Commission: Annual Report (2011-2012). http://www.deczambia.gov.zm/downloads/2011-2012%20ANNUAL%20REPORT.pdf (2014). Accessed 28 Jun 2014.
26. World Health Organisation WHO. Snake Antivenoms. www.who.int/mediacentre/factsheets/fs337/en/ (2010). Accessed 05 Jun 2014.
27. Chang SS, Sterne JA, Wheeler BW, Lu TH, Lin JJ, Gunnell D. Geography of suicide in Taiwan: spatial patterning and socioeconomic correlates. Health Place. 2011;17(2):641–50. doi:10.1016/j.healthplace.2011.01.003.
28. Harriss L, Hawton K. Deliberate self-harm in rural and urban regions: a comparative study of prevalence and patient characteristics. Soc Sci Med. 2011;73(2):274–81. doi:10.1016/j.socscimed.2011.05.011.
29. Mweembaa MJA, Webb E. Residential area as proxy for socio-economic status, paediatric mortality and birth weight in Lusaka. Journal of Tropical Pediatrics: Zambia; 2008.
30. Senarathna L, Buckley NA, Jayamanna SF, Kelly PJ, Dibley MJ, Dawson AH. Validity of referral hospitals for the toxicovigilance of acute poisoning in Sri Lanka. Bull World Health Organ. 2012;90(6):436–A. doi:10.2471/BLT.11.092114.

5

Use of the data system for field management of a clinical study conducted in Kolkata, India

Ju Yeon Park[1], Deok Ryun Kim[1*], Bisakha Haldar[2], Aiyel Haque Mallick[2], Soon Ae Kim[1], Ayan Dey[1], Ranjan Kumar Nandy[2], Dilip Kumar Paul[3], Saugata Choudhury[3], Shushama Sahoo[3], Thomas F. Wierzba[1,4], Dipika Sur[2], Suman Kanungo[2], Mohammad Ali[1,5] and Byomkesh Manna[2]

Abstract

Background: Designing an appropriate data system is important to the success of a clinical study. However, little information is available on this topic. We share our experiences on designing, developing, and implementation of a data system for management of data and field activities of a complex clinical study.

Methods: The data system was implemented aiming at determining the biological basis for the underperformance of oral vaccines, such as polio and rotavirus vaccines in children at a site in Kolkata, India. The system included several functionalities to control data and field activities. It was restricted to authorized users based on their access privileges. A relational database platform was chosen, and Microsoft Visual FoxPro 7.0 (Microsoft Corporation, Seattle, WA, USA) was used to develop the system. The system was installed at the clinic and data office to facilitate both the field and data management activities.

Results: Data were doubly entered by two different data operators to identify keypunching errors in the data. Outliers, duplication, inconsistencies, missing entries, and linkage were also checked. Every modification and users log-in/log-out information was auto-recorded in an audit trail. The system offered tools for preparation of visit schedule of the participants. A visit considered as protocol deviation was documented by the system. The system alerted field staff to every upcoming visit date to organize the field activities and to inform participants which day to come. The system also produced a growth chart for evaluating nutritional status and referring the child to a specialized clinic if found to be severely malnourished.

Conclusion: The data system offered unique features for controlling for both data and field activities, which led to minimize drop-out rates as well as protocol deviations. Such system is warranted for a successful clinical study.

Keywords: Data management, Field management, Database, Data system, Clinical study

Background

Clinical studies play important role for improving human health; therefore, these studies should be managed properly and carefully [1, 2]. Data collection, data cleaning, editing, and management of the data in compliance with regulatory standard and the International Conference on Harmonization Harmonized Tripartite Guideline for Good Clinical Practice (ICH GCP) are important aspects of a clinical study. A data system should ensure that these issues are well addressed in the system design [3]. The design should also ensure that the data are accurate, complete and compliant with regulatory standards and GCP requirements, and the analyses are done using cleaned data sets. Besides, the system should include tools for providing support to the clinic, field and laboratory staff in order to collect data accurately and in a timely manner. Only a few trials goes exactly as initially planned. For instance, a case report form (CRF) may need updating in

*Correspondence: drkim@ivi.int
[1] International Vaccine Institute, Seoul, South Korea
Full list of author information is available at the end of the article

the course of trial, a new trial site may be added, and new technology may emerge [4]. An investigator is, therefore, to worry about installing a data management system that is flexible and compliance with set guidelines and standards.

Although literature is plentiful in describing various aspects of data analysis, little can be found that tells about practical aspects of designing a data system [5–8]. Rarely, a data system includes tools to perform both data and field activities. It is worth mentioning, analyses of the clinical studies can be flawed not only by problems in data acquisition and field methodology, but also by errors in the design of the data system.

Recent hardware and advanced software tools have made it possible to develop an ideal data system for clinical studies [5]. In designing the system, one should consider study objectives, nature of the study site, and the local issues. The design should be flexible to accommodate unanticipated issues in the field and data management. Inclusions of tools for checking data outliers and inconsistencies as well as for queries are essential. Storing other information such as metadata (data dictionary) and audit trail, that tracks all the modifications ever made in the system, must be included in the system. While designing, one should also focus on system specifications, structure of the database, data and field management tools, and performance of the system.

We designed, developed, and implemented a data system for a complex clinical study in Kolkata, India. In the study, the vaccines was given to the participants concomitantly with the EPI routine immunization program for a period of 1 year, and there were multiple visits for specimen collection from the study participants, which could have been well managed with the support from the data system. This paper discusses the design, development, and implementation, as well the performance of the data system.

Methods

The clinical study

The clinical study named provide (Performance of Rotavirus and Oral Polio Vaccine in Developing Countries) was initiated in Kolkata, India with the hypothesis that there are factors for the underperformance of oral vaccines in children living in the developing world. It aimed to determine whether decreased vaccine responsiveness to oral poliovirus or rotavirus vaccines is associated with the presence of tropical enteropathy (TE); and to evaluate whether the impact of an inactivated polio vaccine (IPV) boosted systemic and mucosal immune responses to polio vaccines following vaccination with oral polio vaccine (OPV) in children with and without TE. The study was carried out among infants residing in Kolkata.

The study aim was to recruit 372 children at 6 weeks of age and follow them until they were 53–54 weeks of age. There were 12 visits for each of the participants during the follow-up time including the initial visit. This study was also carried out in accordance with the routine immunization schedule in India. Therefore the participants would have to be vaccinated with other vaccines, such as, BCG, DPT, HepB and Measles.

The data system

A custom-made data system, named INDSys, was designed and developed aiming to turn the information from the participants into data, to transcribe the data into a database without errors, and to manage data delivery from clinics and laboratory efficiently. The design phase focused on defining the database components and the modules and interfaces required for satisfying the need of data and field activities. While developing the system, provisions were kept for accommodating any new data or field related issues into the system. The system was developed using Microsoft Visual FoxPro 7.0 (Microsoft Corporation, Seattle, WA, USA), and the data was managed in a relational database environment. All related data, including clinical, laboratory and other data sets as well as field work schedule, were integrated within the data system.

The data system was restricted to authorized users only such as data managers, data operators, clinical monitors and investigators. There were two levels of restrictions in the system. At the first level, the users required login identification and password to access the system. At the 2nd level, the system functionalities were restricted according to the user's privileges. The functionalities according to the user's role are shown in Table 1. The data entry screens were designed to look similar to the data forms for facilitating the data entry operations. A dual data entry system was designed to avoid keypunching errors in the data [9]. A comprehensive data validation tool was incorporated in order to identify missing values, outliers, duplications, and intra- and inter-record inconsistencies in the data. Errors that cannot be corrected, such as unordinary data or missing laboratory results in the system, were also selected to remain in the database with proper documentation. The data system automatically stored information on changes in the data, users' log-in, log-out, entry, modification, and deletion of the data in an audit trail. Information such as who changed the data and when the changes were made were also stored in the audit trail. Additional information such as a data dictionary, data status, data checking plan and code plans for open-ended questions were accessible through the system. A report generation module was included in the system to monitor the performance of field and data activities.

Table 1 Accessible functionalities according to the user's role

Role	Main responsibilities	Accessible functionalities
Database administrator	Grant permission to a user for accessing system and maintain system and troubleshooting	All functions
Data manager	Supervise data entry, error check, and backup	Entry, view/edit/delete, dual check, error check, report/query, maintenance(backup, change password)
Data operators	Data entry and check dual entry error	Entry, view/edit, dual check, maintenance (change password)
Clinical monitor(s)	View data for monitoring electronic data	View, report/query, maintenance (change password)
Investigator(s)	Supervise all data activities	View, report/query, maintenance (change password)

For the field management, the system design included activities in field office, such as participant's contact, calendar of all visits, participant's discontinuation/drop-outs, growth chart, missing visits, etc. Necessary tools (*vide infra*) were included in the system so that the field management could control the activities easily and smoothly, especially for this complicated schedule of visits. Each participant was to be vaccinated with several vaccines (e.g. DPT, HepB, and Oral Polio Vaccine) in accordance with Expanded Program on Immunization (EPI) in India, and study vaccines (e.g., Rotavirus, Oral Polio Vaccine, or Inactivated Polio Vaccine). If a participant received a vaccine on a day other than the scheduled day, the subsequent date of vaccination as well as scheduled dates of visit for specimen collection would also change to the date of vaccination and a new calendar for the visitation schedule was prepared for the participant accordingly. The data system included tools to generate the new visitation schedule after each visit was made by a participant.

Implementation of the data system

The data system was implemented in standalone computers at the data center and at the field clinic of the National Institute for Cholera and Enteric Disease (NICED). Microsoft Windows was chosen as the operating system to implement the data system. No other software was required to operate the system. The data and field staff of the project were trained on how to operate the data system. Authorized users, had access to the system through assigned identification and password. The staff members at the clinic had access to the system only for management of the field activities. The database at the clinic was continuously updated by the data staff of the project to facilitate field activities with updated data sets.

Ethical considerations

Written informed consent was obtained by mothers of participating children. The study protocol was approved by the scientific advisory committee (SAC), Institutional Ethics Committee of the National Institute

of Cholera and Enteric Diseases (NICED), the Health Ministry Screening Committee of India, and the International Vaccine Institute Institutional Review Board. The protocol was registered at clinical trial registry of India (CTRI/2012/03/002504) and at clinicaltrials.gov (NCT01571505).

Results

Start-up screen

Upon starting the system, a log-in screen appears for accessing the system. After successful log-in, a menu describing the list of activities appears on the screen according to the user's privileges. As a dual data entry system, the system provides options for entering the data either in the 1st or 2nd file according to the user's privileges. If the operator enters a Screening Number for a new recruitment, the system shows the Data Entry Status screen (called start-up screen) of the participant (Fig. 1). In this screen, the data entry status for the different visits of the participant is reflected by color, and the number of successful and missed visits are easily identifiable. Since the screening form is used to assign the Study ID, the user will receive an error message if s/he tries to enter any other forms before entering the screening form. In the event of early termination of a participant, the operators are not allowed to enter any other forms of the participant. When one-year of follow-up of a participant is passed, the system checks for missing visits and specimens, and alerts accordingly. This helps ensure completeness of the data entries of all visits of a participant.

Data entry and editing

The study had two sources of data: clinic and lab. The data from the clinic, such as enrolment, follow-up, and specimen collection were entered into the data system soon after receiving the forms. The lab data were entered and verified by lab scientists following data validation rules and then uploaded onto the system. The embedded data validation process in the system ensures quality of the data after checking for outliers and inconsistencies.

1st Entry: Timeline

Screening Number: 3001   Study Identification: 1001   Exit

Visit Number		01	02	03	04	05	06	07	08	09	10	11	12
Weeks	0 to 6 wks	06 wks	10 wks	14 wks	16 wks	17 wks	18 wks	24 wks	39 wks	40 wks	51 wks	52 wks	54 wks
Screening Form	X												
Mother Enrolment		X											
Infant Enrolment		X											
SES, Water and Sanitation		X											
Follow-Up		X	X	X	X	X	X	X	X	X	X	X	X
Lab Transfer: Breast Milk		X											
Lab Transfer: Mother Blood		X											
Lab Transfer: Infant Blood		X					X			X			X
Lab Transfer: Infant Urine					X					X	X		
Lab Transfer: Infant Stool			X	X	X	X	X					X	X
Referral							X						
Adverse Events							X						
Serious Adverse Events							X						
Early Termination							X						
Subject Summary Report							X						

Fig. 1 The status of data entries of the different forms of a participant (start-up screen)

While entering the data from the clinic, the other functions are inactivated by the system. In the event of a potential error during data entry, the system warns the operator and provides options for correcting it. However, the operator can move on without correcting the data if the correction cannot be made at his/her level. A specific module for data checking is incorporated into the system (vide supra) to trap any error in the database.

The system provides a view screen for reviewing all data forms in one screen. The user can view the data by using navigation keys located on the right side of the page of the screen and selecting the participant ID, or by entering the participant ID in a specified box. If a participant ID is selected, the participant's data form can be viewed by clicking on a specific tab of the form abbreviations.

The lab data, before final submission to data room, were recorded on specific data forms designed for lab results, dually entered in Excel, and further checked by lab personals. The data generated by the laboratory is uploaded onto the system from the soft copy of the data. In this case, the user clicks onto the Upload Lab Result tool to get the list of the file names of all the lab data. If a wrong file name is selected, the system warns the user and prevents him/her from uploading the data.

Unlike clinic data, the lab data are not allowed to edit directly on the screen. If an error is detected in the lab data, the error is sent to the laboratory for correction. After getting the corrected data in a soft copy, the erroneous data was replaced with the corrected one.

Data validation and audit trail

There were two modules in the system for checking accuracy of the data. Firstly, the data are doubly entered to detect keypunching errors. The system provides a list of discrepancies between the two entries including unmatched unique identification of the children between the two entries. Once the keypunching errors in the data are resolved, the user is allowed to move to the second step of data checking which includes outliers, inconsistencies, validity of the dates, and linkage. If the errors generated at the source, the forms along with the type of errors are sent to the field office for resolution. Once the error feedbacks are received, the data are updated accordingly. When an update is done, the user ID, date and time of update, and old and new values are stored in the audit trail. Audit trails are being created incrementally, in chronological order, and in a manner that it does not allow new audit trail information to overwrite existing data. If updates are made multiple times, the users can trace complete history of the updates.

Producing schedule of visits

As mentioned above, there were 12 visits for each participant in a year including the initial visit for consent and screening of the participants. It was necessary to calculate the scheduled dates of visit for each participant during the follow-up period, and remind them to come to the clinic on that date. Since enrolment dates differed from one participant to another and the purpose of visit also differed from one visit to another, keeping track of the schedule dates and purpose of visit would be difficult without having field management tools in the system. Note that the scheduled dates of visit might also change depending on the last date of visit. The system produces a fresh calendar of the scheduled dates of appointments after every visit is made (Fig. 2). This helped Field Supervisors to fill the dates of visit schedule in the Study Identification Card which should be brought when the participants come to the clinic, to remind them by telephone and home visit prior to the schedule date, and to identify whether the visits were made on the planned date or not. The system also produces the list of all visits

to be made on the upcoming clinic day (an example is shown in Fig. 3), so that the field staff can take necessary actions to make those visits successful.

Data backup

Data can be lost by a computer accident or catastrophic loss -such as losing a critical file or experiencing unexplained file corruption, a hard drive crash, or total system loss. The system provides a backup tool to maintain a regular backup at the end of each working day. A backup copy was kept in a separate building away from the data center.

Reporting protocol deviation

One of the most challenging tasks of the clinical study was to manage the scheduled dates of visits of the participants for vaccination and specimen collection. The target visit dates may change depending on the previous date of visit of the participants. For visit week 6–18, participants will be invited to come to the clinic based on the date of his/her last vaccination on account of the mandatory 4 weeks window between vaccinations. For visit week 24–53, participants will be at age of the visit week +7 days, regardless of the date of last vaccination.

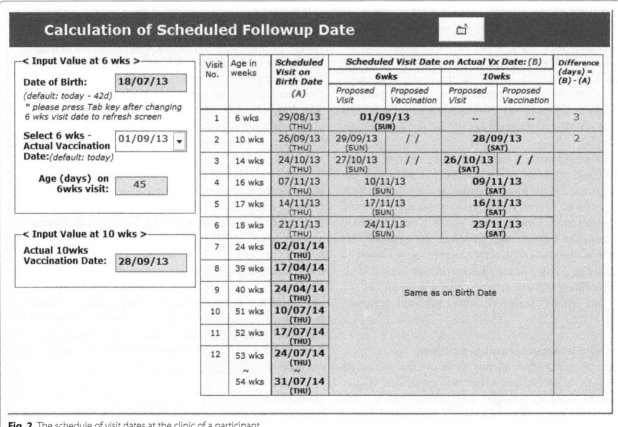

Fig. 2 The schedule of visit dates at the clinic of a participant

Followup Schedule

IVI/PROVIDE STUDY/NICED, INDIA
Proposed Visit / Vaccination Date=26/08/13 (Monday)

SID	Clinic Visit Week	Actual Vx date						Proposed Date		Anthropometry		Vaccination							Specimen Collection				
		6wks (OPV)	10wks (OPV)	14wks (OPV)	17wks (Rota)	39wks (OPV/IPV)	52wks (OPV)	Lower bound	Upper bound	Weight	Length	DTP	HepB	OPV	IPV	Rota	Measles	VitA	Mother BM	Blood	Infant Blood	Urine	Stool
1091	53-54 wks	28/09/12	31/10/12	30/11/12	20/12/12	17/05/13	19/08/13	25/08/13	27/08/13	Y	Y											Y	
1092	53-54 wks	28/09/12	31/10/12	30/11/12	20/12/12	17/05/13	19/08/13	25/08/13	27/08/13	Y	Y											Y	
1093	53-54 wks	28/09/12	31/10/12	30/11/12	20/12/12	17/05/13	19/08/13	25/08/13	27/08/13	Y	Y											Y	
1094	53-54 wks	28/09/12	31/10/12	03/12/12	19/12/12	17/05/13	19/08/13	25/08/13	27/08/13	Y	Y											Y	
1096	53-54 wks	01/10/12	31/10/12	30/11/12	20/12/12	23/05/13	19/08/13	25/08/13	27/08/13	Y	Y											Y	
1097	53-54 wks	01/10/12	31/10/12	03/12/12	21/12/12	23/05/13	19/08/13	25/08/13	27/08/13	Y	Y											Y	
1098	53-54 wks	01/10/12	02/11/12	03/12/12	21/12/12	23/05/13	19/08/13	25/08/13	27/08/13	Y	Y											Y	
1103	52 wks/Day 11	03/10/12	02/11/12	05/12/12	26/12/12	16/05/13	//	25/08/13	27/08/13														Y
1106	52 wks/Day 4	05/10/12	07/11/12	07/12/12	27/12/12	23/05/13	//	25/08/13	27/08/13														Y
1112	52 wks/Day 0	10/10/12	09/11/12	10/12/12	02/01/13	30/05/13	//	23/08/13	26/08/13	Y	Y			Y									Y
1113	52 wks/Day 0	10/10/12	09/11/12	10/12/12	02/01/13	30/05/13	//	23/08/13	26/08/13	Y	Y			Y									Y
1115	51 wks	17/10/12	16/11/12	17/12/12	05/01/13	06/06/13	//	26/08/13	02/09/13	Y	Y											Y	
1200	40 wks	02/01/13	01/02/13	04/03/13	28/03/13	//	//	25/08/13	27/08/13	Y	Y					Y	Y				Y	Y	
1268	24 wks	22/04/13	24/05/13	24/06/13	16/07/13	//	//	26/08/13	02/09/13	Y	Y												
1294	18 wks	30/05/13	01/07/13	31/07/13	//	//	//	25/08/13	27/08/13	Y	Y											Y	
1301	17 wks	07/06/13	08/07/13	07/08/13	//	//	//	26/08/13	02/09/13	Y	Y					Y							
1310	14 wks/Day 0	26/06/13	26/07/13	//	//	//	//	23/08/13	26/08/13	Y	Y	Y	Y	Y									Y
1332	10 wks	26/07/13	//	//	//	//	//	26/08/13	02/09/13	Y	Y	Y	Y	Y		Y							
1333	10 wks	26/07/13	//	//	//	//	//	26/08/13	02/09/13	Y	Y	Y	Y	Y		Y							

Fig. 3 List of the participants to be visited on the upcoming clinic day

If a visit or procedure cannot be made within the specific time period (called window period), then those visits or procedures are treated as protocol deviation. Since this clinical study depends largely on the biological issues, any protocol deviation would have negative impact on the results of the analysis. Therefore, it was important to keep the number of protocol deviations as minimized as possible.

The data system produces how many visits or procedures turned out to be protocol deviation. Note that the system generated protocol deviation is data driven, thus the study could overcome limitation of manually created protocol deviation form, which is prone to error and may differ from the data actually stored in the database. An example of the system generated protocol deviation is shown in Fig. 4. The system also provides the status of all visits, vaccinations, and sample collections with (in red color) and without (in green color) protocol deviation (Fig. 5).

Reporting of severely malnourished children

The study required referring severely malnourished children to a specialized clinic for treatment. Upon request, the system provides an anthropometric data calculator for calculating nutritional status and drawing growth charts of the children, which were evaluated to understand the nutritional status of the children. The system produces two types of growth chart for each participant: weight-for-age and length-for-age. By triggering the participant's ID, the user can instantly get the child's growth status according to the World Health Organization (WHO) child growth standard (http://www.who.int/childgrowth/standards), as shown in Fig. 6. In the figure, the two lines from the bottom were related to malnutrition status. If the child's weight or height is marked below the line of SD2neg (<-2SD), the child is considered malnourished. If the child's weight or height is marked between line of SD2neg and SD3neg, the child is considered moderate malnourished. And, if the child's weight or height is marked below SD3neg (<-3SD), the child is considered severely malnourished. In case of severely malnourished, the child was referred to a specialized clinic for treatment. However, with this growth chart, the user could not get z-scores for anthropometric indicators (weight-for-age and height-for-age) based on the WHO child growth standard. Thus, the list of severely malnourished children generated from the system was just to facilitate field activities (Figs. 7, 8).

Discussion

Running a clinical study smoothly like ours is challenging due to its complex and long duration visit schedule.

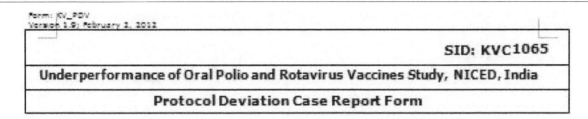

Form: KV_PDV
Version 1.9; February 1, 2011

SID: KVC1065

Underperformance of Oral Polio and Rotavirus Vaccines Study, NICED, India

Protocol Deviation Case Report Form

1	Date of Report	23/08/13	
2	Form completed for	1 = Mother 2 = Infant	2
3	Date of Protocol Deviation	26/07/13	
4	Visit week associated with protocol deviation	01=Enrollment 02=Week 06 03=Week 10 04=Week 14 05=Week 16 06=Week 17 07=Week 18 08=Week 24 09=Week 39 10=Week 40 11=Week 51 12=Week 52 13=Week 53-54 99=Not applicable	12
5	Type of deviation?	01=Missed visit 02=Missed specimen 03=Missed shedding specimen 04=Missed procedure 05=Missed specimen + procedure 06=Blood specimen collected outside visit 07=Urine specimen collected outside visit 08=Stool specimen collected outside visit window 09=Breast milk specimen collected outside visit window 10=Visit occurred outside of window 11=Vaccination outside clinic 12=Incorrectly vaccinated 13=Child received additional dose of OPV 14=Other	02
	5a. If any, please specify	02=Missed specimen: Infant Stool/Day 25	
6	Reason for deviation?	1 = Subject illness 2 = Subject unable 3 = Subject refusal 4 = Clerical 5 = Investigator decision 6 = Other	6
	6a. If any, please specify		
7	Did the deviation result in an adverse event?	1 = Yes 2 = No	2

Fig. 4 A protocol deviation form generated from the data system

In our study, all 372 participants were successfully recruited according to the planned schedule. The dropout rates were only 8 % and protocol deviations stood at 3 %. The reasons for these protocol deviations included: visits occurring outside the window period (44 %), missed specimen (34 %), missed visits (11 %), specimen collected outside the window period (10 %), and missed procedures (1 %). 99 % blood samples, 95 % stool samples, 98 %

Followup Schedule   **SID: KVC** [1001] |◀ ◀ ▶ ▶| 🔍 🖨 📂   Treatment Group Assignment? (A=No IPV, B=With IPV boost): ▮

Field	0	1	2	3	4	5	6	7	8	9	10	11	12
Visit number	0	1	2	3	4	5	6	7	8	9	10	11	12
Age in weeks	Birth	6 wks	10 wks	14 wks	16 wks	17 wks	18 wks	24 wks	39 wks	40 wks	51 wks	52 wks	53-54 wks
Scheduled visit on Birth Date	13/02/12	26/03/12	23/04/12	21/05/12	04/06/12	11/06/12	22/06/12	30/07/12	12/11/12	24/11/12	04/02/13	11/02/13	18/02/13
Scheduled Date on Actual Vx		28/03/12	27/04/12	28/05/12	08/06/12	15/06/12	22/06/12						
1 Date of visit (dd/mm/yy)		28/03/12	27/04/12	30/05/12	12/06/12	15/06/12	22/06/12	30/07/12	17/11/12	23/11/12	04/02/13	11/02/13	25/02/13
2 Weight (Kg)	02.70	3.18	3.83	4.86	5.19	5.14	5.40	6.65	8.52	8.40	9.60	9.35	9.70
3 Length (cm)	999.9	52.2	55.8	58.1	58.7	58.5	59.1	62.5	70.1	70.6	73.5	73.5	74.0

Vaccinations (1=Yes, 2=No)

BCG	1	07/03/12
OPV	1	07/03/12

6 Vaccinations (1=Given on the date of visit, 2=Given on other day, 3=Illness, 4=Absent, 5=Refused, 6=Moved away, 7=Died, 8=Investigator decision, 88=Other, 99=NA)

Field	0	1	2	3	4	5	6	7	8	9	10	11	12
6a. DTP		1	1	1									
6b. HepB		1	1	1									
6c. OPV		1	1	1					1			1	
6d. IPV									99				
6e. Rota		1				1							
6f. Measles										1			
6g. Vit A										88 ilability of			

7 Mother Specimens (use same code as #6)

Field	0	1	2	3	4	5	6	7	8	9	10	11	12
7a. Breast Milk		1											
7b. Blood		1											

8 Infant Specimens (use same code as #6)

Field	0	1	2	3	4	5	6	7	8	9	10	11	12
8a. Blood		1					1			1		1	
8b. Urine				1						1	1		
8c. Stool	(see subtables below)												

8c. Stool — left subtable:

	Scheduled on Actual Vx		Actual
Day 0	30/05/12	1	30/05/12
Day 4	03/06/12	2	02/06/12
Day 11	10/06/12	88	/ /
Day 18	17/06/12	2	15/06/12
Day 25	24/06/12	2	22/06/12

8c. Stool — right subtable:

	Scheduled on Actual Vx		Actual
Day 0	11/02/13	2	08/02/13
Day 4	15/02/13	2	14/02/13
Day 11	22/02/13	2	21/02/13
Day 18	01/03/13	1	01/03/13
Day 25	08/03/13	2	07/03/13

Fig. 5 The status of visits and vaccinations, and sample collections with protocol deviation status generated by the data system

urine samples, and 100 % breast milk samples were successfully collected. Such an excellent performance would have not been possible without having the support provided by the data system.

In addition to manage data activities and generate data reports, our data system provides support for management of the field activities such as preparing visit schedule, alerting next day visit schedule and assessing requirement of the logistics including number of doses of the vaccines, etc. for the next visit schedule. It also ensures a good clinical practice, a legal requirement to conduct clinical trials in many countries. The other advantage in our system is that it generates nutritional status report of the participants at each time point so as to take immediate actions against severely malnourished infants, such as referring to a specialized clinic where proper treatment can be ensured. In the system, the data interoperabilities are limited to Acrobat Reader and Excel, as required by us. However, we have kept provision for the data interoperability in any other standard data format.

Our data system is specific to our study, which is unlikely to match exactly with any other studies. Three-month time of a skilled system designer and programmer was required to design and develop the system. Unlike open source software where many developers have the opportunity to scrutinize the system, our system was scrutinized in-house.

Since many developers scrutinized the open source application, it is hard for bugs to hide in that application. Also, since codes of the open source software are shared among numerous parties, it is typically well structured, which cannot be ensured a single company develops like us [10].

However, our system passes through different courses of action over the time, and we were able to fix the bugs in the system. More importantly, we were able to tailor it specific to the project activities, which may not have been possible in an open source software solution.

The limitation in our system is that it was installed on standalone computers. Therefore, we had to upload of the updated database to the field office computer on a regular basis. Similarly, the data generated at the lab were uploaded manually into the system. This offline mechanism could have been avoided if the computers at the clinic and lab were connected to the data office through a network. However, we could not make it possible in our setting due to limitation of resources.

Still a large part of clinical centers uses their own developed solution or a single solution [11] because

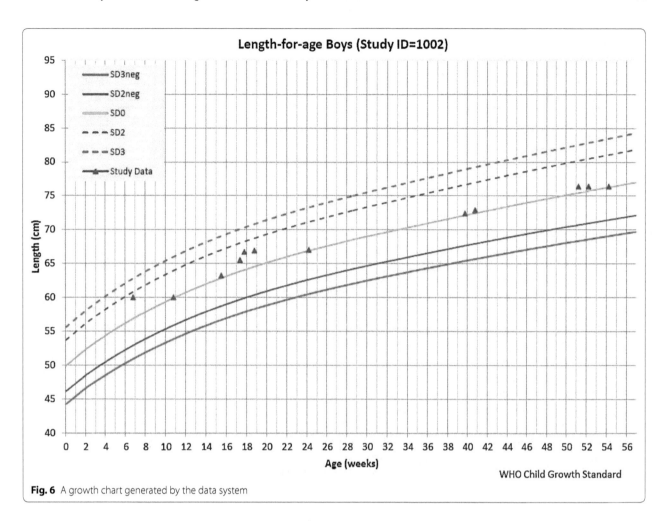

Fig. 6 A growth chart generated by the data system

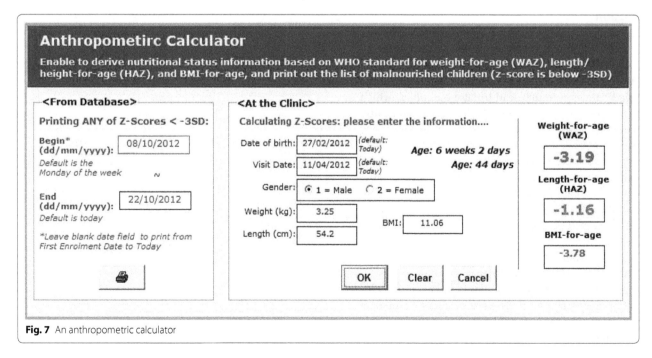

Fig. 7 An anthropometric calculator

List of any Z-Score <-3SD

IVI/PROVIDE STUDY/NICED, INDIA

Study ID	Clinic Visit Week	Gender (1=M;2=F)	Age (days)	Weight (kg)	Length (cm)	BMI	Weight -for-age	Length -for-age	BMI -for-age	Referral Form Exists (1=Yes)	Comments
1152	39 wks	1	276	5.94	60.4	16	-3.614	-5.191	-0.653		
1152	40 wks	1	283	6.02	60.5	16	-3.564	-5.260	-0.508	1	
1312	06 wks	1	44	3.22	52.4	11	-3.246	-2.070	-3.206	1	
1328	06 wks	1	43	3.20	50.3	12	-3.230	-3.076	-2.364	1	
1336	06 wks	1	45	2.86	50.6	11	-4.023	-3.042	-3.722	1	

Fig. 8 The list of participants malnourished children (z-score is below -3SD) generated by the system

clinical data managements are very heterogeneous, and the open source solutions do not play a major role in clinical trial data management [12]. However, because of flexibility, increased innovation, shorter development times, and faster procurement processes, open source software may be attracted by an organization. Also by using open source software, an organization will not be locked into using a proprietary software program. One disadvantage in an open source solution is that, due to the web-based nature of this system, it may pose a challenge for real time data entry because in many developing country settings internet connectivity is a problem. One may also face sluggish response times and system timeouts. Additionally, XML rules may adversely affect the application's response time and therefore other options may need to be explored and used while using open software solution [3].

Conclusion

Clinical data management has evolved and will continue to do so in response to need [13]. Limited literature hinders the capacity of scientists to design and develop a well-managed data system for their studies [14]. An ill-managed data system may lead to false outcomes, which is detrimental for the study; eventually for human health. The concepts and ideas we discussed in this paper may be useful for designing and developing a well-managed data system for the clinical studies. By controlling both the data and field activities in a system, the investigators may overcome the complexities of the visit schedules in their studies. We believe such a system would be useful for the investigators who want to initiate a complex clinical study.

Availability of supporting data

This paper describes the design, development, and implementation of a data system. The source codes of the data system and operators' manual can be made available upon request.

Abbreviations

GCP: good clinical practice; TE: tropical enteropathy; IPV: inactivated polio vaccine; OPV: oral polio vaccine; EPI: expanded program on immunization; ID: identification; WHO: World Health Organization; SD: standard deviation.

Authors' contributions

DRK and MA contributed to the design of the data system. DRK, BM, and MA contributed to the implementation of the system. DRK, BM, SK, BS, AHM, SAK, AD, RKN, DKP, SC, SS, TFW, DS and MA supervised the study activities. JYP, DRK, and MA analyzed the system tools, reviewed the performance of the system, and wrote the first draft of the manuscript. All authors participated in the writing of the manuscript and had access to the data system. All authors read and approved the final manuscript.

Author details

[1] International Vaccine Institute, Seoul, South Korea. [2] National Institute of Cholera and Enteric Diseases, Kolkata, India. [3] B.C. Roy Post Graduate Institute of Pediatric Sciences, Kolkata, India. [4] PATH, Washington, DC, USA. [5] Johns Hopkins Bloomberg School of Public Health, Baltimore, USA.

Acknowledgements

We are grateful to the people of the study area in Kolkata and our field staffs. The study was funded by the Bill & Melinda Gates Foundation. The Foundation had no role in study design, data collection and analysis, decision to publish, or preparation of the manuscript.

Competing interests

The authors declare that they have no competing interests.

References

1. Krishnankutty B, Bellary S, Kumar NBR, Moodahadu LS. Data management in clinical research: an overview. Indian J Pharmacol. 2012;44(2):168–72.
2. La HO. Quality management system of clinical research. Kor J Clin Pharmacol Ther. 2006;14(1):23–8.
3. Ngari MM, Waithira N, Chilengi R, Njuguna P, Lang T, Fegan G. Experience of using an open source clinical trials data management software system in Kenya. BMC Res Notes. 2014;7:845.
4. Ene-Iordache B, Carminati S, Antiga L, Rubis N, Ruggenenti P, Remuzzi G, Remuzzi A. Developing regulatory-compliant electronic case report forms for clinical trials: experience with the demand trial. J Am Med Inform Assoc. 2009;16:404–8.
5. Pradhan EK, Katz J, LeClerq SC, West KP Jr. Data management for large community trials in Nepal. Control Clin Trials. 1994;15(3):220–34.
6. Youngblut JM, Loveland-Cherry CJ, Horan M. Data management issues in longitudinal research. Nurs Res. 1990;39(3):188–9.
7. Goodger WJ, Bennett T, Garcia M, Clayton M, Pelletier J, Eisele C, Thomas C. Development of a database management/analysis system for field

research activities within a coordinated research project. Prev Vet Med. 1999;38(2–3):85–100.

8. Ali M, Park JK, von Seidlein L, Acosta CJ, Deen JL, Clemens JD. Organizational aspects and implementation of data systems in large-scale epidemiological studies in less developed countries. BMC Public Health. 2006;6:86.

9. Cummings J, Masten J. Customized dual data entry for computerized data analysis. Qual Assur. 1994;3:300–3.

10. Baumann B. Overcoming obstacles to successful clinical trials through open source. http://www.appliedclinicaltrialsonline.com/appliedclinicaltrials/article/articleDetail.jsp?id=743711 (2011). Accessed 10 October 2015.

11. Fegan GW, Lang TA. Could an open-source clinical trial data-management system be what we have all been looking for? PLOS Med. 2008;5(3):347–9.

12. Kuchinke W, Ohmann C, Yang Q, Salas N, Lauritsen J, Gueyffier F, Leizorovicz A, Schade-Brittinger C, Wittenberg M, Voko Z, Gaynor S, Cooney M, Doran P, Maggioni A, Lorimer A, Torres F, McPherson G, Charwill J, Hellström M, Lejeune S. Heterogeneity prevails: the state of clinical trial data management in Europe—results of a survey of ECRIN centres. Trials. 2010;11:79.

13. Lu Z, Su J. Clinical data management: current status, challenges, and future directions from industry perspectives. Open Access J Clin Trials. 2010;2:93–105.

14. Roberts RJ, Musick BS, Olley B, Hall KS, Hendrie HC, Oyediran AB. Data management in a longitudinal cross-cultural study. Stat Med. 2000;19(11–12):1645–9.

6

Tobacco is "our industry and we must support it": Exploring the potential implications of Zimbabwe's accession to the Framework Convention on Tobacco Control

E. Anne Lown[*], Patricia A. McDaniel and Ruth E. Malone

Abstract

Background: Zimbabwe is the largest tobacco producer in Africa. Despite expressing opposition in the past, Zimbabwe recently acceded to the World Health Organization's Framework Convention on Tobacco Control (FCTC). We explored why Zimbabwe acceded to the FCTC and the potential implications for tobacco control within Zimbabwe and globally.

Methods: We conducted a qualitative archival case study based on 542 documents collected from 1) the Truth Tobacco Industry Documents; 2) media indexed in the Lexis-Nexis media database; 3) the websites for tobacco growers' associations, tobacco control groups, and international agencies; 4) FCTC reports and Framework Convention Alliance newsletters; 5) Zimbabwe's legal codes; and 6) the peer reviewed scientific literature related to tobacco growing.

Results: Zimbabwe has a long history of tobacco growing. There are currently over 90,000 tobacco farmers, and tobacco growing is prioritized, despite widespread food insecurity and environmental degradation. Zimbabwean government officials have been outspoken FCTC critics; but recently joined the accord to better protect Zimbabwe's tobacco growing interests. FCTC membership obligates nations to implement a variety of tobacco control measures; Zimbabwe has implemented several measures aimed at reducing tobacco demand, but fewer aimed at reducing tobacco supply or protecting the environment. Zimbabwe joins the FCTC amid increased efforts to protect FCTC proceedings from industry interference, to adopt recommendations for alternative crops and livelihoods and reduce environmental damage.

Conclusion: Zimbabwe's decision to accede to the FCTC does not appear to represent a softening of its historical opposition to the treaty. Thus, its status as a Party creates opportunities for it to undermine ongoing efforts to implement and strengthen the treaty. At the same time, however, Zimbabwe's accession could provide much needed international support for Zimbabwe's civic organizations and its Ministry of Health to develop stronger tobacco control measures. How Zimbabwe's participation impacts the work of the FCTC as a whole may ultimately depend on the allegiances of its delegates, and the effectiveness of FCTC measures to limit tobacco industry interference and enforce compliance with FCTC measures.

Keywords: Tobacco industry, Agriculture, Zimbabwe, Developing countries, World Health Organization, FCTC, Global health, Humans, Smoking*/prevention & control, International cooperation

* Correspondence: anne.lown@ucsf.edu
Department of Social and Behavioral Sciences, School of Nursing, University of California, San Francisco, CA 94143-0612, USA

Background

While tobacco use is leveling off in high-income countries such as the US and Britain, the tobacco industry is aggressively marketing to low and middle-income nations [1]. Nonetheless, many African countries still have relatively low rates of tobacco use ([2] pp. 268) suggesting that the tobacco epidemic that killed 100 million in the 20th century, mostly in higher income nations, could still be averted there. Tobacco use is distinguished from many other health problems by the presence of an aggressive, transnational tobacco industry whose goals are fundamentally incompatible with public health [3]. Like other industries, the tobacco industry not only seeks to promote use of its products and expand into new markets, but also seeks to weaken strong tobacco control policies and undermine public health advocacy efforts [4–8].

African nations played an integral role in developing and establishing a strong policy response to the tobacco problem, the United Nations World Health Organization's Framework Convention on Tobacco Control (WHO-FCTC) [9, 10]. The FCTC treaty entered into force in 2005 with 40 signatories. In contrast to most of its African neighbors, Zimbabwe, one of the largest tobacco producers in Africa and the world, [11] was opposed to the FCTC's creation [12, 13]. However, on December 4, 2014, Zimbabwe deposited a signed version of the FCTC treaty to the United Nations and on March 4, 2015 Zimbabwe officially became the 180th Party to the accord [14–16].

It is unknown what positions Zimbabwe will take as a Party to the FCTC. If Zimbabwe uses its influence to obstruct, delay, or diminish FCTC provisions related to tobacco growing, marketing and distribution, its accession would represent a setback for global tobacco control efforts. Adopting the role of obstructionist would also place Zimbabwe at odds with many of its African neighbors, who continue to be actively engaged in implementing the FCTC. However, as a negotiating Party, Zimbabwe may also find itself forced to compromise in ways that ultimately benefit tobacco control efforts within the country and within the region.

This paper describes the role that tobacco plays in Zimbabwe's economy, and why the country acceded to the FCTC. Next, it examines the obligations and privileges associated with FCTC membership, and concludes by considering the possible implications of Zimbabwe's accession to the FCTC for both the international tobacco control movement and for tobacco control within the country.

Methods

In this archival qualitative study we examined data from multiple sources. First, to identify tobacco industry influence in Zimbabwe, the first and second authors searched the Truth Tobacco Industry Documents (TTID) (https://industrydocuments.library.ucsf.edu/tobacco/). The TTID contains over 14 million internal tobacco industry documents released as part of the 1998 Master Settlement Agreement between the attorneys general of 46 U.S. states and the tobacco industry [17]. To locate documents, we used search terms for tobacco growers' associations active in Zimbabwe (e.g., "International Tobacco Growers Association," "Zimbabwe Tobacco Association"), as well as tobacco control activities (e.g., "World No Tobacco Day"), and tobacco industry activity (e.g., "British American Tobacco-Zimbabwe," "Savanna Tobacco," "Courtesy of Choice Campaign") in Zimbabwe. We retrieved and screened over 5,000 documents; after eliminating duplicates and irrelevant materials, we examined in more detail 45 TTIDs.

Because the bulk of tobacco industry documents we found were dated from 1981 to 2000, the first author also searched the Lexis Nexis database for media accounts of the current situation in Zimbabwe. LexisNexis indexes over 26,000 media sources, including local, national and international newspapers, magazines, trade journals, and radio and television broadcast transcripts. She used search terms related to Zimbabwe and tobacco (e.g., "Zimbabwe" AND "tobacco" OR "cigarette" OR "smoking" OR "tobacco control" OR "FCTC") and to political, health, and economic dynamics in Zimbabwe (e.g., "Zimbabwe" AND "sustainable development goals" OR "world tobacco day" OR "deforestation" OR "environment" OR "child labour/labor" OR "tobacco exports" OR "land reform"). She found 168 relevant media items; most were newspaper or magazine articles or transcripts of radio or television broadcasts from news sources in Zimbabwe, the UK, the US, and China.

For the most current information on the activities of tobacco growers' associations and tobacco manufacturers in Zimbabwe, the first and second authors examined their websites (e.g., tobaccoleaf.org, fctobacco.com, bat.com, savanatobacco.com). To understand the history and process of the WHO-FCTC, the first author examined online WHO-FCTC reports (e.g., "Conference of the Parties to the WHO FCTC, No 5, Friday, 17 October 2014") and Framework Convention Alliance (FCA) newsletters and reports. To understand international tobacco issues the first and second authors examined various websites (e.g., the United Nations Development Program), (N = 94) reports (e.g., Food and Agriculture Organization or World Bank) (N = 98), proceedings (e.g., All Africa Conference on Tobacco Control) (N = 4), and books or book chapters (e.g., *Tobacco Control in Africa: People, Politics and Policies*) (N = 7). The authors also examined the text of Zimbabwe's tobacco control law (e.g., Statutory Instrument 264 of 2002). Finally, in order to place our findings in context, the first and second authors examined the peer reviewed scientific literature related to tobacco growing, Africa and/or the FCTC (N = 122). The total number of documents that served as the basis for our analysis was 542.

We followed an approach consistent with a qualitative case study [18]. All relevant documents were downloaded into an Endnote database, notes were added, key words were assigned, and key pieces of information were highlighted (e.g., policies on land use and tobacco growing, comments from Health Ministers about FCTC or tobacco control measures). The documents were organized chronologically and by topic (e.g., FCTC-related statements made over time by Zimbabwe government officials). For validation purposes we asked two experts involved in FCTC negotiations to review the penultimate draft of our report.

Results

Tobacco's role in Zimbabwe's economy

The Zimbabwean government regards tobacco as the "lifeblood of Zimbabwe's economy" [13]. In 2012 the country was the top tobacco-producing nation in Africa, and in 2013 it was the sixth largest tobacco producer in the world [11]. According to Zimbabwe's Tobacco Industry and Marketing Board, 98 % of Zimbabwe's tobacco is exported, making it the country's largest foreign currency generator (accounting for 10–43 % of the country's gross domestic product) [19, 20]. Zimbabwe receives a higher percent of government revenue from tobacco leaf than any other country in the world, except Malawi [21], partly due to a levy system that taxes both growers and buyers [22].

Tobacco is a major source of employment: there are over 90,000 small scale tobacco farmers in Zimbabwe [19, 23], supported by a robust tobacco growing infrastructure. For example, banks dedicate significant revenue for loans to tobacco farmers [24], though small-scale farmers have fewer loan options [25]), land (taken in 2000 from white farmers) is preferentially given to black tobacco farmers by the government [26–28], tobacco companies offer loans for seeds and fertilizer [19, 24], and tobacco farmers receive cash payments upon delivering their crop [29]. As a result, despite widespread hunger in Zimbabwe, farmers are more likely to grow tobacco than grain [19, 24].

Zimbabwe's Ministry of Agriculture and Ministry of Industry and Commerce oversee tobacco industry-related organizations such as The Tobacco Research Board, the Tobacco Industry and Marketing Board, and the Boka Tobacco Auction Floors. Two independent groups that claim to represent tobacco farmers' interests, the Zimbabwe Tobacco Association (ZTA) (and its offshoot, the Farmers Development Trust, recipient of

several US$100,000 grants from Phillip Morris [30]), and the International Tobacco Growers Association (ITGA), are influential in Zimbabwe [31, 32]. The ZTA was founded in 1928 (originally as the Rhodesian Tobacco Association) to "promote and support research and training to ensure the continued development and expansion of the flue-cured tobacco growing industry" [32]. In 1984, the ZTA and representatives of five other tobacco-growing nations founded the ITGA with funding from transnational tobacco companies [33–35]. Previous research has exposed the ITGA as a public relations vehicle for transnational tobacco companies, providing a "human face" and a "grass roots voice" to articulate the positions of tobacco manufacturers [35, 36]. Both groups have publicly criticized the FCTC [12, 13, 32, 34, 37] and both have tried to influence FCTC proceedings [36, 38, 39].

While industry, government, and tobacco grower organizations in Zimbabwe work together to support tobacco growing, their interests and positions sometimes conflict. For example, the ZTA opposed government levies on growers and a land redistribution program in the late 1990s, which resulted in many highly productive white tobacco farmers fleeing to Zambia, South Africa, and Mozambique [40, 41] (where tobacco growing subsequently increased) [11].

Zimbabwe's economy is near collapse due to its US$11 billion debt [42], made worse by continuing corruption [42–44], high unemployment (80–85 %) [42, 45, 46], widespread hunger [47], succession battles [42, 44, 48–51], and a 2014 law that requires all companies to hand over 51 % of shares to black Zimbabweans [52]. In the face of economic strains, tobacco growing is likely to continue to be a major income generator for the government.

Zimbabwe's accession to the FCTC

In the past, Zimbabwe government officials and growers' organizations have been outspoken supporters of tobacco growing and critics of the FCTC [31, 53, 54]. For example, Zimbabwe's President Robert Mugabe expressed support early in his presidency for the tobacco industry saying: "If we sell it, we must grow it as well. It is our industry and we must support it" [31]. In 2000, at the FCTC public hearings in Geneva, the ZTA criticized the work of the FCTC as a "crusading task of drawing up a global tobacco prohibition accord, to be legally imposed upon governments" [12]. (The FCTC does not, in fact, ban tobacco growing [55]). Both the ZTA and the ITGA developed a briefing on the FCTC describing it as a "thoroughly bad and damaging international treaty" which represented an "an attack on [Zimbabwe's] national sovereignty" [32].

By 2010, as the FCTC garnered increasing international support, Zimbabwe appeared to re-assess the value of its outsider status. Joseph Made, Zimbabwe's Minister of Agriculture and close ally of President Mugabe, argued that it was time to join the FCTC because the country's outsider status made it more difficult to protect its tobacco interests and it needed to work in concert with other countries [13]. In 2013, Gavin Foster, ZTA president, appealed to the Zimbabwean government to sign the FCTC accord "so that we can defend not only our tobacco growing industry but that of the entire continent under threat. Lets [sic] us stop non producing and non tobacco [sic] dependent countries; countries and organisations with hidden agendas deciding the future of our industry and livelihoods" [34]!

The need for tobacco control in Zimbabwe

While daily smoking prevalence among women in Zimbabwe is relatively low (5 %), men's smoking prevalence is much higher (33 %) [56], reflecting the growing popularity of smoking among African men [57]. In Africa, civil society organizations have played a key role in spurring government tobacco control [58], but in Zimbabwe only one civic tobacco control organization, the Zimbabwe Framework for Tobacco Control Trust, is apparently active. It applied to attend a recent FCTC meeting but was turned away as it has no website, no identifiable members, and scant media coverage [19, 59]. There is a demonstrable need for tobacco control in Zimbabwe.

FCTC Membership: Obligations and Privileges

In addition to several general obligations, the FCTC requires members to adopt and implement measures that address tobacco control in three domains – tobacco demand reduction, tobacco supply reduction, and protecting the environment – as spelled out in the 18 primary articles that comprise the treaty. Tables 1, 2, 3 and 4 outline how Zimbabwe's current tobacco control policies and practices measure up against FCTC articles.

General obligations for FCTC Parties as outlined in Article 5 require member countries to actively engage in tobacco control work, financing and coordinating the work on a national level (Table 1) [60]. Zimbabwe has few tobacco control measures and one national tobacco control law, Statutory Instrument 264 of 2002 [61]. In 2009 it had a national tobacco control agency (with one employee), and no budget for tobacco control activities [62]. In 2014 Zimbabwe developed national tobacco control objectives [63]. President Mugabe continues to publicly express support for tobacco growing [64].

FCTC Article 5.3 specifies that tobacco control measures should be protected from commercial or other vested interests of the tobacco industry [60]. Just four months after acceding to the FCTC, a Zimbabwean government ministry signed a Memorandum of Understanding accepting a

donation of $527,000 from the British American Tobacco (BAT) to enhance tobacco production by providing training, building tobacco curing barns, and improving access to credit for youth, women, and disabled small farmers [65–67].

Tobacco control activities to reduce demand (Articles 6-16) in Zimbabwe have been minimal (Table 2). Health warnings are required on cigarette packages [56], there are some designated smoke-free settings [68], and cigarettes are taxed at 60 % of the retail price [68]. Beyond that, there are few other regulations. Cigarettes are widely advertised [56, 68], sponsorships by Savanna Tobacco, a local Zimbabwean company, are common [69–73], and single stick cigarette sales are popular to market smoking to the poor [74]. There are no mass education anti-smoking programs [56, 68], and government and tobacco industry officials have publicly minimized the dangers of smoking [34, 53]. For example, in 1994, at a national congress meeting, President Mugabe minimized the risk of tobacco use when he said, "I think WHO has its priorities wrong. Why can they not be more fair with tobacco and start with alcohol" [53]. At the 2013 World Tobacco Day ZTA president Gavin Foster said, "The impact of tobacco on the health of individuals whether on us growers, our workers and families, processors, manufacturers, our end user the smoker and the general populace ranks very low when ranked against the World Health Organisation's deadliest causes of death and diseases such as heart disease, strokes, lower respiratory diseases, HIV, and other NCDs" [34].

Tobacco control activities aimed at reducing the supply of tobacco (Articles 15-17) have been even less vigorously pursued. There are widespread reports of cigarette smuggling to surrounding countries [74–81]. While there are laws to prevent tobacco sales to minors, [61] young urban and rural dwellers report easy access (Table 3) [82]. Article 17 is particularly challenging for Zimbabwe since it involves the "provision of support for economically viable alternative activities" to tobacco growing. Both government and industry officials claim that there are no economically viable alternative crops to replace tobacco, [34, 83] despite evidence to the contrary [84]. Local media reports continue to emphasize the advantages of growing tobacco [85, 86].

Finally, tobacco control efforts aimed at the "protection of the environment and health of persons" (Article 18) represent another hurdle (Table 4) [60]. Deforestation is a particularly significant problem for Zimbabwe [23, 87–93], since flue-cured tobacco requires heat to process the leaves, and wood is used as a fuel supply [87].

A key privilege of joining the FCTC is becoming a voting member at Conference of the Party (COP) meetings [14]. COP is the governing body of the FCTC and is

Table 1 Zimbabwe's 2015 tobacco control policies in relation to FCTC general obligations

FCTC Article [60]	Zimbabwe's tobacco control policies	Zimbabwe's practice
Article 5: Develop and implement tobacco control measures; finance and coordinate the work nationally.	• One law, Statutory Instrument 264 of 2002, outlines smoke-free premises, no smoking signs, tobacco and children, product ingredients disclosures, promotion of tobacco products, and importing tobacco.	• The government rationale for joining the FCTC was: "[w]e cannot fight from outside and win [13]."– Minister of Agriculture (2010) • "We will grow [tobacco] for those who want to smoke it. You should listen to what your doctor says. But if you over smoke, don't blame us [64]."– President Robert Mugabe (April, 2015)• The Minister of Agriculture-Joseph Made described an unusual unity between black and white farmers in order to save tobacco-Zimbabwe's dominant cash crop. "There are no differences between us on this one," he says. "Everyone is working together….[13]" (2010) • Economic problems and corruption [42–44] slow tobacco control implementation and coordination.
Article 5.3: Protect tobacco control policies from commercial and other vested interests of the tobacco industry.	• No laws protect tobacco control policies from tobacco industry interests.	• Media reports credit nepotism for government's failure to act on Zimbabwe's Savanna Tobacco Company smuggling charges. Savanna Tobacco is owned by Mugabe's relative [75, 81]. • "There is need for all of us to be aware of the tobacco industry's activities to undermine tobacco control efforts through advertising, promotion and sponsorship which lure you into believing that tobacco is good…We will not tolerate any interference from the tobacco industry as we go about our duty of forming and enforcing laws that are good for the health of our people [110]."– Minister of Health Madzorera (2013) • Zimbabwe government ministry accepted $527,000 from BAT to support small tobacco farmers [65].

comprised of its 180 Parties [60]. Parties outline, adopt, and amend policies, make decisions on implementation, and discuss compliance with FCTC articles [94]. FCTC rules stipulate that COP meets in regular sessions biennially and that further work happens in regional meetings and designated working groups between COP meetings [95]. Membership in working and regional groups is voluntary. Decision-making is by consensus among Parties (observers can comment), with the caveat that a three-quarter majority rule is acceptable for substantive matters or a simple majority rule for procedural matters [95]. In past practice, consensus has dominated decision-making. Given the preference for consensus and voluntary membership in regional and working groups, there are opportunities for a Party to influence or obstruct FCTC provisions that it finds objectionable. Moreover, as a member of COP, Zimbabwe will be party to negotiations and have access to documents and conversations that would likely be of interest to the tobacco industry.

In acceding to the FCTC, Zimbabwe has joined a club to which 43 of 47 African nations belong. (Only Eritrea, Malawi, and South Sudan have not ratified the FCTC. Mozambique has signed but not ratified the treaty [16, 96]). African regional unity was key to negotiating a strong treaty, with African nations (both tobacco producing and non-producing) voting as a bloc and making alliances with other regional blocs to advance their tobacco

control agenda [9, 10]. Thus, at COP meetings, Zimbabwe may contend with pressure to advance not simply its own interests, but regional interests as well [96].

Future COP meetings are likely to discuss two issues of particular significance for Zimbabwe: strengthening Article 5.3, and reviewing progress on recommendations for implementing Articles 17 and 18. Article 5.3 specifies that tobacco control measures should be protected from commercial or other vested interests of the tobacco industry [60]. Recent COPs have accelerated efforts to comply with Article 5.3 [60] which was first adopted at COP3 [97]. At COP5, Parties requested further discussion about the large number of industry representatives among the public attendees at COP meetings. At COP6, discussion centered on the need for more rigorous and advance vetting of the public (including the media) at future COP meetings and the exclusion of observers at the current meeting, where all Party delegates (not just observers, as before) might be required to file a declaration denying "any form of real, perceived, or potential conflict of interest with the tobacco industry" ([98, 99], pp. 31-32).

Further discussion on minimizing industry influence and accelerating Article 5.3 implementation is likely to occur at COP7 scheduled to take place in New Delhi in late 2016. Specific language to strengthen Article 5.3 could result in the exclusion of media, observers, or

Table 2 Zimbabwe's 2015 tobacco control policies in relation to FCTC measures to reduce demand for tobacco

FCTC Article [60]	Zimbabwe's tobacco control policies & activities	Zimbabwe's practice
Article 6: Price and tax measures to reduce the demand for tobacco	• Tax is 45 % of the retail price of cigarettes. [111]	• Tobacco growers and leaf buyers are also taxed [22].
Article 8: Protection from exposure to tobacco smoke	• 3 smoke-free public places: health care institutions; non-University educational facilities; and public transport [68]. • Fine of Z$500, imprisonment or both for violators [112].	• No/scant enforcement for passive smoking laws-Ministry of Health [113].
Article 9: Regulation of the contents of tobacco products	• No regulations identified.	
Article 10: Regulation of tobacco product disclosures	• Statutory Instrument 264, sec 7 • "Every tobacco product shall bear accurate information on the percentage of the tar and nicotine content and any other ingredients...visible on the package [61]."	
Article 11: Packaging and labeling of tobacco products	• Brand descriptors (e.g.,"light," "low tar") allowed [9, 56]. • 20 % of cigarette package must be covered by health warning [9, 56, 63]. • Packaging must contain one of three health warnings [61].	• Inexpensive, single stick cigarette sales are lucrative marketing strategy in Africa [114, 115] aimed at low income, low education, and young smokers [114]. • Smuggled single stick packages create tobacco control challenges for surrounding countries [74] • BAT-Z accused of selling cigarettes without Zimbabwe's prescribed warnings [116].
Article 12: Education, communication, training and public awareness of tobacco control issues	• No mass education campaigns implemented between 2012-2014 [56, 68]. • World No Tobacco Day has been celebrated in Zimbabwe since 2013 [117, 118].	• Government officials minimize risk of tobacco use [34, 53]. • No whole population media anti-smoking messages [63, 111].
Article 13: Comprehensive ban on tobacco advertising, promotion and sponsorship	• No direct or indirect bans on tobacco advertising, promotion or sponsorship [56, 68], (except,visual entertainment) [9, 56]. • Promotional events are only allowed for adults [61]. • No bans on free cigarette distribution, promotional discounts, sponsored events, or corporate social responsibility activities [56].	• Savanna Tobacco Co. sponsored Miss Zimbabwe contest [70], Zimbabwe's signature musician, Oliver Mtukudzi [71], local soccer teams [72, 73], and proposed $10 million donation for Harare stadium to be named after its Pacific brand [69]. • 63–77 % of youth exposed to tobacco advertising and 69–86 % exposed to brand names at sports events [82]. • Tobacco marketing in Zimbabwe–more aggressive than in high income countries [119].
Article 14: Demand reduction measures concerning tobacco dependence and cessation.	• Nicotine Replacement Therapy (sold with prescription) and/or some smoking cessation services available; costs not covered [68]. No national quitline [111].	

Table 3 Zimbabwe's 2015 tobacco control policies in relation to FCTC measures to reduce supply for tobacco

FCTC Article [60]	Zimbabwe's tobacco control policies & activities	Zimbabwe's practice
Article 15: Eliminate illicit trade in tobacco products.	• No tax stamps, local-language cigarette pack warnings, aggressive enforcement, or penalties in place [120].	• Cigarette smuggling by STC and BAT-Z widely reported in media [75–81].
Article 16: Prohibit sales to and by minors	• Sales of tobacco to under age 18 is prohibited [61]. • Enforcement information unavailable.	• 12 % of youth-current smokers [56] • 28–49 % bought cigarettes in a store [82].
Article 17: Provision of support for economically viable alternate activities	• No government sponsored programs to promote alternative crops.	• Ronald Watts, Zambian agricultural consultant, listed 53 possible alternative crops that could be developed in the region (1993) [84, 121]. • "There are no sustainable, economic [ally] viable alternate crops to tobacco [34]." ZTA chairman (2014) • Government and industry officials say- no economically viable alternative crops exist to replace tobacco [34, 83]. • Incentives for tobacco growing remain strong with increasing acreage devoted to it [122, 123]. • Local media favor stories of successful tobacco growing [85, 86].

Table 4 Zimbabwe's 2015 tobacco control policies in relation to FCTC measure to protect the environment

FCTC Article [60]	Zimbabwe's tobacco control policies & activities	Zimbabwe's practice
Article 18: Due regard for the protection of the environment and the health of persons in respect to tobacco cultivation and manufacture	• Section 4 of Zimbabwe's Environmental Management Act (Chapter 20:27), 2002, describes 4 general environmental rights: 1) Clean healthy environment; 2) Access to environmental information; 3) Environment to be protected for benefit of present and future generations; 4) Right to promote policies to end pollution and environmental degradation, and support sustainable management of resources [124]. • Statutory Instrument 116 of 2012 regulates use and trade of firewood and timber [125].	• Deforestation is widespread [23, 87–92] threatening to denude the country by 2016 [23, 88, 91, 93, 126]. • Zimbabwe is among top 10 countries for largest forest cover loss between 1990 and 2010 [127]. • Child labor on tobacco farms exposes children to harmful pesticides and fertilizers and prevents school attendance [128, 129]. • Tobacco pickers risk nicotine poisoning [130, 131]. • Tobacco industry sponsors Sustainable Afforestation tree planting program [91, 132].

even individual delegates from COP meetings; the mandatory use of new tools to track implementation of Article 5.3; increased transparency regarding industry involvement in Party countries; and the elimination of conflicts of interest for government officials and employees [100].

COP has been working on how best to implement Articles 17 and 18 since 2006. (Article 17 was included in the FCTC to protect tobacco farmers by addressing the possible economic consequences of effective tobacco control policies that could reduce demand for their crop [101].) At COP6 in 2014, an Articles 17/18 working group submitted its report. Although it was 8 years in the making, COP6 decided that the report needed further refinement. Parties quickly established an informal group to provide a brief set of nine recommendations drawn from the report ([99], p 16) COP6 adopted the policy options and recommendations in the full working group report despite divergent views [102] and requested that the Convention Secretariat implement the nine recommendations ([99], p. 79). The working group's mandate was not renewed [99]. At COP7 (New Delhi, 2016), the Secretariat will provide a progress report on the implementation of the recommendations [99]. Issues related to planting alternative crops and reducing environmental and health damage from tobacco growing are contentious and complex and any proposed solutions are likely to pose challenges for Zimbabwe, now officially involved in future discussions.

Discussion

Zimbabwe's current economic hardship, its robust tobacco growing and distribution infrastructure, and continued world demand for tobacco suggest that the government will continue to prioritize tobacco production in the absence of incentives to do otherwise. Its recent decision to accede to the FCTC does not appear to represent a softening of its historical opposition to the treaty, but rather a strategic move to better protect and

defend its tobacco interests in a world with a growing commitment to tobacco control.

Zimbabwe is not the first tobacco-dependent nation to sign on to the FCTC. Brazil, despite its status as one of the world's top tobacco producers, was instrumental in the creation of the FCTC and has been successful in reducing tobacco use by 50 % [103, 104]. Like Zimbabwe, most of its tobacco growing revenue came from exports. Since tobacco control measures that target internal tobacco use cause little conflict with export profits, Brazil was able to meet many of its FCTC obligations [105]. South Africa and Zambia, despite having strong tobacco growing industries, have also been able to advance tobacco control [9, 106].

These examples suggest that Zimbabwe may also be able to implement tobacco control at home [105]. As a member of the FCTC, Zimbabwe's internal tobacco control organizations and the Ministry of Health will now have international support to develop and promote stronger tobacco control measures [19]. Vigorous tracking of compliance with FCTC measures by the FCTC secretariat and public consequences for failure to meet obligations would further support tobacco control efforts in Zimbabwe [107].

Of concern is Zimbabwe's recent acceptance of a financial donation from BAT just months after acceding to the FCTC. This action could jeopardize Zimbabwe's participation in FCTC activities especially if there is stricter FCTC monitoring of compliance with Article 5.3 for "real, perceived, or potential conflict of interests" [99]. Acceptance of the BAT donation is a flagrant act of non-compliance with Articles 5.3, 17, and 18 [67].

Given these alliances Zimbabwe may undermine efforts to implement and strengthen the FCTC. For instance, its delegates could act as the eyes and the ears of the tobacco industry, reporting back on delegates' activities and sharing draft documents. This occurred previously when a Brazilian delegate who made numerous calls to a Brazilian subsidiary of BAT during COP4 meetings [108]. The inclusion of delegates with tobacco industry agendas within FCTC does occur (although it has been declining), and there are no current clear mechanisms to prevent this until a formal vetting process for delegates is in place.

Zimbabwe's status as a Party also offers it the opportunity to influence ongoing discussions about Articles 17 and 18. The FCTC has been slow to agree on a coherent and effective policy around supporting economically viable alternatives to tobacco growing and protecting the environment. Although the working group devoted to these issues no longer exists, discussions about alternative crops are likely to remain active, particularly if demand for tobacco declines. In the interim, Zimbabwe may be dismissive of many of the Articles 17/18 recommendations. Given COP's preference for consensus-based decision-making, it may require little effort by Zimbabwe to further stall progress. Zimbabwe could be aided in this endeavor by its natural alliances with other tobacco growers in the region – particularly in those countries to which white Zimbabwean tobacco farmers emigrated. However, the strong bloc of unified African countries that have a history of support for the FCTC may also hold Zimbabwe in check. Some of Zimbabwe's neighbors have much stronger tobacco control (e.g., Zambia). Zimbabwe's accession to the FCTC may be welcome in the region since membership will provide an obligation for Zimbabwe to take measures to reduce smuggling.

Conclusion

By 2025, much of Africa faces a worsening tobacco epidemic among men [109]. Implementing the FCTC's demand reduction measures has the potential to reverse this outcome. By its own admission, Zimbabwe joined the FCTC as a Party in order to defend its tobacco growing interests, but its status as a Party may open doors for tobacco control. Zimbabwe's participation in the FCTC as a whole, and progress on Articles 5.3, 17, and 18 in particular, may ultimately depend on allegiances that exist between Zimbabwe's delegates and 1) the tobacco industry, 2) the Zimbabwean government, and 3) Parties within the African region, as well as vigorous FCTC monitoring for compliance. To encourage Zimbabwe to be a productive member of the FCTC, it will be necessary to increase pressure on Parties to resist tobacco industry interference and comply with treaty obligations.

Abbreviations

BAT-Z: British American Tobacco Zimbabwe; COP: Conference of Parties; FCA: Framework Convention Alliance; ITGA: International Tobacco Growers Association; WHO FCTC: World Health Organization Framework Convention on Tobacco Control; ZTA: Zimbabwe Tobacco Association.

Competing interests

EAL has no competing interests. REM owns one share of Altria, Philip Morris International, and Reynolds American stock for research and advocacy purposes. REM and PAM served as tobacco industry documents consultants for the Department of Justice in *United States of America v. Philip Morris et al.* REM served as an advisor on the World Health Organization panel making recommendations for the guidelines for implementation of Article 5.3 and attended COP3 as part of the WHO delegation.

Authors' contributions

EAL collected and analyzed data, wrote the first draft of the manuscript, and revised subsequent drafts. PAM collected and analyzed data and edited each version of the manuscript. REM conceived of the study, participated in the design and analysis/synthesis of materials for the study, and edited all versions of the manuscript. All authors read and approved the final manuscript.

Acknowledgements

This research was supported by National Cancer Institute grant R01 CA120138. We would like to thank two anonymous FCTC experts for valuable comments on an earlier draft of this article.

References

1. Eriksen M, Mackay J, Ross H, Schluger N, Islami F, Drope J. The Tobacco Atlas. 5th ed. Atlanta and New York, N.Y: American Cancer Society, World Lung Foundation; 2015. http://3pk43x313ggr4cy0lh3tctjh.wpengine.netdna-cdn.com/wp-content/uploads/2015/03/TA5_2015_WEB.pdf. Accessed 22 Dec 2015.
2. WHO. WHO Report on the Global Tobacco Epidemic, 2008. Geneva: The MPower package; 2008. http://www.who.int/tobacco/mpower/mpower_report_full_2008.pdf. Accessed 21 Dec 2015.
3. WHO FCTC. Guidelines for implementation. Geneva: WHO; 2013. http://www.who.int/fctc/guidelines/adopted/guidel_2011/en/. Accessed 21 Dec 2015.
4. Connolly GN. Worldwide expansion of transnational tobacco industry. J Natl Cancer Inst Monogr. 1992;12:29–35.
5. Gilmore AB, Fooks G, Drope J, Bialous SA, Jackson RR. Exposing and addressing tobacco industry conduct in low-income and middle-income countries. Lancet. 2015;385(9972):1029–43. doi:10.1016/S0140-6736(15)60312-9.
6. McDaniel PA, Intinarelli G, Malone RE. Tobacco industry issues management organizations: creating a global corporate network to undermine public health. Global Health. 2008;4:2. doi:10.1186/1744-8603-4-2.
7. WHO. Tobacco Industry Interference with Tobacco Control. Geneva: World Health Organization; 2008. http://www.who.int/tobacco/publications/industry/interference/en/. Accessed 20 Mar 2015.
8. Yang JS, Malone RE. "Working to shape what society's expectations of us should be": Philip Morris' societal alignment strategy. Tob Control. 2008; 17(6):391–8. doi:10.1136/tc.2008.026476.
9. Tumwine J. Implementation of the framework convention on tobacco control in Africa: current status of legislation. Int J Environ Res Public Health. 2011;8(11):4312–31. doi:10.3390/ijerph8114312.
10. Collin J. Tobacco politics. Development. 2004;47(2):91–6.
11. Food and Agriculture Organization of the United Nations. Food and agriculture organization of the United National Statistics Division. 2015. http://faostat3.fao.org/download/Q/QV/E. Accessed 5 Mar 2015.
12. Zimbabwe Tobacco Association. Response to request by the World Health Organization for submission of comments on a proposed Framework Convention on Tobacco Control for public hearings at the Geneva International Conference Center (CICG)2000 October 12-13 http://www.who.int/tobacco/framework/public_hearings/zimbabwe_tobacco_association.pdf. Accessed 22 Mar 2015.
13. Mutsaka F. Zimbabwe enemies unite on tobacco. Wall Street Journal. 2010; http://online.wsj.com/news/articles/SB100014240527023035509045755616232168076147?mod=googlenews_wsj&mg=reno64-wsj&url=http%3A%2F%2Fonline.wsj.com%2Farticle%2FSB1000142405270230355090457556162321680761407614.html%3Fmod%3Dgooglenews_wsj. Accessed 22 Dec 2015.

14. WHO FCTC, Zimbabwe Accession, Reference: C.N.751.2014.TREATIES-IX.4 (Depositary Notification) (2015).

15. Zim signs tobacco control treaty. The Herald. 2014, July 31; http://www.herald.co.zw/zim-signs-tobacco-control-treaty/. Accessed 1 Aug 2014.

16. WHO FCTC. Status of the WHO Framework Convention on Tobacco Control (FCTC). Geneva: World Health Organization; 2015. http://www.fctc.org/images/stories/docs/ratifications/latest_ratifications.pdf. Accessed 13 Jul 2015.

17. Malone RE, Balbach ED. Tobacco industry documents: treasure trove or quagmire? Tob Control. 2000;9(3):334–8.

18. Yin R. Case study research design and methods. Thousand Oaks, CA: Sage Publications; 1994.

19. Lingui X. Health or cash - Zimbabwe's tobacco dilemma. CoastWeek.com. 2015, April 28; http://www.coastweek.com/3704-culture-05.htm. Accessed 28 Apr 2015.

20. Diao Z, Robinson S, Thomas M, Wobst P. Assessing impacts of declines in the world price of tobacco on China, Malawi, Turkey, and Zimbabwe. 2002 Contract No.: TMD Discussion Paper No. 91http://www.ifpri.org/publication/assessing-impacts-declines-world-price-tobacco-china-malawi-turkey-and-zimbabwe. Accessed 21 Dec 2015.

21. World Bank. Economics of Tobacco Use & Tobacco Control in the Developing World. Brussels: World Bank, World Health Organization and the European Commission; 2003. http://ec.europa.eu/health/archive/ph_determinants/life_style/tobacco/documents/world_bank_en.pdf. Accessed 21 Dec 2015.

22. Food and Agriculture Organization of the United Nations. Issues in the global tobacco economy: Selected case studies. Rome 2003 http://www.fao.org/3/a-y4997e.pdf. Accessed 7 May 2015.

23. Scoones I. Going up in smoke: The environmental costs of Zimbabwe's tobacco boom. Zimbabweland. 2014, January 20, https://zimbabweland.wordpress.com/2014/01/20/going-up-in-smoke-the-environmental-costs-of-zimbabwes-tobacco-boom/. Accessed 22 Dec 2015.

24. Business reporter. Banks offer 60 percent funding for tobacco farming. The Herald. 2014, Nov 3; http://www.herald.co.zw/banks-offer-60pc-funding-for-tobacco-farming/. Accessed 22 Dec 2015.

25. Hungwe B. Plight of Zimbabwe's small-scale tobacco growers. BBC. 2014, 8 March 2014; http://www.bbc.com/news/business-26485084. Accessed 22 Dec 2015.

26. Hawkins T. Farmers face slow recovery hampered by politics, drought and lack of funding; Zimbabwe. The Financial Times limited. 2014, Jan 21; http://www.ft.com/intl/cms/s/0/8fb40e14-5dca-11e3-95bd-00144feabdc0.html#axzz3v4TTR7sc. Accessed 22 Dec 2015.

27. United Nations Country Team, Government of Zimbabwe. Country Analysis Report for Zimbabwe. Harare: United Nations; 2010. http://www.zw.one.un.org/sites/default/files/Country%20Analysis%20Report%20for%20Zimbabwe%202010.pdf. Accessed 21 Dec 2015.

28. Wofford T. Mugabe: Whites can't own land in Zimbabwe. Newsweek. 2014 July 7, http://www.newsweek.com/mugabe-whites-cant-own-land-zimbabwe-257529. Accessed 22 Dec 2015.

29. Integrated Regional Information Networks (IRIN). Zimbabwe: Small-scale farmers choose tobacco over maize. IRIN, Humanitarian News and Analysis. 2011, October 26; http://www.irinnews.org/report/94074/zimbabwe-small-scale-farmers-choose-tobacco-over-maize. Accessed 22 Mar 2015.

30. Zimbabwe Tobacco Association (ZTA), In Support of Tobacco Indigenisation Training Programmes Million Zim Dollar: Donation from Philip Morris, 1998, August. Philip Morris. http://legacy.library.ucsf.edu/tid/zrc08d00. Accessed 01 Jul 2014.

31. Lowe Morna C. Zimbabwe's Tobacco Addiction. 1987, July/August; http://www.multinationalmonitor.org/hyper/issues/1987/07/morna.html. Accessed 22 Mar 2015.

32. Zimbabwe Tobacco Association, International Tobacco Growers Association, Briefing from Zimbabwe Tobacco Association and the International Tobacco Growers' Association, [2000], British American Tobacco. http://legacy.library.ucsf.edu/tid/eur03a99. Accessed 12 Mar 2015.

33. Bloxcidge JA, International Tobacco Growers' Association (ITGA), 1988, 11 Oct. British American Tobacco. http://legacy.library.ucsf.edu/tid/sik47a99. Accessed 1 Jul 2014.

34. Foster G. Zimbabwe Tobacco Association President's World Tobacco Day Speech. Zimbabwe Tobacco Association. 2013. http://protectfarmers.tobaccoleaf.org/wtgd_2013.aspx. Accessed 22 Mar 2015.

35. Must E. ITGA Uncovered: Unravelling the spin–the truth behind the claims: PATH Canada Guide, 2001 June http://www.healthbridge.ca/itgabr.pdf. Accessed 22 Mar 2015.

36. Assunta M. Tobacco industry's ITGA fights FCTC implementation in the Uruguay negotiations. Tob Control. 2012;21(6):563–8.

37. Lovegot T. Farmers Development Trust submission to WHO's first public hearing on tobacco control. WHO, International FCTC public hearings, 2000, October 12-13 http://www.who.int/tobacco/framework/public_hearings/F2610256.pdf. Accessed 22 Dec 2015.

38. van der Merwe F. Zimbabwe: Rights of tobacco farmers under threat. The Standard. 2014, August 10; http://allafrica.com/stories/201408110616.html. Accessed 22 Dec 2015.

39. International Tobacco Growers Association (ITGA). World Health Organization Ploughs on with Bureaucratic Blunder and Slams the Door on 30 Million Farmers. Lisbon, Portugal. 2010. http://www.businesswire.com/news/home/20100921006065/en/ITGA-World-Health-Organization-Ploughs-Bureaucratic-Blunder#.VK7-5SvF-Cm. Accessed 20 Mar 2015.

40. Selby A. Commercial Farmers and the State: Interest Group Politics and Land Reform in Zimbabwe. DPhil Thesis. Oxford, England: 2006.

41. LaFraniere S. Zimbabwe's white farmers start anew in Zambia. New York Times. 2004, March 21; http://www.nytimes.com/2004/03/21/world/zimbabwe-s-white-farmers-start-anew-in-zambia.html. Accessed 3 Jul 2015.

42. Ncube M. Desperate dictator: China refuses Robert Mugabe's request for Zimbabwe bailout. The Christian Science Monitor. 2014, March 10; http://www.csmonitor.com/World/Africa/2014/0310/Desperate-dictator-China-refuses-Robert-Mugabe-s-request-for-Zimbabwe-bailout. Accessed 22 Dec 2015.

43. Muleya D. Zimabwe must shape up. Zimbabwe Independent. 2014, June 6; http://www.theindependent.co.zw/2014/06/06/zimbabwe-must-shape/. Accessed 22 Dec 2015.

44. Tongogara P. As fighting for legitimacy in Zanu (PF) rages, will buffalo sink croc? Radio Voice of the People. 2015, January 14; http://www.radiovop.com/index.php/national-news/11596-as-fighting-for-legitimacy-in-zanu-pf-rages-will-buffalo-sink-dr.html. Accessed 22 Dec 2015.

45. Rotberg R. Zimbabwe: President Mugabe's new attack on white farmers. The Christian Science Monitor. 2014, July 7; http://www.csmonitor.com/World/Africa/Africa-Monitor/2014/0707/Zimbabwe-President-Mugabe-s-new-attack-on-white-farmers. Accessed 22 Dec 2015.

46. Kadirire H. 'It's not my fault'. dailynews. 2014, July 18; http://www.dailynews.co.zw/articles/2014/07/18/it-s-not-my-fault. Accessed 22 Dec 2015.

47. Food and Agriculture Organization of the United Nations. Tobacco in Zimbabwe. 2014. http://faostat.fao.org/CountryProfiles/Country_Profile/Direct.aspx?lang=en&area=181. Accessed 22 Dec 2015.

48. Editor. Allegiance to Mugabe supersedes ability. The Standard. 2014, December 15; http://allafrica.com/stories/201412160361.html. Accessed 22 Dec 2015.

49. Zimbabwe: Mugabe succession game plan exposed. Voice of Africa Radio 2012, May 5, http://www.thestandard.co.zw/2012/05/05/mugabe-succession-game-plan-exposed/. Accessed 22 Dec 2015.

50. Jongwe F. Mugabe succession debate intensifies. news24. 2012, April 12; http://www.news24.com/Africa/Zimbabwe/Mugabe-succession-debate-intensifies-20120412. Accessed 22 Dec 2015.

51. Zimbabwe: Look east or look Chinese? allAfrica. 2007, October 25; http://allafrica.com/stories/200710251237.html. Accessed 22 Dec 2015.

52. Njikizana J. Ex Zimbabwe PM says Mugabe 'out of ideas' to fix the economy. Modern Ghana. 2014, July 7; http://www.modernghana.com/news/554323/1/ex-zimbabwe-pm-says-mugabe-out-of-ideas-to-fix-the.html. Accessed 22 Dec 2015.

53. Parirewa PW, Mugabe on Anti-Smoking Lobby 1994, Sept 27. British American Tobacco http://legacy.library.ucsf.edu/tid/swh10a99. Accessed 07 Aug 2014.

54. Vera I, Zimbabwe Tobacco Industry Faces New Threat from WHO, 2000, 17 Mar. British American Tobacco. http://legacy.library.ucsf.edu/tid/tpr03a99. Accessed 12 Jun 2014.

55. Framework Convention Alliance. Working group on economically sustainable alternatives to tobacco growing (in relation to Articles 17 and 18: provision of support for economically viable alternatives and protection of the environment and the health of persons), COP4. Uruguay: FCA 2010 November 15-20. Report No.: COP/4/7 http://www.fctc.org/images/stories/Policy%20Briefing%20Art%2017and18.pdf. Accessed 22 Mar 2015.

56. WHO. WHO Report on the Global Tobacco Epidemic, 2013-Country Profile-Zimbabwe. Geneva WHO 2013 http://www.who.int/tobacco/surveillance/policy/country_profile/zwe.pdf?ua=1. Accessed 22 Dec 2015.

57. Lopez AD, Collishaw EE, Phia T. A descriptive model of the cigarette epidemic in developed countries. Tob Control. 1994;3:242–7.

58. Drope J. Tobacco Control in Africa: People, Politics and Policies. Anthem: London and New York; 2011.

59. Zvongougy T. ZFTCT endorses WHO framework on tobacco control. Zimbabwe Independent. 2013, September 20; http://www.theindependent. co.zw/2013/09/20/zftct-endorses-framework-tobacco-control/. Accessed 22 Dec 2015.

60. WHO FCTC. WHO Framework Convention on Tobacco Control (FCTC). Geneva WHO 2005 http://whqlibdoc.who.int/publications/2003/9241591013. pdf?ua=1. Accessed 20 Mar 2015.

61. Zimbabwe Government. Statutory Instrument 264. 2002; http://www. tobaccocontrollaws.org/files/live/Zimbabwe/Zimbabwe%20-%202002% 20Regs%20-%20national.pdf. Accessed 22 Dec 2015.

62. WHO Regional Office for Africa. Report card on the WHO Framework Convention on Tobacco Control-Zimbabwe. WHO, Regional Office for Africa. 2010. http://www.google.com/url?sa=t&rct=j&q=&esrc=s&source=web&cd= 2&ved=0CC8QFjAB&url=http%3A%2F%2Fwww.afro.who.int%2Findex. php%3Foption%3Dcom_docman%26task%3Ddoc_download%26gid% 3D5910&ei=UVUWU67WCYT1oASCnYHYCw&usg=AFQjCNGxlYYtml6JPyb S4bmm9x7AeSR_xA&sig2=cmCucsC3ADe79-Z8DJPz0g&bvm=bv.62333050,d. cGU. Accessed 22 Dec 2015.

63. WHO. WHO Report on the Global Tobacco Epidemic, 2015. Geneva: WHO; 2015. http://www.who.int/tobacco/global_report/2015/en/. Accessed 22 Dec 2015.

64. Dzirutwe M. Zimbabwe takes tobacco road to agriculture recovery. Reuters. 2015, April 16; http://www.reuters.com/article/2015/04/16/zimbabwe-tobacco-idUSL5N0XB1N720150416. Accessed 22 Dec 2015.

65. Nyakudya M. Govt, BAT sign MoU. The Herald. 2015, Nov. 9, 2015; http:// www.herald.co.zw/govt-bat-sign-mou/. Accessed 22 Dec 2015.

66. Zimbabwe Government. Ministry signed a Memorandum of Understanding. 2015. http://www.myiee.gov.zw/index.php/news/86-ministry-signed-a-memorandum-of-understanding. Accessed 22 Dec 2015.

67. Makichi T. Zimbabwe: Govt, BAT Sign MoU. AllAfrica. 2015; http://allafrica. com/stories/201511090754.html. Accessed 22 Dec 2015.

68. WHO. WHO Report on the Global Tobacco Epidemic, 2015: Raising taxes on tobacco. Geneva: World Health Organization, 2015 http://apps.who.int/iris/ bitstream/10665/178574/1/9789240694606_eng.pdf?ua=1. Accessed 22 Dec 2015.

69. Ruwende I. Savanna offers to rename Rufaro Stadium. The Herald. 2014, March 10; http://www.herald.co.zw/savanna-offers-to-rename-rufaro-stadium/. Accessed 22 Dec 2015.

70. Machingura M. Zimbabwe: Beauty queens tour Savanna Tobacco. The Herald. 2014, June 5; http://allafrica.com/stories/201406050250.html. Accessed 22 Dec 2015.

71. Staff Reporter. Savanna Tobacco, Sweet smoky music. Business Excellence. 2011, March 23; http://www.bus-ex.com/article/savanna-tobacco. Accessed 22 Dec 2015.

72. Savanna Tobacco. Savanna Tobacco. website. 2014. http://www. savannatobacco.com/. Accessed 22 Dec 2015.

73. Nkiwane B. Savanna, Black Rhinos extend sponsorship deal. Southern Eye. 2014, January 12; http://www.southerneye.co.zw/2014/01/12/savanna-black-rhinos-extend-sponsorship-deal/. Accessed 22 Dec 2015.

74. Times of Zambia, Tma News: 13-Feb-2002 World, 2002, 13 Feb. RJ Reynolds. http://legacy.library.ucsf.edu/tid/niz10d00. Accessed 30 Jun 2014.

75. Staff Reporter. Mugabe's niece linked to cigarette smuggling. Bulawago24. 2014, Dec 29; http://bulawayo24.com/index-id-news-sc-national-byo-40757. html. Accessed 22 Dec 2015.

76. Staff Reporter. Two men arrested for attempting to smuggle 1,000 cigarette boxes. Bulawayo. 2013, February 22; http://bulawayo24.com/index-id-news-sc-regional-byo-26654.html. Accessed 22 Dec 2015.

77. Chitongo P. Police intercept truckload of cigarettes. the Standard. 2014, April 6; http://www.thestandard.co.zw/2014/04/06/police-intercept-truckload-cigarettes/. Accessed 22 Dec 2015.

78. Muronzi C. BAT Zim spying on competitors. Zimbabwe Independent, The Leading Business Weekly. 2012, November 16, http://www. theindependent.co.zw/2012/11/16/bat-zim-spying-on-competitors/. Accessed 22 Dec 2015.

79. Savanna Tobacco refutes cigarette smuggling charge. dailynews. 2014, January 2, http://www.dailynews.co.zw/articles/2014/01/02/savanna-tobacco-refutes-cigarette-smuggling-charge. Accessed 22 Dec 2015.

80. Industrial espionage on the rise in Zimbabwe. Zimbabwe Independent, the Leading Business Weekly. 2012, November 30, 2012; http://www.

theindependent.co.zw/2012/11/30/industrial-espionage-on-the-rise-in-zimbabwe/. Accessed 22 Dec 2015.

81. Staff Reporter. Cigarette smuggling racket exposed. the Zimbabwean. 2014, November 19, http://www.thezimbabwean.co/business/business-analysis/74085/cigarette-smuggling-racket-exposed/. Accessed 22 Dec 2015.

82. Global Youth Tobacco Survey. Report on the Results of the Global Youth Tobacco Survey in Zimbabwe: Harare & Manicaland Regions, 1999-2000: UNICEF-Zimbabwe2000 http://www.who.int/tobacco/surveillance/Zimbabwe%20Report%201999-2000.pdf?ua=1. Accessed 22 Dec 2015.

83. Mambondiyani A. Bittersweet tale of tobacco farming in Zimbabwe. New Zimbabwe. 2014, October 12; http://www.newzimbabwe.com/business-18360-Bittersweet+tale+of+%E2%80%98new+tobacco%E2%80%99+in+Zim/business.aspx. Accessed 22 Dec 2015.

84. Keyser JC. Costs and Profitability of Tobacco Compared to Other Crops in Zimbabwe: Tobacco Free Institute and the World Health Institution, 2002 June, http://siteresources.worldbank.org/HEALTHNUTRITIONANDPOPULATION/Resources/281627-1095698140167/Keyser-TheCostsandProfitability-whole.pdf. Accessed 22 Dec 2015.

85. Moyo J. Zimbabwe's emerging tobacco queens. Zimbabwe Situation. 2014, May 11, http://www.zimbabwesituation.com/news/zimsit_zimbabwes-emerging-tobacco-queens/. Accessed 22 Dec 2015.

86. Mutingwende B. Tobacco farming: Counting the cost for rural poor. New Zimbabwe. 2014, May 19, http://www.newzimbabwe.com/opinion-15818-Tobacco%20Counting%20the%20cost%20for%20rural%20poor/opinion.aspx. Accessed 22 Dec 2015.

87. Chapman S, Yach D, Saloojee Y, Simpson D. All Africa conference on tobacco control. Br Med J. 1994;308(6922):189–91.

88. Christie S. Zimbabwe's forests are going up in smoke. Mail & Guardian. 2013, November 1, http://mg.co.za/article/2013-11-01-00-zimbabwes-forests-are-going-up-in-smoke. Accessed 22 Dec 2015.

89. Geist HJ. Global assessment of deforestation related to tobacco farming. Tob Control. 1999;8(1):18–28.

90. Gogo J. Zimbabwe: Tobacco Boom v. Deforestation. The Herald. 2013, December 16; http://allafrica.com/stories/201312161130.html. Accessed 22 Dec 2015.

91. Mambondiyani A. Tobacco farmers wiping out Zimbabwe's indigenous forests. OpenDemocracy. 2013, August 20; http://www.opendemocracy.net/andrew-mambondiyani/tobacco-farmers-wiping-out-zimbabwe%E2%80%99s-indigenous-forests. Accessed 22 Dec 2015.

92. Staff Reporter. Mugabe warns tobacco farmers against deforestation. New Zimbabwe. 2014, April 21; http://www.newzimbabwe.com/news-15363-Mugabe+threatens+tobacco+farming+ban/news.aspx. Accessed 22 Dec 2015.

93. Thornycroft P. Tobacco farming negatively impacts Zimbabwe's indigenous forests. Voice of America. 2011, December 20, http://www.voanews.com/content/zimbabwe-trees-sacrificed-to-tobacco-farming-135992498/149782. html. Accessed 22 Dec 2015.

94. WHO FCTC. Conference of the Parties to the WHO Framework Convention on Tobacco Control. Geneva. 2014. http://www.who.int/fctc/cop/en/. Accessed 3 Jan 2015.

95. WHO FCTC. Rules of Procedure of the Conference of the Parties. 2014th ed. Geneva: World Health Organization; 2014. http://whqlibdoc.who.int/publications/2006/9789241594554_eng.pdf?ua=1. Accessed 5 Mar 2015.

96. WHO AFRO. Kenya hosts commemoration to accelerate comprehensive implementaion of WHO FCTC in the African Region. World Health Organization-Africa (WHO AFRO). 2015. http://www.afro.who.int/en/media-centre/pressreleases/item/7408-kenya-hosts-commemoration-to-accelerate-comprehensive-implementation-of-who-fctc-in-the-african-region.html. Accessed 22 Dec 2015.

97. WHO FCTC. Conference of the Parties to the WHO Framework Convention on Tobacco Control, COP3 Third session, South Africa, 2008. Punta del Este, Uruguay: WHO FCTC, 2008 November 17-22. Report No.: FCTC/COP/3/DIV/3 http://apps.who.int/gb/fctc/PDF/cop3/FCTC_COP3_REC1-en.pdf. Accessed 20 Mar 2015.

98. Framework Convention Alliance. COP6 daily bulletin (Day 5). Moscow Framework Convention Alliance, 2014 October 17 Contract No.: 127 http://www.fctc.org/images/stories/Moscow_Day_5_page_WEB.pdf. Accessed 20 Mar 2015.

99. WHO FCTC. Report of the sixth session of the Conference of the Parties to the WHO Framework Convention on Tobacco Control, Final Report. Russia

2014 Contract No.: December 15 http://apps.who.int/gb/fctc/PDF/cop6/
FCTC_COP6_Report-en.pdf. Accessed 20 Mar 2015.

100. WHO FCTC Convention Secretariat. Implementation of Article 5.3 of the
WHO FCTC: Evolving issues related to interference by the tobacco industry.
Moscow: World Health Organization Framework Convention on Tobacco
Control, 2014 July 14 Contract No.: FCTC/COP/6/16 http://apps.who.int/gb/
fctc/PDF/cop6/FCTC_COP6_16-en.pdf. Accessed 22 Mar 2015.

101. WHO FCTC. Study group on economically sustainable alternatives to
tobacco growing (in relation to Articles 17 and 18 of the Convention)
COP3. Durban, South Africa: WHO-FCTC2008 September 4 Contract No.:
FCTC/COP/3/11 http://apps.who.int/gb/fctc/PDF/cop3/FCTC_COP3_11-en.
pdf. Accessed 22 Dec 2015.

102. Framework Convention Alliance. FCA Policy Briefing for COP6: Report of the
Article 17/18 Working Group. Moscow: Framework Convention Alliance
2014 October 3 http://www.fctc.org/images/stories/FCA_policy_brief_Art_
1718.pdf. Accessed 19 Feb 2015.

103. Temporao JG. Public Health and tobacco control in Brazil. Cadernos de
saude publica. 2005;21(3):671. 0. doi:10.1590/S0102-311X2005000300001.

104. Lee K, Chagas LC, Novotny TE. Brazil and the framework convention on
tobacco control: global health diplomacy as soft power. PLoS Med. 2010;
7(4):e1000232. doi:10.1371/journal.pmed.1000232.

105. Bialous S, da Costa e Silva VL, Drope J, Lencucha R, McGrady B, Richter AP.
The Political Economy of Tobacco Control in Brazil: Protecting Public Health
in a Complex Policy Environment. Rio de Janeiro and Atlanta: Centro de
Estudos sobre Tabaco e Saude, Escola Nacional de Saude Publica/FIOCRUZ
and American Cancer Society, 2014 http://www.cancer.org/acs/groups/
content/@research/documents/document/acspc-044951.pdf. Accessed
22 Dec 2015.

106. International Tobacco Control Policy Evaluation Project. Zambia needs to
increase tobacco prices and anti-tobacco campaigns including pictorial
health warnings to combat increased threat of tobacco epidemic.
Lusaka, Zambia. 2014. http://www.itcproject.org/node/112. Accessed
22 Dec 2015.

107. Keith LC. Constitutional Provisions for Individual Human Rights (1976-1996):
Are They More than Mere 'Window Dressing'? Political Research Quarterly.
2002;55:111–43.

108. Framework Convention Alliance. Brazen–or clueless–Brazilian official
puts links to tobacco industry in writing Washington: FCA, 2010 July 14
http://www.fctc.org/images/stories/Brazil_5%203%20140711.pdf.
Accessed 22 Dec 2015.

109. Bilano VL. Global trends and projections for tobacco use, 1990-2025: An
analysis of smoking indicators from the WHO Comprehensive Information
Systems for Tobacco Control. Lancet. 2015;385(March 14):966–76.

110. WHO Regional Office for Africa. Zimbabwe commemorates World No
Tobacco Day. Geneva 2013. http://www.afro.who.int/en/zimbabwe/press-
materials/item/5616-zimbabwe-commemorates-world-no-tobacco-day.html.
Accessed 22 Dec 2015.

111. Eriksen M, Mackay J, Ross H, Schluger N, Islami F, Drope J. The Tobacco
Atlas, Fifth Ed. Zimbabwe Country Fact Sheet. Atlanta and New York, N.Y.:
American Cancer Society, World Lung Foundation, 2015 http://www.
tobaccoatlas.org/country-data/zimbabwe/. Accessed 22 Dec 2015.

112. Public smokers to spend 6 months in Zimbabwean jail, or pay $500 fine.
Sowetan Live. 2014, July 28; http://www.sowetanlive.co.za/news/africa/2014/
07/28/public-smokers-to-spend-6-months-in-zimbabwean-jail-or-pay-500-
fine. Accessed 22 Dec 2015.

113. Chideme-Monodawafa A. National Cancer Prevention and Control Strategy
for Zimbabwe 2014-2018. Mutare, Zimbabwe: Hospice & Palliative Care
Association of Zimbabwe, Ministry of Health and Child Care, Epidemiology
& Disease Control Non Communicable Diseases Unit, 2015 September 24,
http://news.isncc.org/national-cancer-prevention-and-control-strategy-for-
zimbabwe/. Accessed 22 Dec 2015.

114. Kluger J. Big tobacco sets its sights on Africa. Time Magazine. 2009 July 24
http://content.time.com/time/health/article/0,8599,1911796,00.html.
Accessed 22 Dec 2015.

115. Transcripts service. Savannah Tobacco moves ahead one cigarette at a time.
Business Day, BDLive. 2012, April 12; http://www.bdlive.co.za/articles/2012/
04/12/savannah-tobacco-moves-ahead-one-cigarette-at-a-time;
jsessionid=CAD52D413F6C09D260D1B920409DEFF4.present1.bdfm.
Accessed 22 Dec 2015.

116. Staff Writer. Police clamp down on tobacco companies. Zimbabwe
Independent. 2014, January 24, http://www.theindependent.co.zw/2014/01/
24/police-clamp-tobacco-companies/. Accessed 22 Dec 2015.

117. WHO Health Harare. Zimbabwe commemorates World No Tobacco Day.
World Health Organization Harare. 2013. http://www.afro.who.int/en/
zimbabwe/press-materials/item/5616-zimbabwe-commemorates-world-no-
tobacco-day.html. Accessed 22 Dec 2015.

118. NewZania. Health ministry steps up tobacco tax push, World No Tobacco
Day. Chronicle. 2014, June 21; http://www.chronicle.co.zw/health-ministry-
steps-up-tobacco-tax-push/. Accessed 22 Dec 2015.

119. Savell E, Gilmore AB, Sims M, Mony PK, Koon T, Yusoff K, et al. The
environmental profile of a community's health: a cross-sectional study on
tobacco marketing in 16 countries. Bull World Health Organ. 2015;93:851–
61G. http://dx.doi.org/10.2471/BLT.15.155846.

120. World Bank. Curbing the epidemic: governments and the economics of
tobacco control. The World Bank. Tob Control. 1999;8(2):196–201.

121. Yach D, Harrison S, Proceedings of the All Africa Conference on Tobacco
Control 1993, November 17. http://legacy.library.ucsf.edu/tid/ddl87a99.
Accessed 30 Jun 2014.

122. Khumalo CCM. Can Farmers Diversify from Growing Tobacco in Zimbabwe?
[Masters]. Uppsala: Swedish University of Agricultural Sciences; 2013. http://
stud.epsilon.slu.se/6277/1/khumalo_c_131114.PDF. Accessed 22 Dec 2015.

123. Mambondiyani A. Zimbabwe farmers fear winter of hunger after poor
tobacco crop. Reuters. 2015, July 22; http://www.reuters.com/article/2015/
07/22/us-zimbabwe-tobacco-idUSKCN0PW1FH20150722. Accessed
22 Dec 2015.

124. Government of the Republic of Zimbabwe. Constitution of the Republic of
Zimbabwe. Harare 2000. http://www.saiea.com/dbsa_handbook_update09/
pdf/16Zimbabwe09.pdf, Accessed 22 Dec 2015.

125. Zimbabwe Government. Statutory Instrument 116. 2012, http://www.cfuzim.
org/index.php/legal-the-law/2720-statutory-instrument-116-of-2012-forest-
control-of-firewood-timber-and-forest-produce-regs-2012. Accessed
22 Dec 2015.

126. Kamuti T. The booming Zimbabwe tobacco sector and massive
deforestation: causes for concern. Zimdev. 2013, August 8, https://zimdev.
wordpress.com/2013/08/08/the-booming-zimbabwe-tobacco-sector-and-
massive-deforestation-causes-for-concern/. Accessed 22 Dec 2015.

127. Tobacco-curing eats up Zimbabwe's forests. IRIN News. 2014, July 31, 2014;
http://www.neurope.eu/article/tobacco-curing-eats-zimbabwes-forests.
Accessed 22 Dec 2015.

128. U.S. Department of Labor. Zimbabwe, 2012 Findings on the Worst Forms of
Child Labor 2012 http://www.dol.gov/ilab/reports/child-labor/zimbabwe.
htm. Accessed 22 Dec 2015.

129. Integrated Regional Information Networks (IRIN). Zimbabwe's ailing
economy fuelling child labour. World News. 2014, January 9; http://www.
irinnews.org/report/99443/zimbabwe-s-ailing-economy-fuelling-child-labour.
Accessed 22 Dec 2015.

130. Gumbo T. Tobacco use in Zimbabwe in spotlight as companies target
Africa. Voice of America/Zimbabwe. 2015, July 13; http://www.
voazimbabwe.com/content/zimbabwe-cigarette-smoking/2860085.html.
Accessed 22 Dec 2015.

131. WHO. Tobacco and Poverty: A Vicious Circle. Geneva: Tobacco Free
Initiative, 2004 http://www.who.int/tobacco/communications/events/wntd/
2004/en/wntd2004_brochure_en.pdf. Accessed 22 Dec 2015.

132. Mambo E. Tobacco companies embark on massive reforestation
programme. the Standard. 2014, Aiprl 13, http://www.thestandard.co.zw/
2014/04/13/tobacco-companies-embark-massive-reforestation-programme/.
Accessed 22 Dec 2015.

7

The use of national administrative data to describe the spatial distribution of in-hospital mortality following stroke in France, 2008–2011

Adrien Roussot[1,2], Jonathan Cottenet[1,2], Maryse Gadreau[3], Maurice Giroud[4], Yannick Béjot[4] and Catherine Quantin[1,2,5,6,7*]

Abstract

Background: In the context of implementing the National Stroke Plan in France, a spatial approach was used to measure inequalities in this disease. Using the national PMSI-MCO databases, we analyzed the in-hospital prevalence of stroke and established a map of in-hospital mortality rates with regard to the socio-demographic structure of the country.

Methods: The principal characteristics of patients identified according to ICD10 codes relative to stroke (in accordance with earlier validation work) were studied. A map of standardized mortality rates at the level of PMSI geographic codes was established. An exploratory analysis (principal component analysis followed by ascending hierarchical classification) using INSEE socio-economic data and mortality rates was also carried out to identify different area profiles.

Results: Between 2008 and 2011, the number of stroke patients increased by 3.85 %, notably for ischemic stroke in the 36–55 years age group (60 % of men). Over the same period, in-hospital mortality fell, and the map of standardized rates illustrated the diagonal of high mortality extending from the north-east to the south-west of the country. The most severely affected areas were also those with the least favorable socio-professional indicators.

Conclusions: The PMSI-MCO database is a major source of data on the health status of the population. It can be used for the area-by-area observation of the performance of certain healthcare indicators, such as in-hospital mortality, or to follow the implementation of the National Stroke Plan. Our study showed the interplay between social and demographic factors and stroke-related in-hospital mortality. The map derived from the results of the exploratory analysis illustrated a variety of areas where social difficulties, aging and high mortality seemed to meet. The study raises questions about access to neuro-vascular care in isolated areas and in those in demographic decline. Telemedicine appears to be the solution favored by decision makers. The aging of the population managed for stroke must not mask the growing incidence in younger people, which raises questions about the development of classical (smoking, hypertension) or new (drug abuse) risk factors.

Keywords: PMSI, Stroke, Geography, In-hospital mortality

Background

The management of stroke is becoming an increasingly heavy burden worldwide for both developed and developing countries. Though the incidence rate of the disease in rich countries has fallen over the last 20 years, prevalence has increased as the quality of stroke management has improved [1, 2]. It is becoming necessary to evaluate responses provided by healthcare systems and then to implement public healthcare actions to cope with the burden of this disease in both the acute and chronic phase.

Since the year 2000, France has been engaged in a battle against stroke, and since 2010, all of the actions in the

*Correspondence: catherine.quantin@chu-dijon.fr
[7] Biostatistics, Biomathematics, Pharmacoepidemiology and Infectious Diseases (B2PHI), Univ. Bourgogne Franche-Comté, Inserm UMR 1181, Dijon 21000, France
Full list of author information is available at the end of the article

management of stroke patients have been incorporated in a "2010–2014 National Stroke Action Plan" [3]. This plan, which was based on a comprehensive 'inventory' requested by the Ministry of Health and which associated researchers, the relevant learned societies and representatives of patients [4], emphasizes the need for a territory-wide stroke-care network. At the regional level, emergency stroke management is centered on stroke units and better coordination between these establishments and follow-up care and rehabilitation departments in the downstream management of stroke.

The national strategy in the fight against stroke also involves the development of epidemiological research in stroke, notably through the increased exploitation of existing information systems: PMSI-MCO (Programme de médicalisation des systèmes d'information) and SNIIR-AM (Système national inter-régime de l'assurance maladie) (action 8 of the Plan). Indeed, a number of studies have been conducted thanks to the availability and long-standing nature of medico-administrative databases. The PMSI-MCO in particular is a precious source of information for studies in epidemiology [5] or healthcare economics [6]. Indeed, the PMSI is the main source of French hospitalisation data. For each patient, it gathers all of the hospital stays during the year and allows patients to be followed over time thanks to a unique data linkage number.

Earlier studies on the incidence and prevalence of stroke conducted using the PMSI-MCO showed that the demographics of the population managed for stroke have changed over the last 20 years. This situation is probably related to the greater efficacy of prevention messages and the earlier involvement of the healthcare system. A study published in 2012 [7] underlined the interest of the PMSI-MCO to elaborate and analyze hospital and follow-up care trajectories. The study highlighted the growing importance of stroke units between 2007 and 2009 and concluded that the overall management of stroke was more effective, with a reduction of the in-hospitality mortality.

This work is a continuation of these observational studies on the results of care in stroke patients, in the context of the deployment of the National Action Plan. In this context, we can make the hypothesis that this decrease may be observable for a larger period and that its spatial distribution in France follows an heterogenic organization. We studied the number of stroke victims at the national level in France between 2008 and 2011 using PMSI-MCO medico-administrative databases, as well as the evolution of the principal characteristics of this population, notably with regard to in-hospital mortality. The analysis presents a map of in-hospital mortality, as well as an exploratory analysis of the territorial distribution

of this mortality with regard to demographic and socio-economic data.

The aim of this analysis was to describe the spatial distribution of in-hospital mortality related to the socio-economic characteristics of the patients' places of residence.

Methods
Source of data and selection criteria
Given the lack of long-term data in the national PMSI databases and the absence of accurate coding to distinguish between first-ever and recurrent stroke, this study analyses the characteristics of patients hospitalized for stroke rather than the in-hospital incidence.

The algorithm used was the same as that used for other French studies conducted using the national PMSI database. All of the hospital stays for patients presenting with a diagnosis of stroke recorded in the national PMSI-MCO databases from 2008 to 2011, whatever their age, were included. The hospital stays were selected according to the principal diagnosis (PD) according to the following ICD10 codes:

- I60, I61, I62.9 for hemorrhagic stroke.
- I63, I64, G46 for ischemic stroke.

In our selection process, we chose to keep patients with a "transfer" admission, that is to say patients who stayed first in one establishment and then moved to a second establishment with a PD of stroke. In these cases of transfer, only the second stay with a diagnosis of stroke was taken into account for the analysis. All hospital stays ending with in-hospital death (discharge code = 9) were included, even when the hospital stay was 0 days. For deceased patients who had accumulated several hospital stays after a stroke, their death was identified in a period of 30 days following the first hospital stay for stroke. For patients who were transferred during their management, the complete duration of the hospital stay was taken into account.

Selection was limited to geographical codes for France. PMSI geographic codes indicate where patients live; in France these places correspond to zip codes. Hospital stays presenting coding errors shown by a return code or an error in the DRG (Diagnosis Related Group) code were removed.

Calculation of standardized in-hospital mortality rates
The mortality rate included all of the in-hospital deaths recorded during the period of the study (2008–2011). It was standardized for age according to the direct method, by using as the reference INSEE (Institut National de la Statistique et des Etudes Economiques: French national census institute data of the 2009 population census at the

level of the PMSI geographic code for the place of residence. These population data were obtained by aggregation of the census data available for each town using the post code and the corresponding PMSI geographic code established by the ATIH (Agence Technique de l'Information Hospitalière: Technical agency for hospital information) in 2010. Mortality rates are expressed for 100,000 inhabitants. The exploratory analysis is based on commune-by-commune INSEE data for Employed persons—active Population from the 2011 census and aggregated according to the post code and PMSI geographic code.

Exploratory analysis: typology of the territories according to their socio-economic and demographic structure related to in-hospital mortality

- The exploratory analysis consisted of a principal components analysis (PCA) followed by an ascending hierarchical classification (AHC) using Ward's step method bearing on several variables of interest at the level of the 5672 PMSI geographic codes of their residence in France. The ascending hierarchical classification (AHC) consisted in gradually aggregating the geographic codes according to their resemblance, which allowed us to predict the cluster of an individual according to the values taken by the predictive variables: Proportion of each occupational category in the active population
- Proportion of unemployed people in the active population
- Proportion of retired or pre-retired people aged 15–64 in the active population
- Proportion of the whole population aged less than 20 years
- Proportion of the whole population aged from 20 to 59 years
- Proportion of the whole population aged more than 60 years
- Standardized rate of in-hospital mortality due to stroke for 100,000 inhabitants

We kept the first three factorial axes from the PCA for the AHC. These allowed us to synthesize 69.2 % of the information. All of the variables selected in the AHC were discriminating for the description and the construction of the different clusters of PMSI geographic areas (cf. Table 5). Only the managers or professional occupations category (SPC n°3) was not retained to describe cluster 4 (p > 0.05). The typology from the AHC was based on 5 classes of affectation for the geographic codes. This apportionment was obtained after interpretation of the associated dendogram, from the cubic clustering criterion (measures the quality of the cluster) and from the

semi-partial R^2 (measures the loss of interclass inertia). The results obtained from the classification are presented in Tables 5 and 6, which present the means of each variable within the clusters, as well as their discriminating power (p < 0.05) for the construction of each cluster. The cartographic results concerning the classification of geographic codes of the place of residence are shown in Fig. 5. For each variable, the legend presents the mean deviation, calculated overall for the geographic codes of the place of residence. The bars on the right of the vertical line represent a positive delta, while those on the left represent a negative delta. The wider the bar, the greater the mean deviation (positive or negative) is.

The description of each cluster can be determined in a complementary manner from Fig. 5, Tables 5 and 6.

SAS 9.3 software was used for all of the analyses. GIS (Geographic Information System) MapInfo 11.0 was used for the cartography.

Results
Hospitalizations for AVC: characteristics of the study population

In France, the number of people hospitalized for stroke increased by 3.9 %, from 96,695 to 100,420 between 2008 and 2011 (c.f. Table 1). There was, however, a slight fall in the number of patients between 2010 and 2011 (fall of 1295 cases). In detail, the greatest increase concerned ischemic stroke (+3.9 %); the number of patients hospitalized for hemorrhagic stroke increased by 3.3 %.

From 2008 to 2011, 97,574 people were hospitalized for stroke in France, 22,327 (22.8 %) presented hemorrhagic stroke and 75,247 (77.2 %) ischemic stroke. The distribution according to the year was stable (Table 1).

More women than men were hospitalized for stroke [203,467 (50.8 %) vs. 197,335 (49.2 %) for the whole period] and whatever the year. The differences between the years were not significant (Table 1). The percentage of women hospitalized for hemorrhagic stroke (51.2 %—Table 2) was greater than that for ischemic stroke (50.6 %—Table 3). The difference was significant ($p = 0.0067$). In addition, for hemorrhagic stroke (Table 2), the proportion of women hospitalized increased between 2008 (50.7 %) and 2011 (51.6 %), the difference was significant (Somers'd = 0.0452).

For all strokes (Table 1), we found an increase in the proportion of people older than 55 hospitalized for stroke from 85.7 % in 2008 to 86.2 % in 2011. The difference was significant (Somers'd = 0.0106). This significant increase occurred in women (88.0 % in 2008 vs 88.6 % in 2011: Somers'd = 0.0013) but not in men (Table 1). This global trend was related (Table 2) to the substantial increase in the proportion of patients older than 55 years hospitalized for hemorrhagic stroke (76.3 % in 2008 vs 78.5 % in

Table 1 Global description of strokes

Strokes	2008		2009		2010		2011		Total		χ^2	Somers'd
	n	%	n	%	n	%	n	%	n	%	p	p
All strokes	97,574		99,398		102,593		101,237		400,802			
Hemorrhagic	22,327	22.9	22,618	22.7	23,426	22.8	23,056	22.8	91,427	22.8	NS	NS
Ischemic	75,247	77.1	76,780	77.3	79,167	77.2	78,181	77.2	309,375	77.2		
Age												
All patients												
≤35	2476	2.5	2491	2.5	2586	2.5	2310	2.3	9863	2.5	0.0005	0.0106
36–55	11,464	11.8	11,395	11.5	12,017	11.7	11,706	11.6	46,582	11.6		
>55	83,634	85.7	85,512	86.0	87,990	85.8	87,221	86.2	344,357	85.9		
Male												
≤35	1220	2.5	1202	2.5	1332	2.6	1127	2.3	4881	2.5	0.0058	NS
36–55	6786	14.1	6728	13.8	7069	14.0	7044	14.1	27,627	14.0		
>55	40,255	83.4	40,867	83.8	42,061	83.4	41,644	83.6	164,827	83.5		
Female												
≤35	1256	2.6	1289	2.6	1254	2.4	1183	2.3	4982	2.5	0.0074	0.0013
36–55	4678	9.5	4667	9.2	4948	9.5	4662	9.1	18,955	9.3		
>55	43,379	88.0	44,645	88.2	45,929	88.1	45,577	88.6	179,530	88.2		
Sex												
Male	48,261	49.5	48,797	49.1	50,462	49.2	49,815	49.2	197,335	49.2	NS	NS
Female	49,313	50.5	50,601	50.9	52,131	50.8	51,422	50.8	203,467	50.8		
In-hospital death (in 30 days)												
All patients	16,178	16.6	16,234	16.3	16,700	16.3	16,249	16.1	65,361	16.3	0.0160	0.0009
% age-sexe-adjusted		16.6		16.2		16.2		15.9				
Male	7389	15.3	7430	15.2	7554	15.0	7285	14.6	29,658	15.0	0.0116	0.0006
% age-adjusted		15.3		15.1		14.9		14.6				
≤35	86	7.1	77	6.4	83	6.2	63	5.6	309	6.3	NS	0.0765
36–55	547	8.1	561	8.3	577	8.2	550	7.8	2235	8.1	NS	NS
>55	6756	16.8	6792	16.6	6894	16.4	6672	16.0	27,114	16.5	0.0206	0.0010
Female	8789	17.8	8804	17.4	9146	17.5	8964	17.4	35,703	17.6	NS	NS
% age-adjusted		17.8		17.4		17.6		17.4				
≤35	62	4.9	49	3.8	51	4.1	46	3.9	208	4.2	NS	NS
36–55	416	8.9	407	8.7	374	7.6	386	8.3	1583	8.4	NS	0.0482
>55	8311	19.2	8348	18.7	8721	19.0	8532	18.7	33,912	18.9	NS	NS

2011: *Somers'd* < 10^{-3}). The trend was observed in both men (*Somers'd* = 0.0012) and women (*Somers'd* < 10^{-3}). This trend was not found for ischemic strokes overall (Table 3) (*Somers'd non-significant*) even though significant differences were found in the distribution of patients by age group ($p = 0.0235$) in the different years. However, the structure by age and sex showed an increase in the proportion of men aged 36–55 years (12.4 % in 2008 vs. 12.8 % in 2011) and a fall in the proportion of those aged more than 55 years (86.1 % in 2008 vs. 85.7 % in 2011: *Somers'd* = 0.0462). We found no statistically significant evolution in the structure according to age group in women.

In contrast (Table 2) the proportion of men aged 36–55 years who presented hemorrhagic stroke fell during the study period (19.6 % in 2008 vs. 18.9 % in 2011) whereas that in patients older than 55 years increased (74.4 % in 2008 vs. 76.2 % in 2011); the differences were significant (*Somers'd* = 0.0012). The same significant trends were observed in women (Table 2) with a decrease in the proportion of women aged less than 36 years (4.8 % in 2008 vs. 4.0 % in 2011) and in those aged 36–55 years (17.2 % in 2008 vs. 15.4 % in 2011) as well as an increase in those aged more than 55 years (78.1 % in 2008 vs. 80.7 % in 2011). These differences were significant (*Somers'd* < 10^{-3}).

Table 2 Description of hemorrhagic strokes

Hemorrhagic strokes	2008		2009		2010		2011		Total		χ^2	Somers'd
	n	%	n	%	n	%	n	%	n	%	p	p
All patients	22,327		22,618		23,426		23,056		91,427			
Age												
All patients												
≤35	1205	5.4	1120	5.0	1169	5.0	1021	4.4	4515	4.9	<10⁻³	<10⁻³
36–55	4093	18.3	3946	17.5	4026	17.2	3935	17.1	16,000	17.5		
>55	17,029	76.3	17,552	77.6	18,231	77.8	18,100	78.5	70,912	77.6		
Male												
≤35	663	6.0	599	5.4	676	5.9	551	4.9	2489	5.6	0.0007	0.0012
36–55	2152	19.6	2106	19.0	2077	18.2	2105	18.9	8440	18.9		
>55	8192	74.4	8365	75.6	8673	75.9	8495	76.2	33,725	75.5		
Female												
≤35	542	4.8	521	4.5	493	4.1	470	4.0	2026	4.3	<10⁻³	<10⁻³
36–55	1941	17.2	1840	15.9	1949	16.2	1830	15.4	7560	16.2		
>55	8837	78.1	9187	79.6	9558	79.7	9605	80.7	37,187	79.5		
Sex												
Male	11,007	49.3	11,070	48.9	11,426	48.8	11,151	48.4	44,654	48.8	NS	0.0452
Female	11,320	50.7	11,548	51.1	12,000	51.2	11,905	51.6	46,773	51.2		
In-hospital death (in 30 days)												
All patients	7153	32.0	7367	32.6	7469	31.9	7438	32.3	29,427	32.2	NS	NS
% age-sexe-adjusted		32.0		32.3		31.6		31.7				
Male	3450	31.3	3511	31.7	3657	32.0	3500	31.4	14,118	31.6	NS	NS
% age-adjusted		31.3		31.5		31.8		31.0				
≤35	72	10.9	58	9.7	68	10.1	58	10.5	256	10.3	NS	NS
36–55	379	17.6	407	19.3	422	20.3	399	19.0	1607	19.0	NS	NS
>55	2999	36.6	3046	36.4	3167	36.5	3043	35.8	12,255	36.3	NS	NS
Female	3703	32.7	3856	33.4	3812	31.8	3938	33.1	15,309	32.7	0.0458	NS
% age-adjusted		32.7		33.1		31.4		32.5				
≤35	47	8.7	44	8.5	39	7.9	39	8.3	169	8.3	NS	NS
36–55	332	17.1	324	17.6	283	14.5	310	16.9	1249	16.5	0.0471	NS
>55	3324	37.6	3488	38.0	3490	36.5	3589	37.4	13,891	37.4	NS	NS

Whatever the type of stroke and year, the mean age of women in the group aged more than 55 years was higher than that in men: (80.39 years [80.35–80.44] vs. 75.01 years [74.97–75.06] p < 10⁻³) and this whatever the type of stroke: hemorrhagic : 78.24 years [78.14–78.35] vs. 70.03 years [73.93–74.14] (p < 10⁻³); ischemic: 80.96 years [80.91–81.00] vs. 75.27 years [75.21–75.32] (p < 10⁻³). Moreover, for this same age group, we found an increase in the mean age from 2008 to 2011 whatever the sex and type of stroke (Figs. 1, 2).

In-hospital mortality

For strokes overall (Table 1), we found a significant fall in the raw in-hospital mortality rate, which fell from 16.6 % in 2008 to 16.1 % in 2011, and in the standardized mortality rate (16.6 vs. 15.9 %). The difference was significant (Somers'd = 0.0009). This fall in in-hospital mortality was especially due to the fall in the lethality of ischemic stroke (12.0 % in 2008 vs. 11.3 % in 2011; Somers'd < 10⁻³) (Table 3), while in-hospital mortality in patients with hemorrhagic stroke (Table 2) remained stable and high (32.0 % in 2008 vs. 32.3 % in 2011; Somers'd NS).

For strokes overall (Table 1), the decrease in the raw and standardized mortality rates was only significant in men (Somers'd = 0.0006). However, the decrease in mortality rates following ischemic stroke over the period was statistically significant for both sexes (Table 3). In men, the raw mortality rate fell from 10.6 % in 2008 to 9.8 % in 2011 (Somers'd < 10⁻³) and in women it fell from 13.4 % in 2008 to 12.7 % in 2011 (Somers'd = 0.038). This decrease concerned all age groups for men and the more than 55 years group for women.

Table 3 Description of ischemic strokes

Ischemic strokes	2008		2009		2010		2011		Total		χ^2	Somers'd
	n	%	n	%	n	%	n	%	n	%	p	p
All patients	75,247		76,780		79,167		78,181		309,375			
Age												
All patients												
≤35	1271	1.7	1371	1.8	1417	1.8	1289	1.7	5348	1.7	0.0235	NS
36–55	7371	9.8	7449	9.7	7991	10.1	7771	9.9	30,582	9.9		
>55	66,605	88.5	67,960	88.5	69,759	88.1	69,121	88.4	273,445	88.4		
Male												
≤35	557	1.5	603	1.6	656	1.7	576	1.5	2392	1.6	0.0347	0.0462
36–55	4634	12.4	4622	12.3	4992	12.8	4939	12.8	19,187	12.6		
>55	32,063	86.1	32,502	86.2	33,388	85.5	33,149	85.7	131,102	85.9		
Female												
≤35	714	1.9	768	2.0	761	1.9	713	1.8	2956	1.9	NS	NS
36–55	2737	7.2	2827	7.2	2999	7.5	2832	7.2	11,395	7.3		
>55	34,542	90.9	35,458	90.8	36,371	90.6	35,972	91.0	142,343	90.8		
Sex												
Male	37,254	49.5	37,727	49.1	39,036	49.3	38,664	49.4	152,681	49.4	NS	NS
Female	37,993	50.5	39,053	50.9	40,131	50.7	39,517	50.6	156,694	50.6		
In-hospital death (in 30 days)												
All patients	9025	12.0	8867	11.6	9231	11.7	8811	11.3	35,934	11.6	0.0002	$<10^{-3}$
% age-sexe-adjusted		12.0		11.5		11.7		11.3				
Male	3939	10.6	3919	10.4	3897	10.0	3785	9.8	15,540	10.2	0.0010	$<10^{-3}$
% age-adjusted		10.6		10.4		10.0		9.8				
≤35	14	2.5	19	3.2	15	2.3	5	0.9	53	2.2	0.0574	0.0088
36–55	168	3.6	154	3.3	155	3.1	151	3.1	628	3.3	NS	0.0493
>55	3757	11.7	3746	11.5	3727	11.2	3629	11.0	14,859	11.3	0.0082	0.0003
Female	5086	13.4	4948	12.7	5334	13.3	5026	12.7	20,394	13.0	0.0023	0.0380
% age-adjusted		13.4		12.7		13.3		12.7				
≤35	15	2.1	5	0.7	12	1.6	7	1.0	39	1.3	NS	NS
36–55	84	3.1	83	2.9	91	3.0	76	2.7	334	2.9	NS	NS
>55	4987	14.4	4860	13.7	5231	14.4	4943	13.7	20,021	14.1	0.0031	0.0466

We found no significant variation in mortality rates according to age group and sex for hemorrhagic strokes (Table 2).

Table 4 shows that, in our population, the risk of dying in hospital in the 30 days following a stroke whatever the type was lower in men than in women (relative risk: male/female (RR): 0.86 [95 % CI 0.84–0.87]). Nonetheless, the RR was different depending on the age group and type of stroke. For both types (hemorrhagic and ischemic), women older than 55 years presented a higher risk of death than men of the same age group (RR: 0.97 [95 % CI 0.95–0.98] for hemorrhagic and RR: 0.78 [95 % CI 0.77–0.80] for ischemic). However, for patients younger than 36 years, the risk was lower in women for both types of stroke (RR: 1.23 [95 % CI 1.02–1.48] for hemorrhagic and RR: 1.68 [95 % CI 1.11–2.53] for ischemic), and for hemorrhagic stroke in women aged 36–55 years (RR: 1.15 [95 % CI 1.08–1.23]).

Spatial analysis of in-hospital mortality

The overall decrease in in-hospital mortality over the 4 years of the study masks stark spatial differences in France (c.f. Fig. 3). The map of the standardized rates illustrates a concentration of high stroke-related mortality along a north-east/south-west diagonal, as well as high rates in Brittany departments. The highest rates are seen in central departments and in Haute-Corse, in north of Corsica. In contrast, the departments of Ile-de-France, Rhône, Isere and Haute-Savoie have the lowest rates.

At the level of geographic codes (c.f. Fig. 4), the map shows clusters with high in-hospital mortality, notably in central Brittany and along a geographical diagonal of high

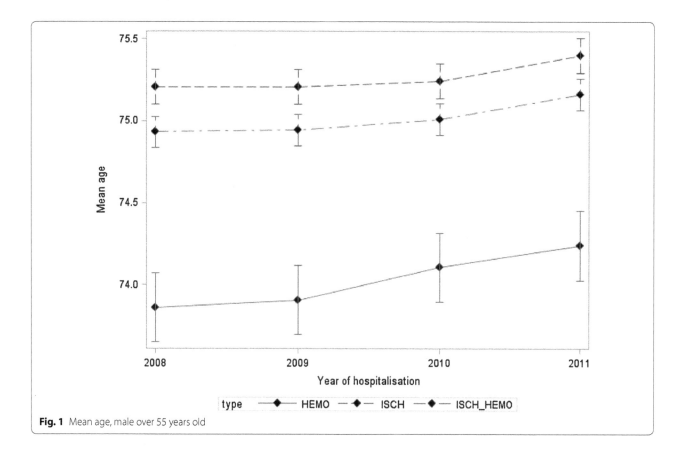

Fig. 1 Mean age, male over 55 years old

mortality through the country, following a north-east/south-west axis. Areas bordering the Rhône and Loire valleys, Alsace and the north-east of the Rhone-Alps region, however, appear to be better protected. In Corsica, areas around the town of Calvi, in the north-west of the island are particularly affected by high mortality.

Tables 5 and 6 present the results of the ascending hierarchical classification at the level of PMSI geographic codes and the characteristics of each cluster. Cluster 1 represents urban areas, near large towns or areas that benefit from the attraction of nearby large towns. Stroke-related mortality is low in these areas; the population is younger than elsewhere, as shown by the lower proportion of over 60 s and pensioners, but the occupational profile was more precarious, with a high proportion of unemployed, intermediate workers and manual workers compared with the low proportion of managers or professional occupations.

Cluster 2, which also represents urban and peri-urban France, has low stroke-related mortality but unlike cluster 1 has a high socio-economic status with a higher proportion of managers and professional occupations and a lower proportion of manual workers and unemployed than in other clusters. This cluster mainly includes peri-urban areas situated in the affluent suburbs of large agglomerations: west of Ile-de-France, Lille, Nancy, Strasbourg, Lyon, Montpellier, Toulouse, Bordeaux, Nantes, Rennes.

Cluster 3 includes dynamic rural areas of the west and east of France. Stroke-related mortality in these areas is relatively low and the population is relatively younger than in other clusters.

The areas in cluster 4 are mostly situated along the coast in the south and south-east of the country in Provence, in the Alps, and Corsica, and are characterized by an aging population, high levels of unemployment and high stroke-related in-hospital mortality.

The spatial distribution of high stroke-related in-hospital mortality seems to follow the north-east/south-west axis (cf. Figs. 3, 4), as shown by the results of the AHC (cf. Fig. 5). Areas with low in-hospital mortality are also those with favorable socio-professional and demographic structures. Areas with high mortality (Fig. 4) corresponded visually with areas in cluster 5, which have low-income occupations, pensioners or pre-retirees and an older population.

For the country as a whole, the spatial distribution of socio-economic and healthcare indicators seems to favor areas around large towns or departmental prefectures. Young people and tertiary-sector professions are concentrated in these main towns (cluster 1), which have a denser healthcare structure and show low stroke-related

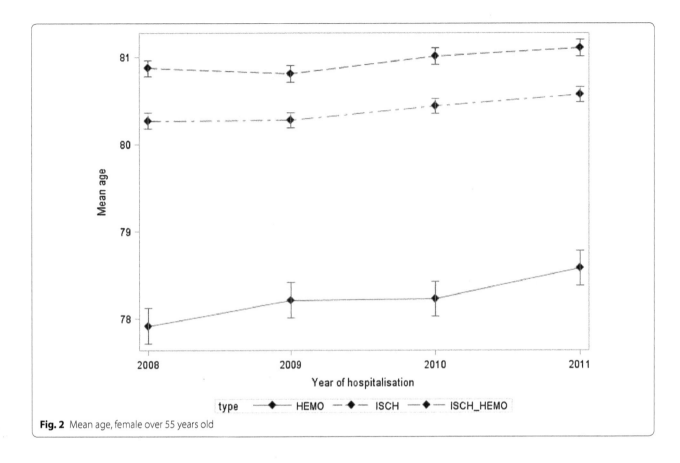

Fig. 2 Mean age, female over 55 years old

Table 4 Relative risk of in-hospital mortality, comparison between males and females

	Relative risk (RR:male:female)								
	Hemorrhagic + ischemic strokes			Hemorrhagic strokes			Ischemic strokes		
	RR	95 % CI		RR	95 % CI		RR	95 % CI	
Age									
≤35	1.51	1.28	1.80	1.23	1.02	1.48	1.68	1.11	2.53
36–55	0.97	0.91	1.03	1.15	1.08	1.23	1.12	0.98	1.27
>55	0.87	0.86	0.88	0.97	0.95	0.99	0.81	0.79	0.82
All	0.86	0.84	0.87	0.97	0.95	0.98	0.78	0.77	0.80

CI confidence interval

mortality. The affluent suburbs of these main towns (cluster 2) are organized in a concentric pattern around these urban centers. Further away, rural areas associated with these urban centers (cluster 3) also have low mortality, but also include large underprivileged areas with aging populations (clusters 4 and 5).

Discussion

The list of diagnostic codes used to select patients corresponded to those used in other studies on stroke mortality, in France [8], and internationally [9].

Different sensitivity and validation analyses have shown the robustness of the methodology [10, 11]. However, following a validation study of PMSI data [8], our selection criteria differed slightly from those of Peretti et al. Our selection of hemorrhagic stroke was based on codes I60 and I61 and notably on code I62.9. We did not use all I62 codes, given their lower sensitivity according to a validation study of PMSI data [8]. Moreover, patients suffering from TIA were not included in our study given the heterogeneous nature of coding practices [12].

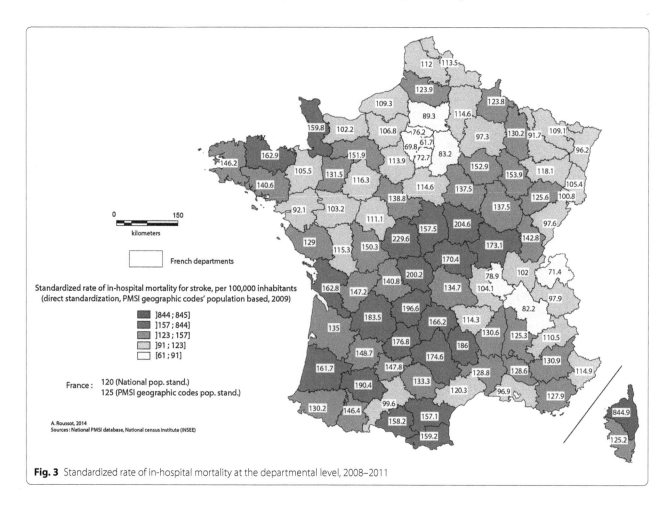

Fig. 3 Standardized rate of in-hospital mortality at the departmental level, 2008–2011

According to the national PMSI databases, overall, the number of patients hospitalized for stroke increased in France from 2008 to 2011, despite a fall between 2010 and 2011. This increase was not homogeneous and depended on the age group. The greatest increases affected patients older than 55 years, which is in line with demographic change: in France according to the INSEE, the number of persons aged over 55 years increased by 2.5 % between 2008 and 2011.

The majority of patients hospitalized following stroke were women, which is in keeping with the results of an earlier study conducted in France [13]. Moreover, our study shows that the increase in the proportion of patients older than 55 years affects women more than men in this his age group. This result agrees with the results of recent study [14], which show that with the increased life expectancy in developed countries, women contribute more than men to the increased prevalence and incidence of stroke in the oldest age group. This increased life expectancy without stroke was shown in an earlier study, which reported a mean increase of 5 years in men and of 8 years in women of stroke in Dijon,

France between 1987 and 2008 [15]. This trend over the same period was also found in Sweden [16] and in New-Zealand [17].

The increase concerning the 36–55 years age group for ischemic stroke, notably in men, is in keeping with recent data, whether from different population registries or from medico-administrative data [7], and with trends observed worldwide [1, 18, 19]. This increase is certainly multifactorial and raises the problem of uncontrolled or increasing risk factors in this population. Such factors include smoking, diabetes, hypercholesterolemia, obesity, or cannabis consumption [18, 20–25]. These results indicate that primary vascular prevention is necessary throughout life and should start in childhood.

At the same time, the characteristics of the hospital stay have changed. First, the mean length of hospital stay decreased and secondly, there was a clear fall in in-hospital mortality. According to a validation study conducted by the Technique de l'Information Hospitaliere (ATIH) and INSEE, the quality of recording in-hospital mortality in the PMSI database has improved. We thus focused a part of our analysis on this indicator of performance

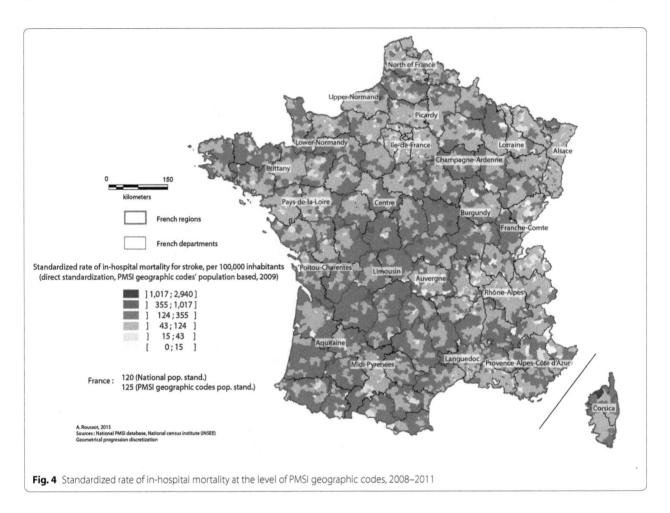

Fig. 4 Standardized rate of in-hospital mortality at the level of PMSI geographic codes, 2008–2011

Table 5 Results of the HAC

Variable	Overall mean	Cluster 1 Prob (test) > 0	Cluster 2 Prob (test) > 0	Cluster 3 Prob (test) > 0	Cluster 4 Prob (test) > 0	Cluster 5 Prob (test) > 0
Farmers (%)	3.30	<0.0001	<0.0001	<0.0001	<0.0001	<0.0001
Craftsmen–storekeepers—entrepreneurs (%)	6.91					
Managers or professional occupations (%)	11.20				0.2305	
Intermediate professions—technicians (%)	22.99				0.0244	
Employees (%)	28.48					
Skilled workers (%)	26.15				<0.0001	
0–20 years old (%)	24.20					
20–60 years old (%)	51.48					
60+ (%)	24.80					
Unemployed persons (%)	10.93					
15–64 years old retired or pre-retired persons (%)	14.84					
Standardized rate of in-hospital mortality for stroke	122.58					

of the healthcare system, especially since this type of analysis is becoming more widespread with the growing use of medico-administrative data [26–28]. The reduced in-hospital mortality observed for hospital stays overall corresponds to observations of a French study, which reported that the proportion of intra-hospital deaths

Table 6 Characteristics of clusters from the HAC

Cluster	1	2	3	4	5
Socio-professional category (mean in each cluster)					
Farmers (%)	1.17	0.57	4.06	1.96	11.02
Craftsmen storekeepers entrepreneurs (%)	5.49	6.26	6.23	9.68	9.39
Managers or professional occupations (%)	9.96	24.65	8.54	NS	6.56
Intermediate professions—technicians (%)	23.41	29.15	21.95	23.32	17.77
Employees (%)	30.96	24.24	26.86	31.53	26.97
Skilled workers (%)	27.69	14.38	31.61	21.32	27.29
Demographic structure (mean in each cluster)					
0–20 years old (%)	25.47	26.24	25.77	20.69	19.45
20–60 years old (%)	53.05	53.91	52.25	48.42	46.95
60+ (%)	21.90	20.07	22.53	31.36	34.30
Sanitary variable (mean in each cluster)					
Unemployed persons (%)	13.15	7.80	9.30	12.94	10.12
15–64 years old retired or pre-retired persons (%)	13.50	11.33	13.77	18.63	19.75
Standardized rate of in-hospital mortality for stroke (per 100,000 inhabitants)	105.13	76.47	114.07	155.41	193.41

during the first hospital stay for stroke had fallen significantly by 0.5 percentage points between 2007 and 2009 [7]. These observations could be related to the better reactivity of hospital emergency departments and the earlier arrival of patients. On this subject, another study pointed out the efficacy of fibrinolysis in patients with ischemic stroke in a context of reinforced on-call duty in specialized neurology units, stroke units [29, 30].

Our results also indicate that raw and standardized mortality rates were significantly higher in women than in men, which was also shown in another study conducted in France [13]. However, this excess mortality following stroke in women was not found at the level of all developed countries, where mortality rates in men are higher than those in women [31]. In our study, however, this excess mortality in women was only found for women aged 56 years and over. Yet, for this age group, the mean age of women was 80 and 5 years older than that of men. As mortality increases with age, this difference in mean ages may explain the excess mortality. In contrast, there was excess mortality in men younger than 56 years for hemorrhagic stroke, and in those younger than 36 years for ischemic stroke. The RR observed in our study for these age groups were of the same order of magnitude as those observed in the United States in young adults [32].

Our spatial study is the first to be conducted at the level of PMSI geographic codes in France. The results using this approach were more accurate than those obtained at the department level. Indeed, earlier studies have already investigated the geographic distribution of stroke prevalence and mortality at the global scale [1, 33]. These studies showed an increase in stroke prevalence associated with a fall in mortality in high-income developed countries, like France. However, we do not have such a small-scale spatial analysis of stroke-related mortality in France. Our work therefore showed the interest of associating medical data with socio-economic data from the national census, which is available at the post-code level. Concerning in-hospital mortality, this association could be used for other diseases and in other countries, depending on the availability of databases and the scale of analysis they allow.

Two major results came out of this study. The map of standardized mortality rates allowed us first of all to illustrate the territorial disparities at the national level, and notably by identifying areas of high mortality from the north-east to the south-west of the country, along the "low population density diagonal". Areas along this diagonal are characterized by aging communities, but the excess mortality cannot be explained by age differences alone as age-standardized mortality was also higher than elsewhere. This zone, which we call the "excess mortality diagonal" had already been pointed out by French geographers, notably in terms of premature death in the population at large [34]. Another hypothesis to explain the high mortality rate could be that these territories are often far from emergency care facilities; this aspect has already been mentioned in several studies [35, 36]. Moreover, if we consider that patients hospitalized for stroke are hospitalized as close as possible to their homes, given that emergency care facilities are supposed to be nearby, these results indicate the location of "protective" and "accidentogenic" zones on a very small scale. Local observations could provide a diagnostic tool for decision-makers to assess the quality of prevention, to evaluate the

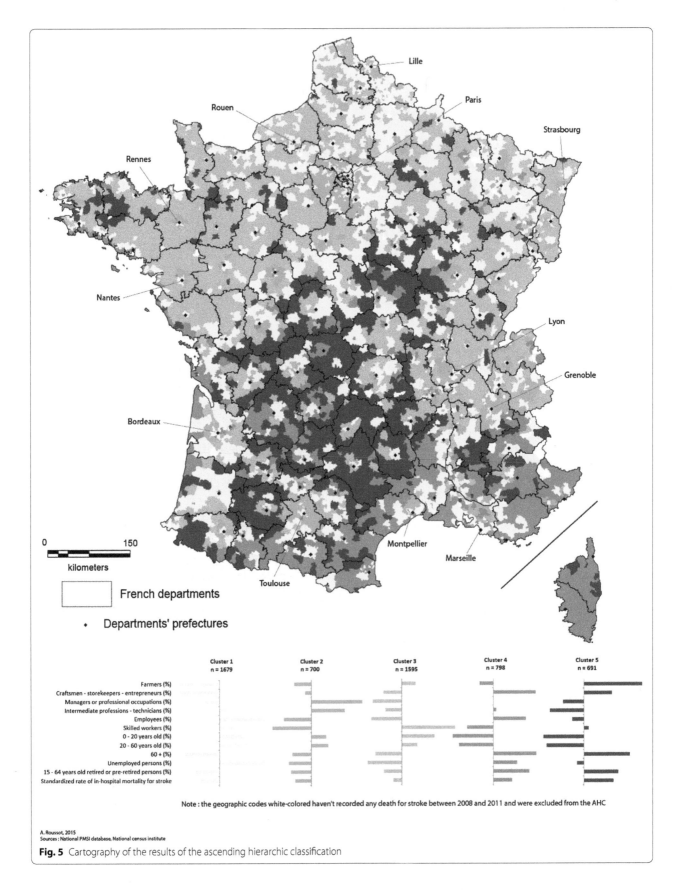

French departments

Departments' prefectures

Note : the geographic codes white-colored haven't recorded any death for stroke between 2008 and 2011 and were excluded from the AHC

A. Roussot, 2015
Sources : National PMSI database, National census institute

Fig. 5 Cartography of the results of the ascending hierarchic classification

efficacy of public healthcare messages and the burden of risk factors in certain areas [37, 38].

The isolation of certain rural areas raises the question of the development of telemedicine in the most serious cases of stroke, which require fibrinolysis. Concerning the management of ischemic strokes, telemedicine makes it possible to link small isolated rural hospitals with major hospitals where neurologists are available round the clock. Teleconsultations allow duty neurologists to help doctors in smaller hospitals to perform thrombolysis when necessary. The deployment of such systems enables the earlier management of stroke victims close to where the stroke occurred and avoids transfers to distant hospitals or stroke units. Telemedicine programs are being deployed in several French regions, notably in Burgundy, a region marked by the isolated rural areas in the centre and recent hospital restructuration. A previous study in the region brought to light the link between the isolation of populations from the healthcare system and poorer results in perinatal care [39]. However, an overall evaluation of these telemedicine programs using national claims data is difficult to achieve, as they are often too recent and because the coding of telemedicine procedures is not consistent. Studies to identify patients who have benefitted from telemedicine are nonetheless under way, but researchers need to go back to patients' medical records at the various establishments [40, 41]. Moreover, several tests were conducted with different variables in the AHC for this study, but we chose to represent the analysis that generated the greatest inertia (69.2 %). The results obtained with variables relative to access to the healthcare system were less satisfactory: these variables were time to reach a stroke unit or a hospital emergency unit, in minutes for each geographic code.

Standardization of mortality rates on a small scale, according to the geographic code of the patient's place of residence, revealed local clusters of high mortality, notably in Brittany. This analysis of local situations, which is more detailed than analyses at the departmental level, highlighted territorial disparities, but cannot replace the results of even smaller scale analyses, at the level INSEE codes for communes, for example. We intend to continue our work using SNIIRAM data, which will allow us to break away from the use of aggregated population data to calculate incidences or comparative indices of mortality. An earlier study underlined the interest of analyzing stroke incidence at the IRIS level (Ilots regroupés pour l'information statistique) using registry data [42, 43]. The analysis established a link between an underprivileged environment and the greater incidence of stroke. Mortality rates were also higher among lower wage earners.

The 5 clusters from the classification divide the territory according to the weight of each variable selected by the AHC. Classification was preferred for this study because it can be used to establish a solid typology that maximizes the resemblance between observations (PMSI geographic codes) within the same cluster. Concerning the ageing population in certain areas, the model presented includes the demographic structure of the geographic codes of the place of residence, as well as the smoothed rate of in-hospital mortality. These variables are treated independently in the classification, which allowed us to contextualize certain high mortality rates. Despite the adjustment for age, areas marked by high mortality were also those with the oldest population. The classification showed that the demographic structure was not the only factor of the socio-territorial organization to affect mortality. Indeed, apart from the age of the population, disparities in mortality also followed the territorial distribution of socio-professional categories. It thus appears that social difficulties and problems linked to the ageing of the population are associated with higher stroke-related mortality than is the case in certain rural or peri-urban areas. The interest of the AHC is justified by the difficulty of linking the healthcare results of a large population with their socio-economic conditions as there are as yet no indicators of this type at the individual level in French medico-administrative databases. Clustering techniques and the geographic approach provided an idea of aggregated healthcare results at a territorial level and illustrated the interplay between the socio-economic environment and healthcare issues, such as, among others, mortality in England and Wales [2] or access to the healthcare system in France [44, 45].

Conclusions

Since the implementation of the National Stroke Plan, most studies have reported better management of patients in France, where the incidence of stroke was amongst the lowest in the world, thanks to the geographic, social and healthcare conditions in the country [46]. In this respect, in-hospital mortality in patients with ischemic stroke has markedly improved thanks to the reinforcement of the stroke units network and the generalization of fibrinolysis and in spite of the increase in the number of people hospitalized. This study makes it easier to understand that the fall in in-hospital mortality was not uniform throughout the country and was accompanied by considerable territorial diversity. We showed that the spatial distribution of healthcare indicator such like in-hospital mortality follows the distribution of demographic and social inequalities. The clustering method showed that areas characterized by unfavorable socio-economic indicators are also affected by high in-hospital mortality. We also know that areas on the "excess mortality diagonal" are often far away from the nearest emergency care facilities. Our study was conducted in the context of a wider program of the territorial organization of healthcare policies to counter the isolation and aging of rural areas. The development of telemedicine programs, another priority axis of the National Stroke Plan, should accelerate the remote management of patients and guarantee better integrated healthcare in these isolated communities.

Ethics approval and consent to participate

This study was approved by the National Committee for data protection (Commission Nationale de l'Informatique et des Libertés, registration number 1576793) and was conducted in accordance with French legislation. The PMSI database was transmitted by the national agency for the management of hospitalization data (ATIH number 2015-111111-47-33).

Consent for publication

Written consent was not needed for this study.

Abbreviations

PMSI-MCO: Programme de médicalisation des systèmes d'information en Médecine, Chirurgie et Obstétrique; SNIIR-AM: Système national inter-régime de l'assurance maladie; ICD 10: International Classification of Diseases, 10th revision; PD: principal diagnosis; DRG: Diagnosis Related Group; INSEE: Institut National de la Statistique et des Etudes Economiques; ATIH: Agence Technique de l'Information Hospitalière; PCA: principal components analysis; AHC: ascending hierarchical classification; GIS: geographic information system; LOS: length of hospital stay.

Authors' contributions

AR: conceptualized and designed the study, conducted the statistical and cartographical analysis, wrote the article. JC: extracted the data, supported the statistical analysis, read back and corrected the article. MG: contributed substantially to the conception of the study and the interpretation of the results. MG: participated in the interpretation of the results and supported the discussion part. YB: participated in the interpretation of the results and supported the discussion part. CQ: designed the study, oversaw the data analysis and interpretation and critically reviewed and revised the manuscript drafts. All authors read and approved the final manuscript.

Authors' information

Catherine Quantin is Professor and head of department of Biostatistics and Medical Informatics in Dijon Teaching Hospital and member of the INSERM U866 team. She works on medical databases in the field of public health and developed new methods in anonymous identification and linkage. She is active in several colleges of medical informatics and epidemiology in France and in the International Society for Clinical Biostatistics (ISCB). She has organized twelve national or international conferences or workshop (IMIA). She is the Editor-in-Chief of the Journal d'Economie et de Gestion Médicales and the lead author/co-author of almost 160 international publications.

Author details

[1] Service de Biostatistique et d'Informatique Médicale (DIM), CHRU Dijon, Dijon 21000, France. [2] Université de Bourgogne, Dijon 21000, France. [3] Laboratoire d'Economie de Dijon, Université de Bourgogne, UMR 6307 CNRS, INSERM U1200, Dijon, France. [4] Registre des AVC dijonnais, EA4184, CHRU, Univ de Bourgogne, Dijon, France. [5] INSERM, CIC 1432, Dijon, France. [6] Clinical Epidemiology/Clinical Trials Unit, Clinical Investigation Center, Dijon University Hospital, Dijon, France. [7] Biostatistics, Biomathematics, Pharmacoepidemiology and Infectious Diseases (B2PHI), Univ. Bourgogne Franche-Comté, Inserm UMR 1181, Dijon 21000, France.

Acknowledgements

This work was supported by the Conseil Regional de Bourgogne. The authors thank M. Philip Bastable for reviewing the English version.

Competing interests

The authors declare that they have no competing interests.

References

1. Feigin VL, Forouzanfar MH, Krishnamurthi R, Mensah GA, Connor M, Bennett DA, et al. Global and regional burden of stroke during 1990–2010: findings from the Global Burden of Disease Study 2010. Lancet. 2014;383(9913):245–54.
2. Wang H, Liddell CA, Coates MM, Mooney MD, Levitz CE, Schumacher AE, et al. Global, regional, and national levels of neonatal, infant, and under-5 mortality during 1990–2013: a systematic analysis for the Global Burden of Disease Study 2013. Lancet. 2014;384(9947):957–79.
3. Plan d'actions national "accidents vasculaires cérébraux 2010–2014", (2010).
4. La prévention et la prise en charge des accidents vasculaires cérébraux en France.: Ministère de la santé et des sportsjuin 2009.
5. Goldberg M, Coeuret-Pellicer M, Ribet C, Zins M. Epidemiological studies based on medical and administrative databases: a potential strength in France. Med Sci (Paris). 2012;28(4):430–4.
6. Chevreul K, Durand-Zaleski I, Gouepo A, Fery-Lemonnier E, Hommel M, Woimant F. Cost of stroke in France. Eur J Neurol. 2013;20(7):1094–100.
7. de Peretti C, Nicolau J, Tuppin P, Schnitzler A, Woimant F. Acute and post-acute hospitalizations for stroke in France: recent improvements (2007–2009). Presse Med. 2012;41(5):491–503.
8. Aboa-Eboule C, Mengue D, Benzenine E, Hommel M, Giroud M, Bejot Y, et al. How accurate is the reporting of stroke in hospital discharge data? A pilot validation study using a population-based stroke registry as control. J Neurol. 2013;260(2):605–13.
9. Kokotailo RA, Hill MD. Coding of stroke and stroke risk factors using international classification of diseases, revisions 9 and 10. Stroke. 2005;36(8):1776–81.
10. Wright FL, Green J, Canoy D, Cairns BJ, Balkwill A, Beral V. Vascular disease in women: comparison of diagnoses in hospital episode statistics and general practice records in England. BMC Med Res Methodol. 2012;12:161.
11. Johnsen SP, Overvad K, Sorensen HT, Tjonneland A, Husted SE. Predictive value of stroke and transient ischemic attack discharge diagnoses in The Danish National Registry of Patients. J Clin Epidemiol. 2002;55(6):602–7.
12. Etude des algorithmes de définition des pathologies dans le système national d'information inter-régimes de l'assurance maladie (SNIIRAM). Rapport CnamTS en cours de publication.
13. De Peretti C. Les risques de décès un an après un accident vasculaire cérébral. Etudes et Résultats. Rapport DREES no. 0939.2015.
14. Feigin VL, Krishnamurthi RV, Parmar P, Norrving B, Mensah GA, Bennett DA, et al. Update on the Global Burden of Ischemic and Hemorrhagic Stroke in 1990–2013: The GBD 2013 Study. Neuroepidemiology. 2015;45(3):161–76.
15. Bejot Y, Gentil A, Biotti D, Rouaud O, Fromont A, Couvreur G, et al. [What has changed for stroke at the beginning of the 21st century]. Rev Neurol (Paris). [Review]. 2009;165(8–9):617–25.
16. Terent A. Trends in stroke incidence and 10-year survival in Soderhamn, Sweden, 1975–2001. Stroke. 2003;34(6):1353–8.
17. Anderson CS, Carter KN, Hackett ML, Feigin V, Barber PA, Broad JB, et al. Trends in stroke incidence in Auckland, New Zealand, during 1981–2003. Stroke. 2005;36(10):2087–93.
18. Bejot Y, Daubail B, Jacquin A, Durier J, Osseby GV, Rouaud O, et al. Trends in the incidence of ischaemic stroke in young adults between 1985 and 2011: the Dijon Stroke Registry. J Neurol Neurosurg Psychiatry. 2014;85(5):509–13.
19. Kissela BM, Khoury JC, Alwell K, Moomaw CJ, Woo D, Adeoye O, et al. Age at stroke: temporal trends in stroke incidence in a large, biracial population. Neurology. 2012;79(17):1781–7.

20. de los Rios F, Kleindorfer DO, Khoury J, Broderick JP, Moomaw CJ, Adeoye O, et al. Trends in substance abuse preceding stroke among young adults: a population-based study. Stroke. 2012; 43(12):3179–83.

21. Dube SR, McClave A, James C, et al. Vital signs: current cigarette smoking among adults aged ≥18 years—United States, 2009. Morbidity Mortality Weekly Report (MMWR). 2010; 59:1135–40.

22. Kanny D, Liu Y, Brewer RD. Vital Signs: Binge drinking among high school students and adults—United States, 2009. Morbidity and Mortality Weekly Report (MMWR). 2010;59(39):1274–9.

23. Kusnik-Joinville O, Weill A, Salanave B, Ricordeau P, Allemand H. Prevalence and treatment of diabetes in France: trends between 2000 and 2005. Diabetes Metab. 2008;34(3):266–72.

24. Marques-Vidal P, Ruidavets JB, Cambou JP, Ferrieres J. Changes and determinants in cigarette smoking prevalence in southwestern France, 1985–1997. Eur J Public Health. 2003;13(2):168–70.

25. Pigeyre M, Dauchet L, Simon C, Bongard V, Bingham A, Arveiler D, et al. Effects of occupational and educational changes on obesity trends in France: the results of the MONICA-France survey 1986-2006. Prev Med. 2011;52(5):305–9.

26. Chang KC, Lee HC, Huang YC, Hung JW, Chiu HE, Chen JJ, et al. Cost-effectiveness analysis of stroke management under a universal health insurance system. J Neurol Sci. 2012;323(1–2):205–15.

27. Lee HC, Chang KC, Huang YC, Hung JW, Chiu HH, Chen JJ, et al. Readmission, mortality, and first-year medical costs after stroke. J Chin Med Assoc. 2013;76(12):703–14.

28. Lee J, Morishima T, Kunisawa S, Sasaki N, Otsubo T, Ikai H, et al. Derivation and validation of in-hospital mortality prediction models in ischaemic stroke patients using administrative data. Cerebrovasc Dis. 2013;35(1):73–80.

29. Raffe F, Jacquin A, Milleret O, Durier J, Sauze D, Peyron C, et al. Evaluation of the possible impact of a care network for stroke and transient ischemic attack on rates of recurrence. Eur Neurol. 2011;65(4):239–44.

30. Nimptsch U, Mansky T. Stroke unit care and trends of in-hospital mortality for stroke in Germany 2005–2010. Int J Stroke. 2014;9(3):260–5.

31. Krishnamurthi RV, Moran AE, Feigin VL, Barker-Collo S, Norrving B, Mensah GA, et al. Stroke prevalence, mortality and disability-adjusted life years in adults aged 20–64 years in 1990–2013: data from the global burden of disease 2013 study. Neuroepidemiology. 2015;45(3):190–202.

32. Poisson SN, Glidden D, Johnston SC, Fullerton HJ. Deaths from stroke in US young adults, 1989–2009. Neurology. 2014;83(23):2110–5.

33. Feigin VL, Mensah GA, Norrving B, Murray CJ, Roth GA. Atlas of the Global Burden of Stroke (1990–2013): the GBD 2013 Study. Neuroepidemiology. 2015;45(3):230–6.

34. Fainzang S, Salem G, Rican S, Jougla E. Atlas de la santé en France, vol. 1 : Les causes de décès. [compte-rendu]. Sciences sociales et santé. 2001;19(2):113–5.

35. Coldefy M, Com-Ruelle L, Lucas-Gabrielli V, Marcoux L. Les distances d'accès aux soins en France métropolitaine au 1er janvier 2007: IRDES2011.

36. Evain F. À quelle distance de chez soi se fait-on hospitaliser ? Etudes et résultats DREES. février 2011;754.

37. Pedigo A, Aldrich T, Odoi A. Neighborhood disparities in stroke and myocardial infarction mortality: a GIS and spatial scan statistics approach. BMC Public Health. 2011;11:644.

38. Pedigo A, Seaver W, Odoi A. Identifying unique neighborhood characteristics to guide health planning for stroke and heart attack: fuzzy cluster and discriminant analyses approaches. PLoS One. 2011;6(7):e22693.

39. Combier E, Charreire H, Le Vaillant M, Michaut F, Ferdynus C, Amat-Roze JM, et al. Perinatal health inequalities and accessibility of maternity services in a rural French region: closing maternity units in Burgundy. Health Place. [Research Support, Non-U.S. Gov't]. 2013;24:225–33.

40. Handschu R, Wacker A, Scibor M, Sancu C, Schwab S, Erbguth F, et al. Use of a telestroke service for evaluation of non-stroke neurological cases. J Neurol. 2015;262(5):1266–70.

41. MasjuanVallejo J. Stroke unit: the best treatment for stroke patients. Neurologia. 2009;24(5):285–7.

42. Grimaud O, Bejot Y, Heritage Z, Vallee J, Durier J, Cadot E, et al. Incidence of stroke and socioeconomic neighborhood characteristics: an ecological analysis of Dijon stroke registry. Stroke. 2011;42(5):1201–6.

43. Grimaud O, Leray E, Lalloue B, Aghzaf R, Durier J, Giroud M, et al. Mortality following stroke during and after acute care according to neighbourhood deprivation: a disease registry study. J Neurol Neurosurg Psychiatry. 2014;85(12):1313–8.

44. Vigneron E. Territorial and social healthcare inequalities in France. Bull Acad Natl Med. 2012;196(4–5):939–52.

45. Ouedraogo S, Dabakuyo-Yonli TS, Roussot A, Dialla PO, Pornet C, Poillot ML, et al. Breast cancer screening in thirteen French departments. Bull Cancer. 2015;102(2):126–38.

46. Sudlow CL, Warlow CP. Comparing stroke incidence worldwide: what makes studies comparable? Stroke. 1996;27(3):550–8.

8

Reporting back environmental exposure data and free choice learning

Monica D. Ramirez-Andreotta[1,3]*, Julia Green Brody[2], Nathan Lothrop[3], Miranda Loh[3,4], Paloma I. Beamer[3] and Phil Brown[5]

Abstract

Reporting data back to study participants is increasingly being integrated into exposure and biomonitoring studies. Informal science learning opportunities are valuable in environmental health literacy efforts and report back efforts are filling an important gap in these efforts. Using the University of Arizona's Metals Exposure Study in Homes, this commentary reflects on how community-engaged exposure assessment studies, partnered with data report back efforts are providing a new informal education setting and stimulating free-choice learning. Participants are capitalizing on participating in research and leveraging their research experience to meet personal and community environmental health literacy goals. Observations from report back activities conducted in a mining community support the idea that reporting back biomonitoring data reinforces free-choice learning and this activity can lead to improvements in environmental health literacy. By linking the field of informal science education to the environmental health literacy concepts, this commentary demonstrates how reporting data back to participants is tapping into what an individual is intrinsically motivated to learn and how these efforts are successfully responding to community-identified education and research needs.

Keywords: Biomonitoring, Exposure assessment, Environmental health literacy, Risk communication, Arsenic, Heavy metals, Informal science education, Free-choice learning

Background

Biomonitoring efforts are widely used in environmental exposures assessments beyond occupational and clinical settings to help identify and assess chemicals observed in the environment and in humans and to inform public-health decisions and regulations [1]. Due to innovations in technology, increased sensitivity in methods, access to resources, and institutional support for community-engaged research, there has been a tremendous increase in the number of human biomonitoring studies [1, 2]. With these types of studies comes an additional level of responsibility to translate the data and findings and address environmental health literacy (EHL) goals.

Using the University of Arizona's Metals Exposure Study in Homes (MESH) extensive report back effort as an example, this commentary highlights how reporting back environmental exposure data is carving out a new informal education setting (learning outside of school classrooms) and is stimulating free-choice learning - learning that is occurring within these settings and that is driven by the needs and interests of the learner rather than an external authority [3]. By taking an in-depth look at exposure study participants' understanding of results and their resulting actions, this commentary contributes to exposure science and expands the concept of EHL and science education by viewing report back as a free-choice learning experience. Lastly, it is proposed that such documentation of learning and action would be an effective method by which to assess report back efforts and, in effect, evaluate a community's EHL.

Literacy

Thus far, scholars have defined literacy in terms of science [4], health [5], critical health [6], public health [7], and the environment [8]. Health literacy implies the achievement of a level of knowledge, personal skills and

* Correspondence: mdramire@email.arizona.edu
[1]Department of Soil, Water, and Environmental Science, University of Arizona, 1177 E Fourth Street, Rm. 429, Tucson, Arizona, USA
[3]Mel and Enid Zuckerman College of Public Health, University of Arizona, Tucson, AZ 85721, USA
Full list of author information is available at the end of the article

confidence to take action to improve personal and community health by changing personal lifestyles and living conditions [5]. Public health literacy is defined as the degree to which individuals and groups can obtain, process, understand, evaluate, and act on information needed to make public health decisions that benefit the community [9]. Environmental literacy is the capacity for individuals and groups to make informed decisions concerning the environment; to be willing to act on these decisions to improve the well-being of other individuals, societies, and the global environment; and to participate in civic life [8]. Recently, efforts have sought to merge existing explanations and define EHL. Thus far, the Society for Public Health Education defines EHL as the ability to "integrate concepts from both environmental literacy and health literacy to develop the wide range of skills and competencies in order to seek out, comprehend, evaluate, and use environmental health information to make informed choices, reduce health risks, improve quality of life and protect the environment" [10].

Literacy as described above, stresses understanding, informed decision-making, and action. However, health literacy efforts traditionally assess basic literacy skills such as reading, writing, and arithmetic, and are geared toward compliance with recommended clinical care. In this context, health literacy is seen as a patient "risk factor" that needs to be managed within the process of providing clinical care [11] and tends to stay within the traditional disciplinary boundaries of medicine and health promotion [6]. This approach does not view health literacy as an asset or a form of health action (personal, social, environmental) and does not focus on or assess individual and/or community efforts regarding knowledge integration, informed choices, actions to improve personal and community health, and methods to reduce risk. When health literacy is viewed as an asset, with roots in public health [11], practitioners can then implement and evaluate "health literacy in action." This is not only defined by functional literacy, but also communicative/interactive and critical literacy, which can then assess whether an individual/community is taking action to improve health, exerting greater control over factors that determine health, reflecting greater autonomy and empowerment, and engaging in a wider range of health actions [6, 11]. These actions include personal behaviors to social action to address the social, economic, and environmental determinants of health. EHL is an evolving concept that spans and synergistically unites various disciplines such as, but not limited to, risk communication, social science, public health, health promotion, and communication [12]. Interestingly the field of science education, specifically the subfield of informal science learning/free-choice learning, has not been part

of the dialogue thus far, and this is a great loss. Efforts to understand how, when and where learning is occurring are at the forefront of informal science education efforts. Measuring these types of changes can be challenging and new methods are needed to improve and evaluate literacy in action, specifically EHL.

Informal science education, defined as science learning opportunities that people experience across their lifespan outside of school [13], contributes greatly to an adult's science learning. In fact, over the course of a lifetime, the average person spends 5 % of their time in school [14] and research suggests that nearly half of the public's science understanding and learning derives from free-choice learning [13]. In a study to determine what sources people relied upon for science and technological information, 74 % of respondents attributed "some or a lot" of their learning to "life experiences," followed by "books and magazines –not for school" [15]. Data indicates that lifelong learning is intrinsically motivated and largely under the choice and control of the learner [13, 15, 16]. It seems ideal to harness the power of free-choice learning to improve EHL.

Free-choice learning in environmentally compromised communities

Informal science education methods are particularly valuable when working with communities impacted by hazardous waste. Communities neighboring contaminated sites are learning on their own about the contaminants of concern at hazardous waste sites and the associated health effects, and this type of learning is a multi-faceted phenomenon that is place-based and socioculturally mediated. As suggested by Falk and Storksdieck (2005), free-choice learning is a cumulative process involving connections and reinforcement among the variety of learning experiences people encounter in their lives [17]. In that way, learning is both a process and a product, suggesting a vibrant and contextual model of learning [17], requiring both creative and innovative evaluation methods [18].

Community-engaged exposure assessment studies as informal education settings

There is already an established infrastructure of organizations providing opportunities for free-choice learning beyond and outside of the formal education system. These include broadcast and print media, libraries, museums, science centers, zoos, aquariums, botanical gardens, environmental centers, and community organizations [13]. Although environmental health issues are discussed broadly and may be addressed in the above organizations, there are no infrastructures dedicated to environmental health, particularly for discussing contaminant fate and transport, exposure assessments, risk characterization, and the challenges of establishing a relationship between exposure(s) and health outcome(s). These topic areas make EHL and free-choice learning especially important to communities neighboring hazardous waste, pollution emissions, and resource extraction activities. Residents of environmentally compromised communities typically want additional information regarding their environmental health, and due to this gap in infrastructure, such communities have begun partnering with research organizations and universities to conduct community-engaged research projects [19, 20]. These partnerships are establishing new informal education infrastructures that support and stimulate free-choice learning. Collaborative research efforts are increasingly directed toward understanding the environmental determinants of chronic disease, and biomonitoring is becoming a key methodology by which to provide the scientific basis for prevention of environmental exposures and motivating action [21].

The need for report back efforts in mining communities

Evaluating exposures and increasing EHL in mining communities is especially crucial. Mining and smelting activities are the primary source of metals entering the environment [22]. In the U.S. alone, approximately 550,000 abandoned mine sites are responsible for generating 45 billion tons of waste, and many of these sites are in arid and semiarid regions [23]. Studies have observed an inverse relationship between the environmental and biomonitoring levels of arsenic and heavy metals and the distance from metal smelters and other mining operations to home or school environments [24, 25]. In an exposure study conducted near the Tar Creek Superfund Site, a former lead and zinc mine, half of the homes sampled had indoor dust concentrations of arsenic, lead, cadmium, and zinc greater than those observed in soil [26]. Due to their common occurrence at hazardous waste sites, toxicity, and potential for human exposure, metals like arsenic, cadmium, and lead are among the Agency for Toxic Substances and Disease Registry's top ten contaminants of concern [27]. Particulate emissions associated with mining operations are commonly associated with significantly elevated levels of one or more of these contaminants [25, 28].

In Arizona alone, there are more than 80,000 abandoned mines [23] and the arid and semi-arid Southwest climate creates great potential for dust emissions and long-range transport of arsenic-contaminated aerosols from these former mining operations [29]. Climate change will exacerbate the risks posed by mining in arid and semi-arid environments, primarily due to land use changes, increased average temperatures, and drought conditions [30]. The Town of Dewey-Humboldt, Arizona, comprised of 3,894 people [31], is sandwiched in between a 153-acre site of legacy mine tailings waste with arsenic and lead concentrations exceeding 3,000 milligram per kilogram and a 189-acre legacy smelter area [32]. Dewey-Humboldt, AZ is home to the Iron King Mine and Humboldt Smelter Superfund Site, a hazardous waste site added to the US Environmental Protection Agency's National Priorities List in 2008. Soon after listing, members of the Dewey-Humboldt, AZ community partnered with the University of Arizona (UAZ) on community-engaged environmental health research initiatives to characterize the extent of anthropogenic and naturally occurring of arsenic and metal contamination in their residential areas (e.g., Gardenroots, [33–35]). The Metals Exposure Study in Homes (MESH) project was developed in response to community concerns about exposure to metal(loid)s such as arsenic, lead, cadmium, nickel, beryllium, aluminum, and chromium. MESH assessed metal concentrations in multiple environmental matrices and their associations with levels of exposure in local children (1–11 years of age) [36]. After the completion of the MESH study and data report back efforts, participants were asked to reflect upon the report back experience, their understanding of results, and actions in response to their results. Not surprisingly, MESH participants described activities that are aligned with the EHL goals. Participants used the MESH data to inform what actions to take to reduce their child's exposure; they posed new research questions; and suggested novel ideas on how to report the data to inform them even further. These outcomes reflect participants' ability to comprehend, evaluate, and use the provided environmental health information to make informed choices and reduce health risks – meeting the EHL literacy goals defined above. Challenges described by the MESH participants included: access to and networking with other participants, more face-to-face engagement with the research team, additional information related to all the metals analyzed, and a spatial representation of the data. Though MESH participants described challenges associated with the report back process, the outcomes of the project are still aligned with EHL goals. Practitioners and researchers can learn from the reported challenges to improve their future report back efforts. These outcomes reflect the findings of past studies designed to take in-depth look at participants' report back experience, their understanding of results, and actions in response to their results [21, 35, 37–40]. These past studies have shown that participants can: learn a great deal [37]; interpret scientific results to affirm lay knowledge; absorb new information regarding other pollutant sources; and gain an understanding of the complex health messages related to environmental quality [35, 38]. Participants can also increase their understanding of environmental science and the scientific method; establish new networks; participate in other environmental projects; and leverage their results to hold government officials to more stringent cleanup standards [35].

Evaluating the outcomes of reporting back environmental exposure data

By evaluating the outcomes of report back efforts, new ways to assess EHL can be illuminated, providing a wider set of parameters to more adequately and successfully reflect health literacy. MESH was one of eight biomonitoring studies selected as part of the Personal Exposure Report-Back Ethics Study, a larger project that examines how: a) researchers report back data; b) Institutional Review Boards evaluate such protocols; and c) participants understand and use results. The PERE research team is among the first to report levels of emerging (i.e. limited toxicological data) and known contaminants to individuals and communities and is leading the field of report back practices and methodologies [21, 35, 37–40]. Frameworks such as clinical ethics, community based participatory approach, and the exposure experience have been applied in the past for analyzing participant responses [21, 38, 39, 40]; based on this work, a set of best practices have been developed to guide academic-community research collaborations [39]. The exposure experience, which builds on the concept of "illness experience" [38], considers how: 1) individuals, communities, and populations are becoming increasingly aware of environmental issues, especially those related to their immediate environment, and are learning about contaminants in their bodies; and 2) the eco-social context, which encompasses participants' past experiences with pollution and how those frame their responses and actions [37]. We know that the distribution of environmental pollution varies across populations and places [41], and these geographic and social differences, and even differences in contaminants of concern, will inform their responses to data about chemicals in their homes and bodies.

In the case of Dewey-Humboldt, AZ, some community members take pride in the mine, which is a large part of their eco-social context. Even the town seal has a graphical depiction of the mine and metal smelter, alongside an agricultural field and the town hall. These idiosyncrasies need to be considered when designing report back efforts and evaluating their effectiveness to raise EHL and see positive changes at individual, programmatic, and community/social-ecological level. For example, a community member who has lived in Dewey-Humboldt her whole life states: "Well I would [have concerns] if we had like a chemical plant, or something like that around here. But, I mean, just the mine. That mine's been there forever." In a recent assessment at the Iron King Mine and Humboldt Smelter Superfund Site after

MESH and "Gardenroots: The Dewey-Humboldt Arizona Garden Project" [33–35], Ramirez-Andreotta et al. (2015): evaluated community inquiries at the time the site was listed and five years later; assessed what community members were most concerned about at a site; whether these concerns changed; and if these concerns were adequately addressed through accessible sources of information. Further, it was hypothesized that the changes in concern and inquiry over time would demonstrate a progression of the community's environmental health understanding (transitioning from knowledge acquisition to application) as a result of the community involvement and engaged research efforts [42]. Key findings of this study were that a cross-sectional analysis at multiple points in time can better describe the social–ecological developments within a community and that changes in concern can demonstrate broader community recognition of the fundamentals of environmental health research (i.e., from understanding the source to potential exposure pathways and exposure mitigation) [42]. Researchers showed how community concerns changed over time as a result of the US Environmental Protection Agency's outreach and UAZ's community-engaged research activities; and that such documentation at contaminated sites is a novel method in which to assess EHL efforts.

Conclusions

A recent national study observed that 29 % of former lead smelters are located in areas prone to natural disasters (floods, earthquakes, tornadoes, and hurricanes), and these locations are at high risk for (re)dispersing toxic chemicals during such an event [43]. The recent Gold King Mine Spill near Silverton, Colorado, where three million gallons of water and waste (e.g. cadmium, copper, lead, arsenic) were inadvertently released into Cement Creek, a tributary of the 126-mile long Animas River [44], reminds us that these mining sites and the wastes they contain are not latent. Legacy mining sites may appear to be dormant, and it is crucial to work with communities to characterize the fate and transport of pollutants off site and to report exposure assessment data back to residents in order for them to translate the results into action. Using the MESH study as an example, this commentary contributes to exposure science and expands the concept of EHL and science education by describing how community-engaged partnerships are creating a new informal learning setting, where report back efforts are supporting free-choice learning. In these newly carved out settings, free-choice learning is occurring at the local level and is a product of conversations taking place between environmental health researchers and community members regarding their personal exposure data. These efforts are building a foundation for a sustainable and informal learning continuum, while meeting the most crucial steps in EHL efforts – empowerment, intervention, and increasing awareness. Free-choice learning is responsible for over 50 % of an adult's learning - it is time for EHL efforts to recognize the role of free-choice learning and to build upon the intrinsic motivation that individuals have to ultimately protect their environmental health.

Abbreviations

EHL: Environmental Health Literacy; MESH: Metals Exposure Study in Homes; UAZ: University of Arizona.

Competing interests

The authors declare that they have no competing interests.

Authors' contributions

MDRA prepared and drafted the commentary. JGB and PB designed the overall Personal Exposure Report-Back Ethics Study and contributed to the writing. ML and PIB are MESH Investigators. NL, ML, and PIB created the report back materials for the MESH participants. All authors read, provided comments, and approved the final manuscript.

Acknowledgements

The Personal Exposure Report-Back Ethics work was supported by NIEHS grant number R01ES017514 and the Metals Exposure in Homes Study was supported by NIEHS P42 ES04940. The authors are grateful to the members of the Dewey-Humboldt, Arizona community for welcoming us in their homes to conduct the interviews.

Author details

[1]Department of Soil, Water, and Environmental Science, University of Arizona, 1177 E Fourth Street, Rm. 429, Tucson, Arizona, USA. [2]Silent Spring Institute, Newton, MA, USA. [3]Mel and Enid Zuckerman College of Public Health, University of Arizona, Tucson, AZ 85721, USA. [4]Institute of Occupational Medicine, Edinburgh, UK. [5]Department of Sociology and Anthropology and Department of Health Sciences, Northeastern University, Boston, MA, USA.

References

1. National Research Council. Committee on Human Biomonitoring for Environmental Toxicants. Human Biomonitoring for Environmental Chemicals, Washington, DC: National Academy Press; 2006.
2. Morello-Frosch R, Varshavsky J, Liboiron M, Brown P, Brody JG. Communicating results in post-Belmont era biomonitoring studies: lessons from genetics and neuroimaging research. Environ Res. 2015;136:363–72. doi:10.1016/j.envres.2014.10.001. Epub 2014 Nov 25.
3. Falk JH. Free-Choice Science Learning: Framing the issues. In: Falk J, editor. Free-Choice Science Education: How We Learn Science Outside of School. New York, NY: Teacher's College Press, Columbia University; 2001.
4. National Research Council. National science education standards. Washington, DC: National Academy Press; 1996.
5. Institute of Medicine. Health literacy: a prescription to end confusion. Washington DC: National Academies Press; 2004.
6. Chinn D. Critical health literacy: A review and critical analysis. Soc Sci Med. 2011;73(1):60–7.
7. Gazmararian JA, Curran JW, Parker RM, Bernhardt JM, DeBuono BA. Public health literacy in America. Amer J Prev Med. 2005;28(3):317–22.
8. North American Association for Environmental Education. http://naaee.org/sites/default/files/envliteracyexesummary.pdf. Accessed 6 June 2015.
9. Freedman DA, Bess KD, Tucker HA, Boyd DL, Tuchman AM, Wallston KA. Public Health Literacy Defined. Am J Prev Med. 2009;36(5):446–51.
10. Society for Public Health Education. What is Environmental Health Literacy? 2007. http://www.sophe.org/environmentalHealth/key_ehl.cfm. Accessed 4 May 2015.
11. Nutbeam D. The evolving concept of health literacy. Soc Sci Med. 2008;67(12):2072–8.
12. Hoover A. Connecting Disciplines to Inform and Develop the Emerging Field of Environmental Health Literacy. 2014. http://www.niehs.nih.gov/research/supported/translational/peph/webinars/health_literacy/ Accessed May 5 2015.
13. National Research Council. Learning Science in Informal Environments: People, Places, and Pursuits. Committee on Learning Science in Informal Environments. In: Bell P, Lewenstein B, Shouse AW, Feder MA, editors. Board on Science Education, Center for Education. Division of Behavioral and Social Sciences and Education. Washington, DC: The National Academies Press; 2009.
14. Falk JH, Dierking LD. The 95 Percent Solution School is not where most Americans learn most of their science. Am Sci. 2010;98(6):486–93.
15. Falk JH. The Contribution Of Free-Choice Learning to Public Understanding of Science. Interciencia. 2002;27(2):62–5.
16. Falk JH, Storksdieck M, Dierking LD. Investigating public science interest and understanding: evidence for the importance of free-choice learning. Public Underst Sci. 2007;16:455–69.
17. Falk JH, Storksdieck M. Using the Contextual Model of Learning to understand visitor learning from a science center exhibition. Sci Educ. 2005;89:744–78.
18. Dierking LD, Falk JH, Rennie L, Anderson D, Ellenbogen K. Policy Statement of the "Informal Science Education" Ad Hoc Committee. 2003. J Res Sci Teach. 2003;40(2):108–11.
19. Brown P, Brody JG, Morello-Frosch R, Tovar J, Zota AR, Rudel RA. Measuring the Success of Community Science: The Northern California Household Exposure Study. Environ Health Persp. 2012;120(3):326–31.
20. Silka L, Renault-Caragianes P. Community-University Research Partnerships: Devising a Model for Ethical Engagement. J High Educ Outreach Engagem. 2007;11(2):171–83.
21. Morello-Frosch R, Brody JG, Brown P, Altman RG, Rudel RA, Pérez C. Toxic ignorance and right-to-know in biomonitoring results communication: a survey of scientists and study participants. Environ Health, 2009;8(6). doi:.10.1186/1476-069X-8-6
22. Lee JS, Chon HT, Kim KW. Human risk assessment of As, Cd, Cu and Zn in the abandoned metal mine site. Environ Geochem Health. 2005;27:185–91.
23. U.S. Environmental Protection Agency. 2004. Abandoned mine lands team: Reference Notebook. http://itepsrv1.itep.nau.edu/itep_course_downloads/TWRAP/15_tlefSuperfund/FedGuidanceMatl/AMLinfoAMLTeam.pdf. Accessed 1 May 2011.
24. Sullivan S. Tainted Earth: Smelters, Public Health and the Environment. NJ: Rutgers University Press; 2014.
25. Meza-Figueroa D, Maier RM, de la O-Villanueva M, Gomez-Alvarez A, Moreno-Zazueta A, Rivera J. The impact of unconfined mine tailings in residential areas from a mining town in a semi-arid environment: Nacozari, Sonora, Mexico. Chemosphere. 2009;77:140–7.
26. Zota AR, Schaider LA, Ettinhger AS, Wright RO, Shine JP, Spengler JD. Metal sources and exposures in the home of young children living near a mining-impacted Superfund site. J Expo Sci Environ Epidemiol. 2011;21:495–505.
27. Agency for Toxic Substances and Disease Registry. 2013. Available: http://www.atsdr.cdc.gov/spl/. Accessed 15 July 2014.
28. Csavina J, Field J, Taylor MP, Gao S, Landázuri A, Betterton EA, et al. A review on the importance of metals and metalloids in atmospheric dust and aerosol from mining operations. Sci Total Environ. 2012;433:58–73.
29. Sorooshian A, Csavina J, Shingler T, Dey S, Brechtel FJ, Sáez AE, et al. Hygroscopic and Chemical Properties of Aerosols Collected near a Copper Smelter: Implications for Public and Environmental Health. Environ Sci Tech. 2012;46(17):9473–80.
30. MacDonald GM. Water, climate change, and sustainability in the southwest. Proc Natl Acad Sci. 2010;107(50):21256–62.
31. U.S. Census Bureau 2010 Census. http://factfinder.census.gov/faces/nav/jsf/pages/community_facts.xhtml. Accessed 04 May 2015.
32. EA Engineering, Science, and Technology, Inc. Remedial investigation report iron King Mine Humboldt smelter superfund site. Dewey–Humboldt, Yavapai County, Arizona. 2010. Available: http://yosemite.epa.gov/r9/sfund/r9sfdocw.nsf/3dc283e6c5d6056f88257426007417a2/9ff58681f889089c882576fd0075ea2f!OpenDocumen. Accessed 28 April 2015.
33. Ramirez-Andreotta MD, Brusseau ML, Beamer P, Maier RM. Home gardening near a mining site in an As-endemic region of Arizona: Assessing As exposure dose and risk via ingestion of home garden vegetables, soils, and water. Sci Total Environ. 2013;454–455:373–82.

34. Ramirez-Andreotta MD, Brusseau ML, Artiola JF, Maier RM. A Greenhouse and Field-Based Study to Determine the Accumulation of Arsenic in Common Homegrown Vegetables. Sci Total Environ. 2013;443:299–306.

35. Ramirez-Andreotta MD, Brusseau ML, Artiola JF, Maier RM Gandolfi AJ. Building a co-created citizen science program with gardeners neighboring a Superfund site: The Gardenroots case study. Int Public Health J. 2014;7(1):139–53.

36. Beamer PI, Sugeng AJ, Kelly MD, Lothrop N, Klimecki W, Wilkinson ST, et al. Use of dust fall filters as passive samplers for metal concentrations in air for communities near contaminated mine tailings. Environ Sci Process Impacts. 2014;16(6):1275–81.

37. Altman RG, Morello-Frosch R, Brody JB, Brown P. Pollution Comes Home and Gets Personal: Women's Experience of Household Chemical Exposure. J Health Soc Behav. 2009;49(4):417–35.

38. Adams C, Brown P, Morello-Frosch R, Brody JG, Rudel R, Zota A, et al. Disentangling the exposure experience: the roles of community context and report-back of environmental exposure data. J Health Soc Behav. 2011;52:180–96.

39. Brody JG, Dunagan SC, Morello-Frosch R, Brown P, Patton S, Rudel RA. Reporting individual results for biomonitoring and environmental exposures: lessons learned from environmental communication case studies. Environ Heal. 2014;13(40):1–8.

40. Brody JG, Morello-Frosch R, Brown P, Rudel RA, Altman RG, Frye M, et al. Improving disclosure and consent: "Is It safe?": new ethics for reporting personal exposures to environmental chemicals. Am J Public Health. 2007;97:1547–54.

41. Morello-Frosch R, Pastor M, Porras C, Sadd J. Environmental justice and regional inequality in Southern California: implications for future research. Environ Health Perspect. 2002;110 Suppl 2:149–54.

42. Ramirez-Andreotta M, Lothrop N, Wilkinson S, Root R, Artiola J, Klimecki W, et al. Analyzing Patterns of Community Interest at a Legacy Mining Waste Site to Assess and Inform Environmental Health Literacy. J Environ Stud Sci, doi:10.1007/s13412-015-0297-x.

43. Wang Y, Kanter RK. Disaster-related environmental health hazards: former lead smelting plants in the United States. Disaster Med Public Health Prep. 2014;8(1):44–50.

44. USEPA. Emergency Response to August 2015 Release from Gold King Mine. Available: http://www2.epa.gov/goldkingmine. Accessed 5 November 2015.

9

Intima-media thickness and arterial function in obese and non-obese children

Heidi Weberruß[1*], Raphael Pirzer[2], Birgit Böhm[1], Robert Dalla Pozza[2], Heinrich Netz[2] and Renate Oberhoffer[1]

Abstract

Background: Obesity is an independent cardiovascular risk factor that contributes to the development of atherosclerosis. Subclinical forms of the disease can be assessed via sonographic measurement of carotid intima-media thickness (cIMT) and distensibility – both may already be altered in childhood. As childhood obesity increases to an alarming extent, this study compares vascular data of obese with normal weight boys and girls to investigate the influence of obesity on cIMT and distensibility of the carotid arteries.

Methods: cIMT and distensibility of 46 obese children (27 girls) aged 7–17 years were compared with measures of 46 sex- and age-matched normal weight controls. cIMT and distensibility were measured by B- and M-mode ultrasound and expressed as standard deviation scores (SDS). Arterial distensibility was defined by arterial compliance (AC), elastic modulus (Ep), stiffness index β (β), and local pulse wave velocity β (PWV β).

Results: Obese girls had significantly stiffer arteries compared with normal weight girls (Ep SDS 0.64 ± 1.24 vs. 0 ± 1.06, β SDS 0.6 ± 1.17 vs. -0.01 ± 1.06 $p < .01$, PWV β 0.54 ± 1.2 vs. -0.12 ± 1.05 $p < .05$). No significant differences were observed for boys. In multiregression analysis, BMI significantly influenced Ep, β and PWV β but not cIMT and AC.

Conclusions: Obese girls seemed to be at higher cardiovascular risk than boys, expressed by stiffer arteries in obese girls compared with normal weight girls. Overall, BMI negatively influenced parameters of arterial stiffness (Ep, β and PWV β) but not compliance or cIMT.

Keywords: Arterial stiffness, Cardiovascular disease, Pediatrics, Prevention, Ultrasound

Background

Childhood obesity increases rapidly in modern developed countries, which leads to adverse effects on children's health [1]. Regarding the cardiovascular system, childhood obesity is claimed as metabolic fundament for atherosclerosis in adulthood [2, 3]. Subclinical indicators of atherosclerosis, like an increased carotid intima-media thickness (cIMT) and impaired arterial distensibility, can already be detected in childhood via ultrasound. Most studies report a significantly increased cIMT in obese children and adolescents compared with normal weight controls [4]. For arterial distensibility, findings are contradictory. Several studies report impaired parameters, hence increased arterial stiffness and reduced compliance [5–7], while others observed lower stiffness and higher compliance in obese children compared with normal weight controls [8–11].

So far, none of these studies addressed sex differences of cIMT and arterial distensibility in obese children. In the normal weight population, girls are reported to have higher arterial stiffness parameters than boys during prepuberty, as well as women after menopause compared with men [12–14]. According to these findings, this study's purpose was to investigate the influence of obesity on cIMT and distensibility in boys and girls.

Methods

Data collection was part of the prevention project "Sternstunden der Gesundheit", a prospective cross-sectional study conducted from October 2012 to July 2013 in the area of Berchtesgadener Land, Germany. 1017 healthy children (483 boys/534 girls) aged 7–18 were examined to establish reference values for cIMT and parameters of arterial distensibility [15]. Children

* Correspondence: heidi.weberruss@tum.de
[1]Institute of Preventive Pediatrics, Technische Universität München, Georg-Brauchle-Ring 60/62, Campus D, 80992 Munich, Germany
Full list of author information is available at the end of the article

had no history of chronic disease or signs of acute infection. The study was approved by the ethics committee of the Technische Universität München (5490/12), written informed consent was obtained from parents and from parents and children ≥ 14 years.

Out of the total study population, $n = 46$ children (27 girls) were obese, according to German reference values which define obesity as BMI SDS above the 97th percentile [16]. Obese children were compared with $n = 46$ sex- and age-matched normal weight controls.

Anthropometric measurements were performed by trained staff according to standardized guidelines [17]. Body weight was measured without shoes, wearing light clothes to the nearest 0.1 kg, body height was measured with a stadiometer (seca 799, seca, Hamburg, Germany), standing upright without shoes to the nearest 0.1 cm. Body-Mass-Index (BMI) was calculated from the ratio of mass (kg) to height^2 (m^2).

cIMT and distensibility were assessed using semi-automated B- and M-Mode ultrasound, (ProSound Alpha 6, Aloka/Hitachi Medical Systems GmbH, Wiesbaden, Germany) with a high frequency linear array probe (5–13 MHz). After 15 min rest patients were examined in supine position, the neck slightly extended and their head turned 45° opposite the site being scanned. cIMT was measured in B-Mode according to the Mannheim consensus [18] on the common carotid artery (CCA) far wall, 1 cm proximal to the bulb at end-diastolic moment. The cardiac cycle was simultaneously controlled with a 3 lead ECG. Of each subject, four measurements were performed, two on the left and two on the right CCA and calculated as average mean value of four measurements.

Distensibility was assessed in real time M-Mode with high precision vascular echo tracking at the same location than cIMT. Two tracking gates were placed on the CCA near and far wall which followed vessel wall motion, thereby calculating diameter change during heart cycles. Four video loops of at least five heart cycles were stored, two for the left and two for the right CCA. Distensibility parameters were calculated as average mean value of four measurements. As distensibility is pressure dependent [19], blood pressure (BP) was measured oscillometrically on the left arm (Mobil-O-Graph®, I.E.M., Stolberg, Germany) after 10 min rest, and applied in the calculation. Hypertension was defined as BP SDS above the 95th percentile according to German reference values [20].

CCA distensibility was defined by arterial compliance (AC), elastic modulus (Ep), stiffness index β (β) and local pulse wave velocity (PWV β) according to following formulae [21]:

$$AC = \pi(D_{max^2} - D_{min^2})/[4(BP_{max} - BP_{min})]$$

AC defines the ability of an artery to increase its volume in response to a given increase in blood pressure and is the inverse of arterial stiffness. It is calculated from changes in blood vessel cross-sectional area (D) and BP.

$$Ep = (BP_{max} - BP_{min})/[(D_{max} - D_{min})/D_{min}]$$

Ep increases with increasing vessel stiffness. The parameter is affected by BP.

$$\beta = ln(BP_{max} / BP_{min})/[(D_{max} - D_{min})/D_{min}]$$

Like Ep, β increases with increasing vessel stiffness, but is low in BP dependency.

$$PWV\beta = \sqrt{((\beta * BP_{min})/(2\rho))}$$

In general, PWV is the speed at which the forward pressure wave is transmitted from the aorta through the vascular tree. In this study, PWV β is assessed as CCA local pulse wave velocity, calculated from β.

All measurements were performed by two experienced examiners. The coefficient of variation (CV) between both examiners, assessed in 27 subjects, was 4.79 for cIMT, and 3.54 % for distensibility, calculated as average CV of AC (4.47 %), Ep (3.42 %), β (4.92 %) and PWV β (1.37 %).

BMI, BP, cIMT and distensibility measures were expressed as sex- and age-dependent standard deviation scores (SDS), calculated as follows:

$$SDS = \frac{\left(\frac{x}{M}\right)^{L-1}}{L \, x \, S} \text{ for } L \neq 0 \quad \text{or} \quad SDS = \frac{\ln\left(\frac{x}{M}\right)}{S} \text{ for } L = 0$$

Data was analyzed using IBM SPSS statistics for Windows, version 21.0 (SPSS, Inc., Chicago, IL, USA). After testing for normal distribution, differences between obese and normal weight children were analyzed by independent samples t-test or Mann–Whitney U-test, for boys and girls separately. The independent influence of BMI and BP on vascular data was analyzed by multivariate stepwise linear regression, and the association with BMI by bivariate correlation, controlled for sex, age, and BP. A P-value of <0.05 was considered to be statistically significant.

Results and discussion

This subsample of 46 obese children and 46 sex- and age-matched controls was part of the prevention project "Sternstunden der Gesundheit", a cross-sectional prospective study to establish reference values for cIMT and distensibility measures [15]. Out of the total study population ($n = 1017$ children), measurements of intima-media thickness and arterial distensibility were performed in 656 children (353 girls) of which 46 children (7 %) were obese (27 girls). Anthropometric and vascular data for normal weight and obese boys and girls are displayed in Table 1. Weight, BMI, and BMI SDS differed significantly between

Table 1 Anthropometric and arterial status of normal weight and obese boys and girls

| | Male (19/19) | | | | | | Female (27/27) | | | | | |
	Normal weight			Obese			Normal weight			Obese		
AGE [yrs]	11.82	±	2.51	11.81	±	2.51	12.68	±	2.84	12.68	±	2.84
HEIGHT [cm]	149.83	±	14.38	157.73	±	16.34	153.71	±	14.62	155.45	±	10.12
WEIGHT [kg]	40.14	±	13.35**	69.91	±	21.99**	42.34	±	12.19**	70.17	±	17.83**
BMI SDS	−0.37	±	0.69**	2.22	±	0.25**	−0.56	±	0.52**	2.35	±	0.5**
BP systolic SDS	0.68	±	1.01	1.23	±	1.05	1.14	±	1.33	1.07	±	1.38
BP diastolic SDS	−0.14	±	1.32	0.55	±	1.02	0.08	±	1.19	0.15	±	1.26
IMT SDS	−0.05	±	0.94	0.03	±	1.39	0.07	±	1.09	0.23	±	0.83
AC SDS	−0.35	±	1.19	0.25	±	0.77	−0.15	±	0.92	0.04	±	1.47
Ep SDS	0.08	±	1.31	0.36	±	1.10	0.00	±	1.06*	0.64	±	1.24*
β SDS	0.23	±	1.28	0.23	±	1.00	−0.01	±	1.06**	0.60	±	1.17**
PWV β SDS	−0.04	±	1.19	0.34	±	1.00	−0.12	±	1.05*	0.54	±	1.2*

*p < .05, **p < .01

normal weight and obese boys and girls (p < .01), there were no significant differences in age, height and BP. Elevated systolic BP levels were present in 24 children (14 girls), elevated diastolic BP levels in 5 (1 girl) and both, elevated systolic and diastolic levles in 2 children (1 girl). 14 children with elevated systolic BP were obese (8 girls) and 10 were normal weight (6 girls). 4 children with elevated diastolic BP were obese (1 girl), and both subjects with elevated systolic and diastolic BP levels were obese.

cIMT SDS did not differ significantly between normal weight and obese boys and girls. Mean cIMT SDS in normal weight boys were −0.05 ± 0.94 compared with 0.03 ± 1.39 in obese boys and 0.07 ± 1.09 in normal weight girls compared with 0.23 ± 0.83 in obese girls. In boys, distensibility parameters did not differ significantly between normal weight and obese participants. Obese girls, on the contrary had significantly increased stiffness parameters compared with normal weight controls (Table 1).

Multivariate stepwise linear regression revealed no significant independent influence of BMI and BP on cIMT. AC was affected by BP but not BMI. Measures of arterial stiffness (Ep, β and PWV β) were influenced by body dimensions, indicating stiffer arteries at a higher BMI (Table 2). In bivariate correlation, parameters of arterial stiffness were also significantly correlated to BMI after

controlling for sex, age, and BP (Ep SDS: $r = 0.26$ β SDS: $r = 0.25$ and PWV β SDS: $r = 0.25$, $p < .05$).

This study compared the vascular status of 46 obese children to 46 age- and sex-matched normal weight controls, separately for boys and girls. Contrary to other studies [4], we did not observe significant higher cIMT values in obese boys and girls. In accordance to findings of Tounian et al. [5], Aggoun et al. [22], and Di Salvo et al. [23] our sample consisted of healthy children with no history of chronic disease. BP levels did not differ significantly between obese and normal weight children, none of the children was diagnosed with manifest hypertension.

The extent of obesity within the sample was 2.22 SDS in boys and 2.35 SDS in girls. Dangardt et al. [8] included obese children with BMI measures > 3 SDS, a significantly higher systolic and significantly lower diastolic BP, and found higher radial artery intimal thickening in obese participants. Giannini et al. [3] included participants with a BMI > 2 SDS and significantly higher systolic and diastolic BP than in lean controls. The coexistence of two risk factors, like hypertension and obesity [24] may lead to a higher increase in cIMT compared to healthy normal weight controls, which can explain nonsignificant differences in our study with obesity as only risk factor.

Table 2 Stepwise multiregression analysis for measures of arterial distensibility with BMI and BP SDS

| | AC SDS $R^2 = 0.43$ | | | Ep SDS $R^2 = 0.3$ | | | β SDS $R^2 = 0.35$ | | | PWV β SDS $R^2 = 0.18$ | | |
	Beta ± SE	β	P	Beta ± SE	β	P	Beta ± SE	β	P	Beta ± SE	β	P
Constant	0.54 ± 0.12		.005	−0.37 ± 0.16		.02	0.19 ± 0.14		.2	−0.3 ± 0.16		.05
BMI SDS				0.18 ± 0.07	0.23	.013	0.16 ± 0.07	0.21	.019	0.17 ± 0.07	0.22	.025
Systolic BP SDS	−0.64 ± 0.08	−0.68	<.001	0.52 ± 0.1	0.54	<.001	0.38 ± 0.09	0.41	<.001	0.32 ± 0.09	0.35	<.001
Diastolic BP SDS	0.48 ± 0.08	0.5	<.001	−0.37 ± 0.1	−0.38	.001	−0.58 ± 0.9	−0.61	<.001			

BMI indicates Body Mass Index, BP Blood Pressure. All measures are expressed as Standard Deviation Scores

Significant differences in parameters of arterial stiffness in contrast to findings on cIMT may be explained with an earlier alteration of an artery's function compared to its structural status [25]. Ep, β and PWV β were independently affected by BMI to a similar extent (Table 2), indicating stiffer arteries with increasing BMI values. AC in our sample, was higher in obese boys and girls compared to controls but did not reach statistical significance. These results are in accordance with Chalmers et al. [9], Tryggestad et al. [11], and Lurbe et al. [10] who also observed increased compliance in obese children. Dangardt et al. [8] explain this higher compliance as chronic vasodilation caused by initial adaptation of the arterial system to a larger blood volume, generated by increased body fat mass. Tryggestad et al. [11] add that childhood obesity may cause an earlier peak in vascular compliance by obesity related acceleration of pubertal development. Chalmers et al. [9] claim the significantly higher pubertal status in their obese participants to be responsible for higher circulating insulin, leading to chronic vasodilation. According to the authors, this status remains until other risk factors contribute to the development of atherosclerosis – at this point the vessel wall surpasses a point of natural adaptation that results in decreased compliance and increased stiffness.

In this study, stiffness parameters in obese girls differed significantly from those in normal weight sex- and age-matched controls which is not the case in male participants. Marlatt et al. [26] did not find significantly sex differences for arterial stiffness parameters in normal weight children. Ahimastos et al. [13] took pubertal-status of children into account and found significantly stiffer arteries in pre-pubertal girls compared to age-matched males, but not in post-pubertal boys and girls. Sex steroid hormones are known to influence vessel structure and function. Hence, authors hypothesize a modulating effect of male and female sex steroids, causing a reduction in arterial stiffness in girls and an increased stiffness in boys during puberty. This may result in non-significantly different post-pubertal stiffness measures. For aortic PWV, Hidvegi et al. [27] have shown a steep increase during puberty in boys and girls, which starts about 2 years earlier in girls than in boys. This earlier development in girls and presence of obesity might be the reason for significantly higher stiffness measures in obese girls in our study and identifies them as being at higher risk for early signs of atherosclerosis. Though, results of our study support a sex specific approach to arterial distensibility with obese girls being at higher risk to develop early atherosclerosis.

Equivalent to aforementioned results, cIMT and AC were not significantly correlated to BMI, whereas arterial stiffness parameters (Ep, β and PWV β) were positively associated with BMI. This reveals Ep, β and PWV β as more sensitive parameters regarding overweight and obesity in children. An increased stiffness represents a functional impairment of the arterial wall, which occurs earlier than structural alterations, defined by an increased cIMT [28]. Increased arterial stiffness is present in children with familial hypercholesterolemia, diabetes, and severe obesity [29–31]. Of all risk factors, the most obvious in the invisible atherosclerotic process is the growing number of overweight and obese children [32].

Conclusion

Detected early in life – by one single risk factor named obesity – children can immediately improve their vascular health by losing weight [8, 12]. A reduction in BMI slows the yearly increase in cIMT and improves CVD risk factors [33, 34]. Juonala et al. [35] reported age-appropriate cIMT values in normal weight adults, who had been obese in youth but lost overweight in adulthood. This study shows a significant association between BMI and parameters of arterial stiffness, especially in girls. As obesity tracks from child- into adulthood [36], with a strong association between childhood BMI and CVD in adulthood [2, 7, 37], it is of highest priority to start prevention as early as possible. Our results support a sex-based approach to prevention programmes, as obese girls are at higher risk than normal weight controls.

Abbreviations
β: stiffness index β; AC: arterial compliance; BMI: body-mass-index; BP: blood pressure; CCA: common carotid artery; cIMT: carotid intima-media thickness; CV: coefficient of variation; Ep: elastic modulus; PWV β: local pulse wave velocity β; SDS: standard deviation scores.

Competing interests
The authors declare that they have no competing interests.

Author's contribution
HW contributed in cIMT measurement, data management, data analysis, drafting of manuscript. RP contributed in cIMT measurement and data management. BB contributed in study conception, cIMT teaching, critical revision of data analysis and manuscript. RDP contributed in study conception and design, critical revision. HN contributed in study conception and design, critical revision. RO contributed in study conception and design, critical revision. All authors have read and approved the final version of the manuscript.

Acknowledgments
Funding
The study was funded by Sternstunden e.V. (non-profit organization) and the district office Berchtesgadener Land.

Author details
[1]Institute of Preventive Pediatrics, Technische Universität München, Georg-Brauchle-Ring 60/62, Campus D, 80992 Munich, Germany. [2]Department of Pediatric Cardiology, Ludwig-Maximilians-University, Marchioninistraße 15, 81377 Munich, Germany.

References

1. Herouvi D, Karanasios E, Karayianni C, Karavanaki K. Cardiovascular disease in childhood: the role of obesity. Eur J Pediatr. 2013;172(6):721–32. doi:10.1007/s00431-013-1932-8.

2. Srinivasan SR, Bao W, Wattigney WA, Berenson GS. Adolescent overweight is associated with adult overweight and related multiple cardiovascular risk factors: the Bogalusa Heart Study. Metab Clin Exp. 1996;45(2):235–40.

3. Giannini C, de Giorgis T, Scarinci A, Ciampani M, Marcovecchio ML, Chiarelli F, et al. Obese related effects of inflammatory markers and insulin resistance on increased carotid intima media thickness in pre-pubertal children. Atherosclerosis. 2008;197(1):448–56. doi:10.1016/j.atherosclerosis.2007.06.023.

4. Lamotte C, Iliescu C, Libersa C, Gottrand F. Increased intima-media thickness of the carotid artery in childhood: a systematic review of observational studies. Eur J Pediatr. 2011;170(6):719–29. doi:10.1007/s00431-010-1328-y.

5. Tounian P, Aggoun Y, Dubern B, Varille V, Guy-Grand B, Sidi D, et al. Presence of increased stiffness of the common carotid artery and endothelial dysfunction in severely obese children: a prospective study. Lancet. 2001;358(9291):1400–4. doi:10.1016/s0140-6736(01)06525-4.

6. Joo Turoni C, Maranon RO, Felipe V, Bruno ME, Negrete A, Salas N, et al. Arterial stiffness and endothelial function in obese children and adolescents and its relationship with cardiovascular risk factors. Horm Res Paediatr. 2013;80(4):281–6. doi:10.1159/000354991.

7. Dangardt F, Chen Y, Berggren K, Osika W, Friberg P. Increased rate of arterial stiffening with obesity in adolescents: a five-year follow-up study. PLoS One. 2013;8(2):e57454. doi:10.1371/journal.pone.0057454.

8. Dangardt F, Osika W, Volkmann R, Gan LM, Friberg P. Obese children show increased intimal wall thickness and decreased pulse wave velocity. Clin Physiol Funct Imaging. 2008;28(5):287–93. doi:10.1111/j.1475-097X.2008.00806.x.

9. Chalmers LJ, Copeland KC, Hester CN, Fields DA, Gardner AW. Paradoxical increase in arterial compliance in obese pubertal children. Angiology. 2011;62(7):565–70. doi:10.1177/0003319711399117.

10. Lurbe E, Torro I, Garcia-Vicent C, Alvarez J, Fernandez-Fornoso JA, Redon J. Blood pressure and obesity exert independent influences on pulse wave velocity in youth. Hypertension. 2012;60(2):550–5. doi:10.1161/HYPERTENSIONAHA.112.194746.

11. Tryggestad JB, Thompson DM, Copeland KC, Short KR. Obese children have higher arterial elasticity without a difference in endothelial function: the role of body composition. Obesity. 2012;20(1):165–71. doi:10.1038/oby.2011.309.

12. Cote AT, Harris KC, Panagiotopoulos C, Sandor GG, Devlin AM. Childhood obesity and cardiovascular dysfunction. J Am Coll Cardiol. 2013;62(15):1309–19. doi:10.1016/j.jacc.2013.07.042.

13. Ahimastos AA, Formosa M, Dart AM, Kingwell BA. Gender differences in large artery stiffness pre- and post puberty. J Clin Endocrinol Metab. 2003;88(11):5375–80. doi:10.1210/jc.2003-030722.

14. Rossi P, Frances Y, Kingwell BA, Ahimastos AA. Gender differences in artery wall biomechanical properties throughout life. J Hypertens. 2011;29(6):1023–33. doi:10.1097/HJH.0b013e328344da5e.

15. Weberruss H, Pirzer R, Bohm B, Elmenhorst J, Pozza RD, Netz H, et al. Increased intima-media thickness is not associated with stiffer arteries in children. Atherosclerosis. 2015;242(1):48–55. doi:10.1016/j.atherosclerosis.2015.06.045.

16. Kromeyer K, Wabitsch M, Kunze D, Geller F. Perzentile für den Body-Mass-Index für das Kindes- und Jugendalter unter Heranziehung verschiedener deutscher Stichproben. Monatsschrift Kinderheilkunde. 2001;149:807–18.

17. WHO. Waist Circumference and Waist-Hip Ratio: Report of a WHO Expert Consultation. Geneva Switzerland: World Health Organization; 2008.

18. Touboul PJ, Hennerici MG, Meairs S, Adams H, Amarenco P, Bornstein N, et al. Mannheim carotid intima-media thickness consensus (2004–2006). An update on behalf of the Advisory Board of the 3rd and 4th Watching the Risk Symposium, 13th and 15th European Stroke Conferences, Mannheim, Germany, 2004, and Brussels, Belgium, 2006. Cerebrovasc Dis. 2007;23(1):75–80. doi:10.1159/000097034.

19. O'Rourke MF, Staessen JA, Vlachopoulos C, Duprez D, Plante GE. Clinical applications of arterial stiffness; definitions and reference values. Am J Hypertens. 2002;15(5):426–44.

20. Neuhauser HK, Thamm M, Ellert U, Hense HW, Rosario AS. Blood pressure percentiles by age and height from nonoverweight children and adolescents in Germany. Pediatrics. 2011;127(4):e978–88. doi:10.1542/peds.2010-1290.

21. Aloka. Aloka Prosound a7. How to use. 2008.

22. Aggoun Y, Farpour-Lambert NJ, Marchand LM, Golay E, Maggio AB, Beghetti M. Impaired endothelial and smooth muscle functions and arterial stiffness appear before puberty in obese children and are associated with elevated ambulatory blood pressure. Eur Heart J. 2008;29(6):792–9. doi:10.1093/eurheartj/ehm633.

23. Di Salvo G, Pacileo G, Del Giudice EM, Natale F, Limongelli G, Verrengia M, et al. Abnormal myocardial deformation properties in obese, non-hypertensive children: an ambulatory blood pressure monitoring, standard echocardiographic, and strain rate imaging study. Eur Heart J. 2006;27(22):2689–95. doi:10.1093/eurheartj/ehl163.

24. Iannuzzi A, Licenziati MR, Acampora C, Renis M, Agrusta M, Romano L, et al. Carotid artery stiffness in obese children with the metabolic syndrome. Am J Cardiol. 2006;97(4):528–31. doi:10.1016/j.amjcard.2005.08.072.

25. Stein JH, Korcarz CE, Hurst RT, Lonn E, Kendall CB, Mohler ER. Use of carotid ultrasound to identify subclinical vascular disease and evaluate cardiovascular disease risk: a consensus statement from the American Society of Echocardiography Carotid Intima-Media Thickness Task Force. Endorsed by the Society for Vascular Medicine. J Am Soc Echocardiogr. 2008;21(2):93–111. doi:10.1016/j.echo.2007.11.011. quiz 89–90.

26. Marlatt KL, Kelly AS, Steinberger J, Dengel DR. The influence of gender on carotid artery compliance and distensibility in children and adults. J Clin Ultrasound. 2013;41(6):340–6. doi:10.1002/jcu.22015.

27. Hidvegi EV, Illyes M, Benczur B, Bocskei RM, Ratgeber L, Lenkey Z, et al. Reference values of aortic pulse wave velocity in a large healthy population aged between 3 and 18 years. J Hypertens. 2012;30(12):2314–21. doi:10.1097/HJH.0b013e328359562c.

28. Urbina EM, Williams RV, Alpert BS, Collins RT, Daniels SR, Hayman L, et al. Noninvasive assessment of subclinical atherosclerosis in children and adolescents: recommendations for standard assessment for clinical research: a scientific statement from the American Heart Association. Hypertension. 2009;54(5):919–50. doi:10.1161/HYPERTENSIONAHA.109.192639.

29. Aggoun Y, Bonnet D, Sidi D, Girardet JP, Brucker E, Polak M, et al. Arterial Mechanical Changes in Children With Familial Hypercholesterolemia. Arterioscler Thromb Vasc Biol. 2000;20(9):2070–5. doi:10.1161/01.atv.20.9.2070.

30. Giannattasio C, Failla M, Piperno A, Grappiolo A, Gamba P, Paleari F, et al. Early impairment of large artery structure and function in type I diabetes mellitus. Diabetologia. 1999;42(8):987–94. doi:10.1007/s001250051257.

31. Iannuzzi A, Licenziati MR, Acampora C, Salvatore V, Auriemma L, Romano ML, et al. Increased carotid intima-media thickness and stiffness in obese children. Diabetes Care. 2004;27(10):2506–8.

32. Engelen L, Ferreira I, Stehouwer CD, Boutouyrie P, Laurent S. Reference Values for Arterial Measurements C. Reference intervals for common carotid intima-media thickness measured with echotracking: relation with risk factors. Eur Heart J. 2013;34(30):2368–80. doi:10.1093/eurheartj/ehs380.

33. Markus RA, Mack WJ, Azen SP, Hodis HN. Influence of lifestyle modification on atherosclerotic progression determined by ultrasonographic change in the common carotid intima-media thickness. Am J Clin Nutr. 1997;65(4):1000–4.

34. Tounian P, Frelut ML, Parlier G, Abounaufal C, Aymard N, Veinberg F, et al. Weight loss and changes in energy metabolism in massively obese adolescents. Int J Obes Relat Metab Disord. 1999;23(8):830–7.

35. Juonala M, Raitakari M. J SAV, Raitakari OT. Obesity in youth is not an independent predictor of carotid IMT in adulthood. The Cardiovascular Risk in Young Finns Study. Atherosclerosis. 2006;185(2):388–93. doi:10.1016/j.atherosclerosis.2005.06.016.

36. Berenson GS. Bogalusa Heart Study g. Health consequences of obesity. Pediatr Blood Cancer. 2012;58(1):117–21. doi:10.1002/pbc.23373.

37. Baker JL, Olsen LW, Sorensen TI. Childhood body-mass index and the risk of coronary heart disease in adulthood. N Engl J Med. 2007;357(23):2329–37. doi:10.1056/NEJMoa072515.

10

Patients' willingness to participate in clinical trials and their views on aspects of cancer research: results of a prospective patient survey

Sing Yu Moorcraft[2,1], Cheryl Marriott[2,1], Clare Peckitt[2,1], David Cunningham[2,1], Ian Chau[2,1], Naureen Starling[2,1], David Watkins[2,1] and Sheela Rao[1,2]*

Abstract

Background: Recruitment to clinical trials can be challenging and slower than anticipated. This prospective patient survey aimed to investigate the proportion of patients approached about a trial who agree to participate, their motivations for trial participation and their views on aspects of cancer research.

Methods: Patients who had been approached about participation in any clinical trials in the Gastrointestinal and Lymphoma Unit at the Royal Marsden were invited to complete a questionnaire. The statistical analysis is mainly descriptive, with percentages being reported. Univariate logistic regression analysis was used to determine any associations between patient characteristics and patient responses.

Results: From August 2013–July 2014, 276 patients received 298 clinical trial patient information sheets and were asked to complete the questionnaire. The majority of patients (263 patients, 88 %) consented to a clinical trial and 249 of the 263 patients (95 %) completed the questionnaire. Multiple factors influenced decisions to participate in clinical trials, with patients stating that the most important reasons were that the trial offered the best treatment available and that the trial results could benefit others. Of the 249 questionnaire respondents, 78 % would donate their tissue for genetic research, 75 % would consider participating in studies requiring a research biopsy and 75 % felt that patients should be informed of trial results. Patients treated with palliative intent and those who had received multiple lines of treatment were more willing to consider research biopsies. Of the patients approached about a clinical trial of an investigational medicinal product, 48–50 % would have liked more information on the study drugs/procedures.

Conclusion: The majority of patients approached about a clinical trial consented to one or more trials. Patients' motivations for trial participation included potential personal benefit and altruistic reasons. A high proportion of patients were willing to donate tissue for research and to consider trials involving repeat biopsies. The majority of patients feel that participants should be informed of trial results and there is a group of patients who would like more detailed trial information.

Keywords: Patient attitudes, Biopsies, Cancer research, Clinical trial recruitment, Consent, Patient feedback, Patient information, Trial ineligibility

* Correspondence: sheela.rao@rmh.nhs.uk
[1]The Royal Marsden NHS Foundation Trust, London, UK
[2]The Royal Marsden NHS Foundation Trust, Sutton, UK

Background

Recruitment to clinical trials can be challenging, leading to 1 in 10 cancer trials registered on ClinicalTrials.gov between 2005 and 2011 being closed prematurely due to poor accrual and other trials taking longer than anticipated to complete recruitment [1–3]. This is a major problem for oncologists, not only from a scientific perspective, but also due to the implications of failing to meet recruitment targets. For example, in the United Kingdom (UK), clinical trial performance metrics include meeting certain government targets, such as recruiting the first study patient within 70 days of receiving a valid research application [4]. Although the UK has one of the highest clinical trial participation rates in the world, with more than 1 in 5 adult cancer patients participating in clinical trials [5], the proportion of patients with whom cancer research is discussed ranges from 10–61 % depending on the hospital trust [6].

Patients' decisions regarding trial participation may be influenced by the information they receive. Trials are becoming larger and increasingly complex, incorporating translational research (including research biopsies), adaptive designs and biomarker selection/stratification [7, 8]. However, the level of scientific and health literacy in the general population remains poor, with a third of older adults in England having difficulty in reading and understanding basic health-related information [9] and previous studies have shown that patients can have misconceptions about aspects of research, such as the risk of side effects, the trial's aims and the likelihood of personal benefit [10–12]. Therefore, there is concern that clinical trial patient information sheets (PIS) may not be fit-for-purpose. In addition, there are concerns that mandatory research biopsies may deter patients from participating in trials and, therefore, adversely affect trial recruitment [13, 14].

A better understanding of patients' motivations for participating in cancer research and their opinions of trial information and the consent process may lead to changes that facilitate trial recruitment and improve patient satisfaction with the recruitment process. We therefore conducted a prospective patient survey of patients treated at the Royal Marsden (RM) for gastrointestinal (GI) cancers or lymphoma in order to investigate patients' willingness to participate in clinical trials and their views on aspects of cancer research.

Methods

The patient survey was approved by the Royal Marsden Committee for Clinical Research and patients verbally consented to participate in the survey. This survey was designed as a 'service evaluation', to evaluate patients' experiences of clinical trials at our institution and thereby investigate if aspects of this process could be improved.

Ethical review by an external review board was, therefore, not required. The primary endpoint was the proportion of patients approached about a clinical trial who agreed to participate in a trial. Secondary endpoints included reasons why patients consented to/declined trials, the proportion of patients who were happy to be approached about participating in research, the proportion of patients who would consider trials involving genetic research or research biopsies and patients' views of the consent process, the trial information provided and feedback of study results to participants.

Study subjects

All patients who had been approached about a trial between August 2013 and July 2014 in the GI and Lymphoma unit at the RM (a specialist cancer centre) were eligible to participate in this patient survey. Clinical Trials of an Investigational Medicinal Product (CTIMP) and non-CTIMP trials were included, as well as pre-screening studies. The CTIMP trials included trials investigating targeted therapies, immunotherapies, chemotherapy, the optimal duration of chemotherapy and the scheduling of chemotherapy and surgery (e.g. peri-operative chemotherapy versus post-operative chemotherapy).

Patients were invited to participate in the survey by the unit research nurses or doctors when they notified staff about their decision regarding participation in a trial. They were also informed that the survey aimed to improve the experiences of patients with regards to clinical trials and that participation in the survey was voluntary with no obligation to take part.

Questionnaires

Two paper questionnaires were developed based on a literature review and the authors' experiences of trial recruitment. The questionnaires were comprised of Likert, multiple choice and free-text questions. Patients who consented to a trial were given the 25-question Questionnaire A (Additional file 1), which included questions on their reasons for deciding to participate in the trial. Patients who declined a trial received the 21-question Questionnaire B (Additional file 2), which included questions regarding their reasons for declining the trial. Patients who consented/declined more than one trial were asked to complete one questionnaire per trial. The questionnaires could be completed in clinic or taken home and returned at the patients' next clinic appointment.

Each patient was allocated a unique survey ID number, which was written on their completed questionnaires and on a demographic sheet completed by the research nurse looking after the patient. The researchers analysing the survey responses were not able to identify the patients from their survey ID numbers. The questionnaire was, therefore, anonymous to the researchers analysing the survey results, unless the patient chose to complete an optional section of the questionnaire and provided their details so that they could be contacted about future surveys.

SYM and CM compared patients' free-text answers to the question: 'what type of cancer do you have?', with the data collected on the demographic sheet and scored the answers as being correct if the patient had clearly identified the site of their primary tumour.

Collection of demographic and trial-related information

Demographic information was collected by research nurses from patients' electronic medical records. Social class was characterised according to the National Readership Survey (NRS) classification [15] by SYM and CM according to the patients' recorded occupation. The percentage of households in poverty in the patients' postcode area was determined using data available from the Office for National Statistics, UK [16], and used as a marker of social deprivation. Data on clinical trial characteristics, PIS characteristics, whether the patient agreed to complete the questionnaire and subsequent trial registration (including reason for trial ineligibility) was also recorded.

Statistical analysis

The majority of the statistical analysis is descriptive, with percentages being reported. The statistical analysis was performed using Stata v13.1 (StataCorp, College Station, TX, USA). Univariate logistic regression analysis was used to determine any associations between patient characteristics and patient responses and between trial characteristics and PIS features. Patient characteristics included in the univariate analysis were age, gender, performance status (PS), number of previous lines of treatment, previous trial participation, aim of treatment (curative versus palliative) and type of trial.

Results

Clinical trial portfolio and patient recruitment

Between August 2013 and July 2014, 36 trials recruited one or more patients (see Table 1). Two hundred and seventy-six patients received 298 PIS for a clinical trial (271 GI, 27 lymphoma), with 257 patients receiving 1 PIS, 16 patients receiving 2 PIS and 3 patients receiving 3 PIS. Patient demographics are shown in Table 2. Two hundred and sixty-three patients (88 %) consented to a trial and 249 (95 %) of these 263 patients completed the questionnaire (see Fig. 1). Ten patients were ineligible for the trial at the time they returned for consent (e.g. due to

Table 1 Characteristics of trials in the Gastrointestinal and Lymphoma Unit ($n = 36$)

Trial characteristic	Number of trials (%) ($n = 36$)
Study type	
CTIMP	24 (67 %)
Non-CTIMP	9 (25 %)
Pre-screening	3 (8 %)
Sponsor	
Royal Marsden	9 (25 %)
Other academic institution	11 (31 %)
Pharmaceutical company	16 (44 %)
Phase	
I	2 (6 %)
II	10 (28 %)
II/III	2 (6 %)
III	13 (36 %)
Not applicable	9 (25 %)
Trial setting	
Neoadjuvant	3 (8 %)
Adjuvant	3 (8 %)
Advanced	16 (44 %)
Any	5 (14 %)
Lymphoma[a]	9 (25 %)
Randomised trial	
Yes	20 (56 %)
No	16 (44 %)
Molecular screening	
Yes	10 (28 %)
No	26 (72 %)
Number of PIS (e.g. separate pharmacodynamics or imaging sub-studies)	
1	20 (56 %)
2	11 (31 %)
3	4 (11 %)
5	1 (3 %)

Key: CTIMP = Clinical Trial of an Investigational Medicinal Product, pre-screening = molecular pre-screening to determine potential eligibility for a specific CTIMP study, PIS = patient information sheet
[a]Lymphoma trials were considered separately as the intent of lymphoma treatment is to induce remission and, therefore, the treatment paradigms differ from that of gastrointestinal malignancies

clinical deterioration) and were, therefore, ineligible for the patient survey.

Reasons for trial ineligibility

Thirty-eight (14 %) of the 263 patients who consented to a clinical trial were not subsequently registered for the trial, including 36 (36 %) of the 101 patients who

Table 2 Patient demographics

Characteristic	N (%)
	(n = 276)
Gender	
Male	188 (68 %)
Female	88 (32 %)
Age	
Median (range)	64 years (19–85)
Native English speaker	252 (91 %)
Ethnicity	
White	238 (86 %)
Asian	21 (8 %)
Black	8 (3 %)
Other	9 (3 %)
Marital status	
Married/partner	194 (70 %)
Single	35 (13 %)
Separated/divorced	15 (5 %)
Widowed	14 (5 %)
Unknown	18 (7 %)
Social class	
Grade A/B (upper middle/middle class)	56 (20 %)
Grade C1/2 (lower middle/skilled working class)	34 (12 %)
Grade D (working class)	48 (17 %)
Grade E (retired)	109 (40 %)
Grade E (unemployed)	5 (2 %)
Unknown	24 (9 %)
Percentage of households in poverty in the patient's postcode area	
≥ 27.61 %	20 (7 %)
22.01–27.6 %	43 (16 %)
17.91–22 %	48 (17 %)
14.41–17.9 %	51 (18 %)
≤ 14.4 %	112 (41 %)
Not in England[a]	2 (1 %)
Type of cancer	
Colorectal	117 (42 %)
Oesophagogastric	100 (36 %)
Pancreatic	18 (7 %)
Hepatobiliary	11 (4 %)
Carcinoma of unknown primary/other GI	3 (1 %)
Hodgkin's lymphoma	10 (4 %)
Non-Hodgkin's lymphoma	17 (6 %)
Treatment aim	
Curative	96 (35 %)
Palliative	180 (65 %)

Table 2 Patient demographics *(Continued)*

Number of previous lines of treatment	
0	133 (48 %)
1	87 (32 %)
2	39 (14 %)
3	13 (5 %)
≥ 4	3 (1 %)
Unknown	1 (1 %)
Performance status	
0	106 (38 %)
1	130 (47 %)
2	20 (7 %)
3	3 (1 %)
Unknown	17 (6 %)

[a]No comparable poverty statistics available for regions outside of England
GI gastrointestinal

consented to CTIMP/pre-screening trials. The main reason for trial ineligibility was that their molecular profile (e.g. human epidermal growth factor receptor 2 (HER2) status) did not meet the study requirements (n = 22). Other reasons for patient ineligibility included: no available tissue for molecular testing (n = 3), further investigations revealed a change in disease extent: e.g. from localised to metastatic disease (n = 3), blood results outside of a specific range (n = 3), deterioration in PS (n = 2) and non-measurable disease on imaging (n = 1).

Reasons for trial participation

Multiple factors influenced patients' decisions to participate in a clinical trial (see Table 3). When patients were asked to indicate their main reason for trial participation, a belief that 'the trial offered the best treatment available' or that 'the trial results could benefit others' were the most frequent responses (see Fig. 2). A univariate analysis was used to determine any associations between patient characteristics and patients' main reason for trial participation. Patients were more likely to state that their main reason for participation was 'the trial offered the best treatment available', if they were being treated with palliative rather than curative intent (33 % versus 19 %, odds ratio 2.11, 95 % CI 1.09–4.08, p = 0.026), had a worse PS (19 % for PS 0, 34 % for PS 1, odds ratio 2.12, 95 % CI 0.97–8.79, p = 0.027) or had not previously participated in a clinical trial (32 % (no) versus 8 % (yes) for previously participated, odds ratio 5.14, 95 % CI 1.51–17.5, p = 0.009). Patients were more likely to state that their main reason for participation was 'the trial results could benefit others' if they were < 65 years compared to ≥ 65 years (64 % versus 39 %, odds ratio 2.77, 95 % CI 1.62–4.74, p < 0.001), being treated with curative rather than palliative

Patients' willingness to participate in clinical trials and their views on aspects of cancer...

93

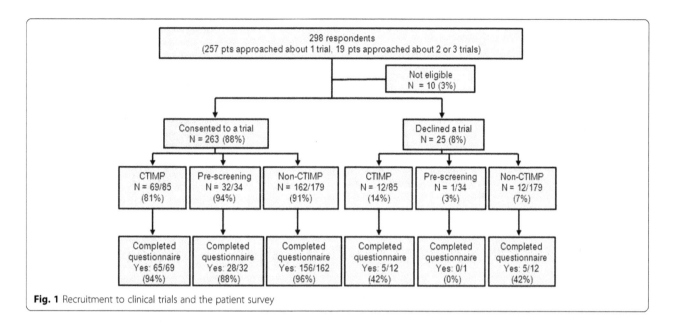

Fig. 1 Recruitment to clinical trials and the patient survey

intent (63 % versus 47 %, odds ratio 1.97, 95 % CI 1.23–3.46, $p = 0.017$) or had previously participated in a clinical trial (72 % (yes) versus 50 % (no) for not participated, odds ratio 2.65, 95 % CI 1.21–5.83, $p = 0.012$). Gender and number of previous lines of treatment did not significantly influence patients' main reason for trial participation.

Patients who declined a clinical trial

Ten of the 25 patients who declined a clinical trial completed the questionnaire. There was no pattern to the types of trial declined and no demographic differences between the patients who consented and those who declined. Reasons for declining a trial included: unwillingness to take the study drug/placebo or have additional research procedures, decision not to have

any further treatment, general anxiety about cancer diagnosis/treatment and a belief that the standard treatment was more effective. Nine of the 10 patients stated that they were glad to have been approached about participating in cancer research.

Patients' views on cancer research and biopsies

Two hundred and twenty-one patients (96 %) who completed Questionnaire A were happy to have been approached about participating in cancer research and 225 out of 228 patients (99 %) believed that cancer research would help doctors better understand and treat cancer.

Fifteen patients (7 %) agreed/strongly agreed, 43 patients (19 %) were neutral and 164 patients (74 %) disagreed/strongly disagreed with the statement:

Table 3 Factors which influenced patients' decision to participate in a clinical trial

Reason	CTIMP	Pre-screening	Non-CTIMP	All
	N (%)	N (%)	N (%)	(n = 241)
	(n = 63)	(n = 28)	(n = 150)	
Patient felt the trial offered the best available treatment	49 (78 %)	16 (57 %)	57 (39 %)	122 (51 %)
Patient felt the trial result could benefit others	53 (84 %)	24 (86 %)	143 (96 %)	220 (92 %)
Patient wanted to contribute to scientific research	37 (59 %)	16 (57 %)	111 (74 %)	164 (68 %)
Patient felt they would be monitored more closely	28 (44 %)	9 (32 %)	42 (28 %)	79 (33 %)
Patient felt they would have better quality care	20 (32 %)	5 (18 %)	24 (16 %)	49 (20 %)
Patient's family were keen for patient to participate	24 (38 %)	8 (29 %)	20 (13 %)	52 (22 %)
Patient trusted the doctor treating them	38 (60 %)	10 (36 %)	73 (49 %)	121 (50 %)
Patient felt that otherwise their cancer will get worse	17 (27 %)	3 (11 %)	13 (9 %)	33 (14 %)
Other reason	4 (6 %)	0 (0 %)	8 (5 %)	12 (5 %)

Key: CTIMP = Clinical Trial of an Investigational Medicinal Product, pre-screening = molecular pre-screening to determine potential eligibility for a specific CTIMP study

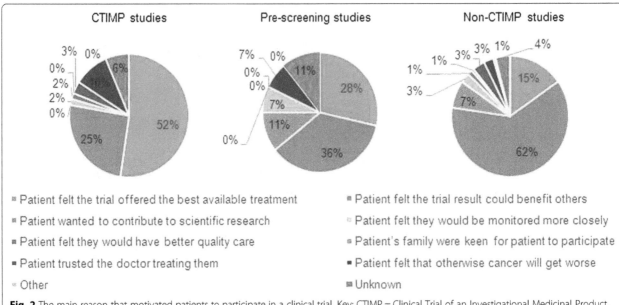

Fig. 2 The main reason that motivated patients to participate in a clinical trial. Key: CTIMP = Clinical Trial of an Investigational Medicinal Product, pre-screening = molecular pre-screening to determine potential eligibility for a specific CTIMP study

'I have concerns about the use and storage of blood and tissue samples for research'. Regarding genetic research, 173 patients (78 %) agreed/strongly agreed, 25 patients (11 %) were neutral and 25 patients (11 %) disagreed/strongly disagreed with the statement: 'I would agree to donate tissue for genetic research even if I was not told my genetic results'.

In response to the question: 'would you participate in a trial that required you to have a repeat biopsy?' 78 patients (34 %) answered 'yes', 95 patients (41 %) answered 'maybe', 48 patients (21 %) answered 'no' and 10 patients (4 %) did not answer the question. The results of a univariate analysis of patient factors and their association with patients' views of research biopsies is shown in Table 4.

Patients' understanding of their cancer diagnosis
One hundred and eighty-three patients (79 %) correctly stated their diagnosis, 14 patients (6 %) wrote an incorrect answer (mainly indicating a metastatic site as their type of cancer) and 34 patients (15 %) did not answer the question. Patients under the age of 65 years were more likely to answer the question correctly (87 % versus 71 %, odds ratio 2.69, 95 % CI 1.38– 5.25, $p = 0.004$).

Patients' views on the written trial information
The mean PIS length was 17 pages (median 4 pages, range 3–50 pages) and was influenced by trial type (CTIMP: 23 pages, non-CTIMP: 8 pages, pre-screening: 5 pages, $p < 0.001$). Two hundred and fifteen patients (90 %) felt the PIS was easy to understand and 22 patients (9 %) felt the PIS was too long

(see Fig. 3). One patient admitted to not having read the information. There was a poor correlation between PIS length and patients' views on whether the PIS was too long (see Fig. 4). All 10 patients who declined a study and completed the questionnaire believed the PIS was easy to understand and none of these patients felt the PIS was too long.

Patients' views on the content of the PIS are shown in Fig. 5. Thirty-six patients (15 %) looked up additional information about the trial (CTIMP: 32 %, pre-screening: 14 %, non-CTIMP: 7 %). Some patients wrote free-text comments requesting additional information: e.g. 'more stats on the progress of the trial' and 'I found reading the actual trial protocol particularly useful'.

Patients' views on the verbal explanation, trial discussions and the consent process
The verbal explanation of the trial was rated as excellent, good, fair or poor by 100 (40 %), 124 (50 %), 14 (6 %) and 1 (0.4 %) patients respectively. All 10 patients who declined a study and completed the questionnaire rated the verbal explanation as excellent/good.

Two hundred and nineteen patients (88 %) discussed the trial with 1 or more people (CTIMP: 97 %, pre-screening: 96 %, non-CTIMP: 83 %), usually a family member (see Table 5). Two hundred and thirty-one patients (93 %) felt they had been given enough time to consider whether they wished to participate in the trial. Twenty-two pre-screening trial patients (79 %), 103 non-

Table 4 Univariate analysis of factors influencing patients' views on whether they would participate in a trial involving a research biopsy

Patient characteristic	Yes N (%) (n = 78)	Odds ratio (95 % CI)	p value[a]
Age			
< 65 years	37 (57 %)	1.0	
≥ 65 years	41 (67 %)	1.55 (0.75–3.21)	0.236
Gender			
Male	59 (64 %)	1.0	
Female	19 (56 %)	0.71 (0.32–1.58)	0.398
Tumour type			
Colorectal	30 (60 %)	1.0	
Oesophagogastric	37 (73 %)	1.76 (0.76–4.06)	0.184
Performance status (PS)			
0	30 (67 %)	1.0	
1	36 (59 %)	0.72 (0.32–1.61)	0.423
2	7 (70 %)	1.17 (0.26-5.16)	0.839
Previously participated in a clinical trial			
Yes	13 (65 %)	1.0	
No	64 (61 %)	1.19 (0.44–3.23)	0.733
Number of previous lines of treatment			
0	24 (47 %)	1.0	
1	31 (67 %)	2.33 (1.02–5.31)	0.045
2+	22 (79 %)	4.13 (1.43–11.9)	0.009
Type of treatment			
Palliative	60 (69 %)	1.0	
Curative	18 (46 %)	0.39 (0.18–0.84)	0.015
CTIMP			
No	44 (60 %)	1.0	
Yes	19 (53 %)	0.74 (0.33–1.65)	0.457

[a]p values compare the proportion of patients who answered 'yes': e.g. 67 % for PS0 versus 59 % for PS1 and 70 % for PS2

Key: CTIMP = Clinical Trial of an Investigational Medicinal Product, pre-screening = molecular pre-screening to determine potential eligibility for a specific CTIMP study

CTIMP trial patients (66 %) and 35 CTIMP trial patients (54 %) would have been willing to consent to the trial on the same day they received the PIS.

Feedback of study results

One hundred and seventy-three patients (75 %) felt patients should be told trial results, 13 patients (6 %) felt they should not be told and 40 patients (17 %) were unsure. A higher proportion of CTIMP trial patients felt participants should be told trial results (88 % versus 68 % for non-CTIMP trials, odds ratio 3.29, 95 % CI 1.46–7.45, p = 0.004). One hundred and ten patients (52 %) felt results should be provided by post, 91 patients (42 %) felt these should be discussed

in clinic, 33 patients (16 %) thought via a website and 2 patients added free-text comments suggesting via Email.

Discussion

The majority of patients in our survey were happy to be approached about participating in cancer research and were keen to participate in clinical trials. We chose to develop our own survey as existing surveys, such as the UK National Cancer Experience Survey, cover a broad range of topics and only include a few questions on clinical trials. Although our survey was less well-validated, it allowed us to determine the proportion of patients who consented to a clinical trial as well as investigate

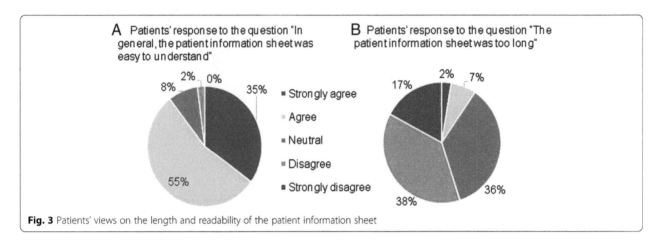

Fig. 3 Patients' views on the length and readability of the patient information sheet

patients' views on cancer research in more detail. Re-assuringly, our results were consistent with the UK National Cancer Experience Survey, which reported that 95 % of patients who had research discussed with them were happy to have been asked and 53 % of patients with whom research was not discussed would have been happy to have been asked [17]. However, patients who have just started their first treatment for cancer are less likely to participate in cancer research and it appears that as time increases from diagnosis, patients are more positive about engaging with research [6, 18]. This may reflect the availability of clinical trials, but may also be influenced by factors such as the psychological impact of a recent cancer diagnosis. Patients were particularly willing to consent to non-CTIMP trials, possibly due to the less interventional nature of these studies. We had originally planned to compare the characteristics of the patients who consented to a trial with those who declined a trial, but this was not possible due to the small number of patients who declined a trial.

However, although a high proportion of patients consented to a trial, 36 % of patients subsequently failed screening for CTIMP/pre-screening trials. Screen failures may become increasingly problematic due to the growing number of biomarker selected/stratified trials. Twenty-eight percent of our trial portfolio involved tissue analysis prior to patient randomisation (either to determine eligibility or for stratification), resulting in 66 % of screen failures being caused by patients' molecular profiles or a lack of tissue for analysis. This has important logistical and workload implications, as staff time is required for trial set-up, patient recruitment and specimen coordination, even though many patients are subsequently ineligible for the trial.

In agreement with other studies, we found that patients' decisions to participate in research are influenced by multiple factors including altruism, trust in their treating physician and beliefs that they would receive superior treatment, closer monitoring and better quality

care [11, 12, 19–23]. However, the 'most important' reason varied according to factors such as trial type and treatment intent. Although 52 % of patients consenting to CTIMP trials were motivated by a belief that the trial was the best treatment option available, 25 % of patients participated for altruistic reasons. Interestingly, 15 % of non-CTIMP trial respondents felt that the trial offered the best treatment available. For some trials (e.g. molecular profiling trials), this was a logical response. However, other trials had no direct patient benefit and, therefore, some patients seem to have misunderstood the trials' aims. Other studies have shown that patients can misunderstand the potential personal benefit from clinical trials [13, 20] and it is important to ensure that patients clearly understand the purpose of any trial and any trial-related procedures.

Translational research is increasingly important and patients' opinions of tissue and genetic research should be considered by researchers and ethics committees when assessing translational research protocols. Reassuringly, only 7 % of our patients had concerns about the use and storage of blood/tissue samples for research, and indeed, many patients strongly felt that this was not

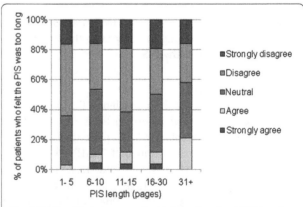

Fig. 4 Relationship between patient information sheet (PIS) length and patients' views on PIS length

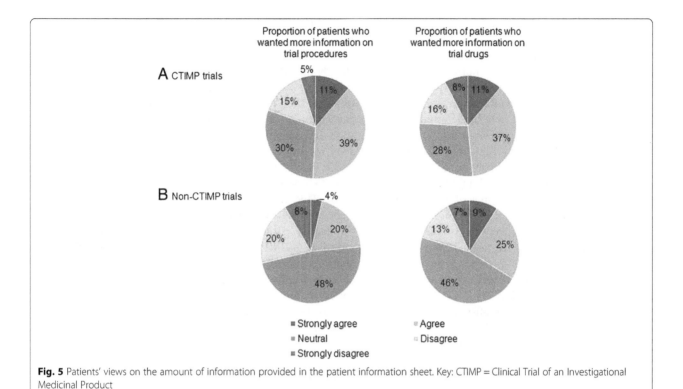

Fig. 5 Patients' views on the amount of information provided in the patient information sheet. Key: CTIMP = Clinical Trial of an Investigational Medicinal Product

an issue. This is supported by the results of other studies, which demonstrate that the majority of cancer patients would allow the use of their tissue for research [13, 24, 25]. In our survey, 78 % of patients would agree to donate tissue for genetic research, even if they were not told their genetic results, indicating patient support for genomic research into cancer. However, these results should be interpreted with caution as no information was provided in our questionnaire regarding the potential implications of genetic results, so patients' understanding and knowledge of any potential issues is unknown.

Biopsies are becoming an increasingly common component of clinical trials and 42 % of our trials involved an optional or mandatory biopsy. There have been ethical concerns about mandatory research biopsies: e.g. a lack of alternative treatment options and patients' understanding of biopsy risks and the purpose of the biopsy [14, 26–28]. Although some patients would not participate in trials involving a biopsy, it is important to highlight that 75 % of our patients stated they would consider participating in a trial involving a repeat biopsy. This is significant as staff and ethics committee assumptions regarding patients' attitudes to biopsies may not be accurate. For example, a survey of patients, medical oncologists and Institutional Review Board (IRB) members on the issue of mandatory research biopsies demonstrated that oncologists and IRB members may overestimate the anxiety associated with biopsies and that

patients would accept a higher risk of biopsy-related complications than oncologists/IRB members [13]. Furthermore, staff may be reluctant to discuss biopsies with older-aged patients or patients with a poorer PS due to assumptions that these patients would not wish to undergo any additional procedures. Interestingly, age and PS did not significantly impact on the willingness of our patients to consider a biopsy and we feel that these factors need not be a barrier to discussing biopsies with patients, allowing them to make their own decisions.

Patients being treated with palliative intent and patients who have received more lines of treatment appear

Table 5 People with whom patients discussed participation in a clinical trial

Person	N (%)
	(n = 249)
Spouse/partner	171 (68 %)
Son/daughter	64 (26 %)
Sibling	56 (23 %)
Friend	37 (15 %)
Parent	16 (6 %)
GP	13 (5 %)
Grandchild	7 (3 %)
Other[a]	11 (4 %)

[a]Other included: other family members, work colleague/boss, other doctors, Macmillan nurse, nutrition advisor/mind coach and their insurance company. Many patients discussed trial participation with more than one person

to be more willing to consider a repeat biopsy. This could be due to a number of reasons, including willingness to participate in anything that could potentially benefit them, increasing altruistic motives or a better understanding of cancer and its treatment. Patients with a recent diagnosis of cancer are often keen to start treatment as soon as possible, and may be deterred by concerns regarding potential biopsy-related delays, may feel psychologically overwhelmed by their diagnosis and, as previously mentioned, are less likely to engage in research [18]. However, these results should be interpreted with caution due to the small number of patients in the subgroup analyses and because trials in more advanced lines of treatment were more likely to contain a biopsy component. Further research is needed into patients' views on biopsies, particularly as it has been suggested that previous negative biopsy experiences may discourage patients from future biopsies [29].

Lengthy trial information can be off-putting to patients [22] and healthcare staff may feel that patients are overwhelmed by the amount of information provided, particularly as they have often also received information about their cancer and their standard treatment options. In addition, lengthy trial information can lead to a poor recall of risks and it has been suggested that shorter information leaflets might lead to better informed consent [30]. Indeed, one patient admitted to not having read the PIS, and this is not unique to our study [31]. PIS are often reviewed/tested by patients prior to submission to ethics committees, and this can result in amendments to their wording and layout that make the final version easier to understand [32]. However, even though the average PIS length was 17 pages, 55 % of patients clearly stated they did not feel it was too long and 48–50 % of patients approached about CTIMP studies would have liked more information on the study drugs/procedures. Therefore, there does seem to be a group of patients who wish to know more details about the trial, and indeed many of the free-text comments expressed a desire for more detailed information. The majority of patients discussed the trial with family members, and so patients' relatives may also wish to have more detailed trial information.

However, approximately 20–28 % of our patients did not want more information on the trial drugs/procedures and other studies have shown that patients feel that the amount of information provided is sufficient [11]. A one-size-fits-all approach is, therefore, unlikely to suit the needs of every patient, and strategies to tailor information according to the individual patient's wishes should be explored. Fifteen percent of patients looked up additional information (rising to 32 % for CTIMP studies) and, therefore, one strategy could be to provide a link in the PIS to a website containing further trial information. This would have the advantage of providing a resource for interested patients without overloading patients who are satisfied with the level of information already provided.

Patients who enrol quickly into clinical trials may not feel that they fully understand the implications of trial participation [33] and, therefore, ethics applications may state that patients will be given at least 24 hours to consider the information provided. However, some patients find it inconvenient to return specifically to sign consent and do not wish to delay screening procedures/treatment. This can be a particular issue for pre-screening trials, which involve biomarker testing of archival tissue to identify patients who might be eligible for corresponding CTIMP trials. As 79 % of patients approached about pre-screening trials would have been willing to consent on the same day as receiving the PIS, perhaps patients who wish to consent on the same day should be able to do so (with the important caveat of ensuring patients do not feel pressurised into signing consent).

Although 75 % of patients in our survey (rising to 89 % for CTIMP trials) felt participants should be informed of trial results, these are not always effectively communicated to patients. The question was specifically worded to highlight the fact that results may not be available for many years, although it did not directly state that patients may be deceased at the point when final study results are available. Our results are comparable to those from other studies [22, 34–36], indicating that the majority of patients feel they should be offered the trial results, not only for their personal interest and satisfaction, but also out of respect for their contribution to the trial [22]. One of the concerns regarding the feedback of trial results is the potential for psychological distress (e.g. due to randomisation to an arm with inferior outcomes) [35, 36]. However, although receiving results can be distressing [37, 38], this does not necessarily lead to regret at receiving results and some patients suggested that the satisfaction of knowing the results outweighed the potential distress of hearing bad news [36]. Indeed, one study demonstrated that 84 % of patients would like to receive results from a negative trial [36] and receiving study results may improve participants' research experience [39]. Furthermore, not receiving results may deter patients from participating in future trials [34].

However, the optimal content, timing and method of providing results to participants is currently unclear, with our patients being divided as to whether results should be provided in clinic or via a letter. Some patients wish to know their personal results, others want the overall study results and many wish to know both [36]. In addition, patients are keen to receive regular updates on the trial's progress [22, 36, 40]. Many sponsors provide participating sites with newsletters providing progress updates, so one strategy could be to provide a lay version of these newsletters to interested patients as well as a lay summary when the results are available.

When considering the applicability of our results to other patient populations, there are a number of factors that should be considered. Firstly, the structure of the UK health service (which is not dependent on patients' health insurance) may facilitate trial participation [41]. Secondly, our patients were predominantly white, middle-class men with low levels of social deprivation. Although we did not specifically assess the educational level or health literacy of our patients, it is likely that our patients are more highly educated than patients from more deprived socioeconomic backgrounds, and issues such as lack of support, financial worries and difficulties with transport may be less problematic for our patients in comparison to patients from socially deprived areas [42]. Despite this, it is concerning that 21 % of patients either did not correctly state their diagnosis or left this question blank. It is uncertain whether the patients who did not answer the question accidentally missed the question or did not know what to write. If patients have not accurately understood their diagnosis, then they are less likely to fully understand the trial information. In addition, this survey only included patients with GI malignancies or lymphoma, and their views (particularly on biopsies) may differ from patients with other types of cancer. Also, the trial portfolio was heterogeneous in nature and the characteristics of the individual trials (e.g. palliative versus curative, study phase) and PIS may have influenced patients' responses.

In addition, whether patients' answers to the questionnaire truly reflect their views on the PIS is uncertain. Patients' responses may be influenced by 'social desirability': i.e. they may give a socially desirable response if they know someone else will read their answers [43]. Furthermore, patients may falsely believe they have understood the PIS. For example, 93 % of patients in one phase I study stated they understood most or all of the information provided, but only 33 % were able to state the purpose of the trial in which they were participating [12]. Additionally, some of the questions were hypothetical in nature for some patients, as they were not relevant to the type of trial for which they had received a PIS and this may have influenced their responses.

However, it is important to highlight that although RM is a specialist cancer centre and patients referred from elsewhere in the UK for consideration of clinical trials may be more motivated to participate in cancer research, the majority of patients in our survey lived locally and were not referred to RM specifically for a trial. In addition, one of the main strengths of this survey is that a high proportion of patients who consented to a trial also completed the questionnaire (thereby minimising any potential bias between questionnaire responders and non-responders).

Conclusions

In summary, this survey provides an insight into the views of patients on cancer research. The majority of patients were happy to have been approached about participating in clinical trials, and only a small proportion of patients declined a clinical trial. Although a major motivating factor was the possibility of improving their own treatment, many patients were also keen to help others and to contribute to scientific research. This extends to the use of tissue samples for research and to the consideration of research biopsies. We recommend that clinical trials and research biopsies are discussed with potentially eligible patients (including older-aged patients), to provide interested patients with the opportunity to participate in research. New strategies for tailoring the information needs to the individual patient, methods for disseminating trial results to participants and incorporating options for feedback of results into the initial trial consent process should be considered.

Abbreviations
CTIMP: Clinical Trial of an Investigational Medicinal Product; GI: gastrointestinal; HER2: human epidermal growth factor receptor 2; IRB: Institutional Review Board; NIHR: National Institute for Health Research; NRS: National Readership Survey; Non-CTIMP: clinical trial not involving an investigational medicinal product; PIS: patient information sheet; PS: performance status; RM: Royal Marsden; UK: United Kingdom.

Competing interests
None of the authors have any conflicts of interest to declare.

Authors' contributions
SYM designed the survey, collected and entered the data, assisted with data interpretation and drafted the manuscript. CM collected and entered the data and assisted with data interpretation. CP performed the statistical analysis. DC, IC, NS and DW recruited patients and assisted with data interpretation. SR conceived the survey, participated in the survey design, recruited patients, assisted with data interpretation and helped to draft the manuscript. All authors read and approved the final manuscript.

Acknowledgments
We acknowledge support from the National Institute for Health Research (NIHR) RM/ICR Biomedical Research Centre. We would like to thank our research nurses D Bottero, L Caley, K Chandler, S Cruse, J Duncan, L Jell, V Pitkaaho, G Smith, J Thomas, A Turner, J Webb and L Wedlake and our clinical trial administrator C Grant.

References

1. Schroen AT, Petroni GR, Wang H, Gray R, Wang XF, Cronin W, et al. Preliminary evaluation of factors associated with premature trial closure and feasibility of accrual benchmarks in phase III oncology trials. Clin Trials. 2010; 7(4):312–21. doi:10.1177/1740774510374973.

2. Schroen AT, Petroni GR, Wang H, Thielen MJ, Gray R, Benedetti J, et al. Achieving sufficient accrual to address the primary endpoint in phase III clinical trials from U.S. Cooperative Oncology Groups. Clin Cancer Res. 2012; 18(1):256–62. doi:10.1158/1078-0432.CCR-11-1633.

3. Stensland K, McBride R, Wisnivesky J, Asma Latif A, Hendricks R, Roper N, et al. Premature termination of genitourinary cancer clinical trials. J Clin Oncol. 2014;32 Suppl 4:abstr 288).

4. National Institute for Health Research. Performance in Initiating and Delivering Research. 2015 http://www.nihr.ac.uk/policy-and-standards/Performance-in-initiating-anddelivering-research.htm. Accessed on 08.01.16.

5. Cancer Research UK. Our research on clinical trials and new treatments. 2014. http://www.cancerresearchuk.org/our-research/our-research-by-cancersubject/our-research-on-clinical-trials-and-new-treatments. Accessed on 08.01.16.

6. Quality Health. Cancer Patient Experience Survey 2014 National Report. 2014.

7. Kay A, Higgins J, Day AG, Meyer RM, Booth CM. Randomized controlled trials in the era of molecular oncology: methodology, biomarkers, and end points. Ann Oncol. 2012;23(6):1646–51. doi:10.1093/annonc/mdr492.

8. Booth CM, Cescon DW, Wang L, Tannock IF, Krzyzanowska MK. Evolution of the randomized controlled trial in oncology over three decades. J Clin Oncol. 2008;26(33):5458–64. doi:10.1200/JCO.2008.16.5456.

9. Bostock S, Steptoe A. Association between low functional health literacy and mortality in older adults: longitudinal cohort study. BMJ. 2012;344, e1602. doi:10.1136/bmj.e1602.

10. Joffe S, Cook EF, Cleary PD, Clark JW, Weeks JC. Quality of informed consent in cancer clinical trials: a cross-sectional survey. Lancet. 2001;358(9295): 1772–7. doi:10.1016/S0140-6736(01)06805-2.

11. Godskesen T, Hansson MG, Nygren P, Nordin K, Kihlbom U. Hope for a cure and altruism are the main motives behind participation in phase 3 clinical cancer trials. Eur J Cancer Care. 2014. doi:10.1111/ecc.12184.

12. Daugherty C, Ratain MJ, Grochowski E, Stocking C, Kodish E, Mick R, et al. Perceptions of cancer patients and their physicians involved in phase I trials. J Clin Oncol. 1995;13(5):1062–72.

13. Agulnik M, Oza AM, Pond GR, Siu LL. Impact and perceptions of mandatory tumor biopsies for correlative studies in clinical trials of novel anticancer agents. J Clin Oncol. 2006;24(30):4801–7. doi:10.1200/JCO.2005.03.4496.

14. Pentz RD, Harvey RD, White M, Farmer ZL, Dashevskaya O, Chen Z, et al. Research biopsies in phase I studies: views and perspectives of participants and investigators. IRB. 2012;34(2):1–8.

15. National Readership Survey. Social grade. http://www.nrs.co.uk/nrs-print/lifestyle-and-classification-data/social-grade/.Accessed on 08.01.16.

16. Office for National Statistics. Households in poverty: model-based estimates at MSOA level, 2007–08. 2008. http://neighbourhood.statistics.gov.uk/HTMLDocs/poverty.html. Accessed on 08.01.16.

17. Department of Health. Cancer Patient Experience Survey 2011/2012 National Report. 2012.

18. Quality Health . National Cancer Patient Experience Survey 2012–13 National Report. 2013.

19. Comis RL, Miller JD, Aldige CR, Krebs L, Stoval E. Public attitudes toward participation in cancer clinical trials. J Clin Oncol. 2003;21(5):830–5.

20. Garcea G, Lloyd T, Steward WP, Dennison AR, Berry DP. Differences in attitudes between patients with primary colorectal cancer and patients with secondary colorectal cancer: is it reflected in their willingness to participate in drug trials? Eur J Cancer Care. 2005;14(2):166–70. doi:10.1111/j.1365-2354.2005.00535.x.

21. Jenkins V, Fallowfield L. Reasons for accepting or declining to participate in randomized clinical trials for cancer therapy. Br J Cancer. 2000;82(11):1783–8. doi:10.1054/bjoc.2000.1142.

22. Locock L, Smith L. Personal experiences of taking part in clinical trials – a qualitative study. Patient Educ Couns. 2011;84(3):303–9. doi:10.1016/j.pec.2011.06.002.

23. Nurgat ZA, Craig W, Campbell NC, Bissett JD, Cassidy J, Nicolson MC. Patient motivations surrounding participation in phase I and phase II clinical trials of cancer chemotherapy. Br J Cancer. 2005;92(6):1001–5. doi:10.1038/sj.bjc.6602423.

24. Baer AR, Smith ML, Bendell JC. Donating tissue for research: patient and provider perspectives. J Oncol Pract/Am Soc Clin Oncol. 2011;7(5):334–7. doi:10.1200/JOP.2011.000399.

25. Karapetis C, Kumar R, Timothy Q, Sukumaran S, Kichenadasse G, Dua D, et al. What do patients with cancer think of the use of their tumor tissue for medical research? J Clin Oncol. 2013;31(Suppl):abstr 6541).

26. Olson EM, Lin NU, Krop IE, Winer EP. The ethical use of mandatory research biopsies. Nat Rev Clin Oncol. 2011;8(10):620–5. doi:10.1038/nrclinonc.2011.114.

27. Peppercorn J, Shapira I, Collyar D, Deshields T, Lin N, Krop I, et al. Ethics of mandatory research biopsy for correlative end points within clinical trials in oncology. J Clin Oncol. 2010;28(15):2635–40. doi:10.1200/JCO.2009.27.2443.

28. Saggese M, Dua D, Simmons E, Lemech C, Arkenau H. Research biopsies in the context of early phase oncology studies: clinical and ethical considerations. Oncol Rev. 2013;7, e5.

29. Seah DS, Scott SM, Najita J, Openshaw T, Krag K, Frank E, et al. Attitudes of patients with metastatic breast cancer toward research biopsies. Ann Oncol. 2013;24(7):1853–9. doi:10.1093/annonc/mdt067.

30. Fortun P, West J, Chalkley L, Shonde A, Hawkey C. Recall of informed consent information by healthy volunteers in clinical trials. QJM. 2008;101(8): 625–9. doi:10.1093/qjmed/hcn067.

31. Zaric B, Perin B, Ilic A, Kopitovic I, Matijasevic J, Andrijevic L, et al. Clinical trials in advanced stage lung cancer: a survey of patients' opinion about their treatment. Multidiscip Respir Med. 2011;6(1):20–7. doi:10.1186/2049-6958-6-1-20.

32. Knapp P, Raynor DK, Silcock J, Parkinson B. Can user testing of a clinical trial patient information sheet make it fit-for-purpose? – a randomized controlled trial. BMC Med. 2011;9:89. doi:10.1186/1741-7015-9-89.

33. Stryker JE, Wray RJ, Emmons KM, Winer E, Demetri G. Understanding the decisions of cancer clinical trial participants to enter research studies: factors associated with informed consent, patient satisfaction, and decisional regret. Patient Educ Couns. 2006;63(1–2):104–9. doi:10.1016/j.pec.2005.09.006.

34. Sood A, Prasad K, Chhatwani L, Shinozaki E, Cha SS, Loehrer LL, et al. Patients' attitudes and preferences about participation and recruitment strategies in clinical trials. Mayo Clin Proc. 2009;84(3):243–7. doi:10.1016/S0025-6196(11)61141-5.

35. Shalowitz DI, Miller FG. Communicating the results of clinical research to participants: attitudes, practices, and future directions. PLoS Med. 2008;5(5), e91. doi:10.1371/journal.pmed.0050091.

36. Cox K, Moghaddam N, Bird L, Elkan R. Feedback of trial results to participants: a survey of clinicians' and patients' attitudes and experiences. Eur J Oncol Nurs. 2011;15(2):124–9. doi:10.1016/j.ejon.2010.06.009.

37. Schulz CJ, Riddle MP, Valdimirsdottir HB, Abramson DH, Sklar CA. Impact on survivors of retinoblastoma when informed of study results on risk of second cancers. Med Pediatr Oncol. 2003;41(1):36–43. doi:10.1002/mpo.10278.

38. Partridge AH, Wong JS, Knudsen K, Gelman R, Sampson E, Gadd M, et al. Offering participants results of a clinical trial: sharing results of a negative study. Lancet. 2005;365(9463):963–4. doi:10.1016/S0140-6736(05)71085-0.

39. Darbyshire JL, Price HC. Disseminating results to clinical trial participants: a qualitative review of patient understanding in a post-trial population. BMJ open. 2012;2(5). doi:10.1136/bmjopen-2012-001252.

40. Tolmie EP, Mungall MM, Louden G, Lindsay GM, Gaw A. Understanding why older people participate in clinical trials: the experience of the Scottish PROSPER participants. Age Ageing. 2004;33(4):374–8. doi:10.1093/ageing/afh109.

41. Sinha G. United Kingdom becomes the cancer clinical trials recruitment capital of the world. J Natl Cancer Inst. 2007;99(6):420–2. doi:10.1093/jnci/djk140.

42. Reed N, Siddiqui N. Trials and tribulations: obstacles to clinical trial recruitment. Br J Cancer. 2003;89(6):957–8. doi:10.1038/sj.bjc.6601233.

43. Streiner DN, Norman GR. Health measurement scales. A practical guide. Oxford: Oxford Medical Press; 1989.

11

The usefulness of school-based syndromic surveillance for detecting malaria epidemics: experiences from a pilot project in Ethiopia

Ruth A. Ashton[1,2*], Takele Kefyalew[3], Esey Batisso[4], Tessema Awano[4], Zelalem Kebede[3], Gezahegn Tesfaye[3], Tamiru Mesele[5], Sheleme Chibsa[6], Richard Reithinger[2,7] and Simon J. Brooker[2]

Abstract

Background: Syndromic surveillance is a supplementary approach to routine surveillance, using pre-diagnostic and non-clinical surrogate data to identify possible infectious disease outbreaks. To date, syndromic surveillance has primarily been used in high-income countries for diseases such as influenza – however, the approach may also be relevant to resource-poor settings. This study investigated the potential for monitoring school absenteeism and febrile illness, as part of a school-based surveillance system to identify localised malaria epidemics in Ethiopia.

Methods: Repeated cross-sectional school- and community-based surveys were conducted in six epidemic-prone districts in southern Ethiopia during the 2012 minor malaria transmission season to characterise prospective surrogate and syndromic indicators of malaria burden. Changes in these indicators over the transmission season were compared to standard indicators of malaria (clinical and confirmed cases) at proximal health facilities. Subsequently, two pilot surveillance systems were implemented, each at ten sites throughout the peak transmission season. Indicators piloted were school attendance recorded by teachers, or child-reported recent absenteeism from school and reported febrile illness.

Results: Lack of seasonal increase in malaria burden limited the ability to evaluate sensitivity of the piloted syndromic surveillance systems compared to existing surveillance at health facilities. Weekly absenteeism was easily calculated by school staff using existing attendance registers, while syndromic indicators were more challenging to collect weekly from schoolchildren. In this setting, enrolment of school-aged children was found to be low, at 54 %. Non-enrolment was associated with low household wealth, lack of parental education, household size, and distance from school.

Conclusions: School absenteeism is a plausible simple indicator of unusual health events within a community, such as malaria epidemics, but the sensitivity of an absenteeism-based surveillance system to detect epidemics could not be rigorously evaluated in this study. Further piloting during a demonstrated increase in malaria transmission within a community is recommended.

Keywords: Malaria, Syndromic surveillance, Schools, Epidemics, Absenteeism

* Correspondence: rashton@tulane.edu
[1]Malaria Consortium, London, UK
[2]Faculty of Infectious and Tropical Diseases, London School of Hygiene & Tropical Medicine, London, UK
Full list of author information is available at the end of the article

Background

Infectious diseases inherently exhibit marked spatial and temporal trends [1–4], which can manifest as epidemics. Epidemics are broadly defined as unusual increases in the burden of illness, that are clearly in excess of normal expectancy [5]. Definitions of "normal" burden vary, but upper and lower limits of normality are often defined as being two standard deviations around the mean number of cases for a facility in a defined time period, after excluding previous epidemic periods [6]. Comprehensive surveillance systems are crucial to enable the timely identification of unusual increases in disease incidence, to minimise onward spread through early detection and treatment of affected individuals and to effectively target control measures. Detection of individuals with an epidemic-prone infectious disease is typically based on clinical or biological diagnosis. Another approach to detecting individuals with disease is the use of pre-diagnostic or surrogate indicators, described as syndromic surveillance.

School absenteeism is one such surrogate indicator. School absenteeism is appealing as an indicator for syndromic surveillance since it utilises an existing and well-established source of data in the form of daily school attendance registers, and has a fine temporal resolution. The primary application of school absenteeism for syndromic surveillance has been for detection of influenza epidemics in high-income countries [7–10], where school enrolment and attendance is generally high and thus schoolchildren are expected to be representative of the wider population. Prior studies using school absenteeism as an indicator of infectious disease outbreaks in resource-poor settings are few. In China, a web-based surveillance system incorporated primary school absenteeism, health facility syndromic data and pharmacy medication sales [11, 12]. In Cambodia, an approach using school absenteeism data submitted by short message service (SMS) to a central server was found to be feasible and acceptable [13].

School absenteeism is a recognised consequence of malaria epidemics that occur in the highlands of East Africa [14], where malaria transmission varies in time and space. Ethiopia has seen some of the largest malaria epidemics in the region with very high case fatality rates [15]. While no severe epidemics have been observed in Ethiopia since 2004, and more recent district-level outbreaks have been successfully contained, both small and large scale epidemics continue to be a significant health threat [16]. As per WHO guidance [17], routine detection of epidemics in Ethiopia is based on health facilities plotting weekly total confirmed malaria cases against a threshold calculated using five years' historical data [18], but this method fails to account for temporal variations in peak transmission [19]. Furthermore, delays in data reporting and incomplete or inaccurate data limit application of the health facility-based epidemic detection system [20–22]. While these limitations persist, alternative tools or strategies that can bridge these gaps and facilitate early identification of epidemics are needed. The need for community-based approaches to malaria surveillance and response, tailored to the local setting, have also been highlighted as a priority in achieving malaria elimination [23]. The dramatic increase in primary school enrolment in Ethiopia and other African countries [24], suggests that school-level malariometric indicators such as prevalence by rapid diagnostic test (RDT) are increasingly representative of the wider population [25]. Febrile illness may be an additional useful indicator for identification of malaria epidemics. While a large proportion of infections in low transmission settings such as Ethiopia are of low parasite density and asymptomatic [26–28], it is hypothesised that during an epidemic symptomatic illness would increase, due to the substantial increase in the total number of *Plasmodium* infections.

The current study was designed to explore the usefulness of a syndromic surveillance approach to identify unusual increases in malaria at community-level in a low-income country, Ethiopia. The specific objectives were to: (i) assess the feasibility of different approaches to routinely collect and analyse indicators from rural primary schools in areas at risk of malaria epidemics; (ii) assess the correlation between changes in these surrogate and syndromic indicators with parasitological indicators of malaria burden within the wider population through cross-sectional surveys and passive health facility case detection; and (iii) specifically investigate the reasons for school absenteeism in this environment and, therefore, the potential of absenteeism as a surrogate surveillance indicator.

Overview of syndromic surveillance approaches

Syndromic surveillance refers to the use of pre-diagnostic health indicators to allow timely detection and investigation of potential infectious disease outbreaks [29] as a supplementary approach to routine public health surveillance, by enabling early identification of clusters of illness before confirmatory data are available. In addition to use of clinical (syndrome) data, syndromic surveillance can be expanded to include surrogate non-clinical data indicating early illness, through mining of available data to track changes in infectious diseases in the population. Surrogate data sources include prescription and over-the-counter drug sales, internet search terms and social media [30–36] and school absenteeism [7–10, 37]. The latter is an alternative indicator of population health that has been applied to monitor influenza outbreaks in high-income countries, but yet to be fully explored as an approach for infectious disease surveillance in resource poor settings. Syndromic surveillance systems piloted in resource poor settings have to date used clinical signs among patients attending health facilities as their indicators [38–42], but two examples of school absenteeism being used as early warning of outbreaks of respiratory and gastrointestinal diseases are available from Cambodia and rural China [11, 13, 43]. The key surveillance studies using school absenteeism for outbreak detection, as well as classic applications of syndromic surveillance utilising data on clinical morbidities are presented in Table 1, to demonstrate the various settings, indicators, temporal resolution and complexity of these syndromic surveillance systems.

Methods

Study design

The study was conducted in Southern Nations, Nationalities and People's Regional State (SNNPRS), Ethiopia, and divided into two phases. Phase 1 comprised cross-sectional school- and household-based surveys at six sites during the minor malaria transmission season (March–May 2012), collection of routinely recorded school attendance data, and weekly summary of clinical and confirmed malaria cases at health facilities serving the study sites. Phase 1 activities aimed to define appropriate indicators for further piloting as part of a syndromic surveillance approach. Two school-based syndromic surveillance approaches were implemented as Phase 2 of the study during the peak transmission season (October 2012 to January 2013), each system being piloted at 10 sites in SNNPRS (Fig. 1).

Cross-sectional surveys at school- and community-level (Phase 1)

Six woredas (districts) were chosen purposively from those designated as "hotspot" woredas by the SNPPRS Regional Health Bureau, indicating epidemic risk and higher malaria burden relative to other woredas (Fig. 2). All sites were located at 1850–2000 metres altitude, along the Rift Valley. Sites included flatlands with savannah-type vegetation, where the main crops are teff and pepper, and highland slopes with abundant vegetation where the main cash crop is coffee. Coverage of health facilities in the areas was in line with the national policy for a "primary health care unit" of one health centre and five satellite health posts for each 25,000 people. In practice, each kebele (municipality) tends to have at least one health post and each woreda at least one health centre [44].

From each woreda, one kebele was purposively chosen as the study site, with inclusion criteria being: government primary school with at least 100 children attending; a health post; <200 metres altitude range; and, accessibility during the rainy season. "School-aged" in the current study was defined as age seven to 16 years, since national policy is for children to enrol in school at seven years of age [45].

Eight repeat school and community surveys were conducted at approximately ten-day intervals from March to May 2012. Due to lack of prior data describing likely range of syndromic indicators of interest, no sample size calculation was completed, but sample size was maximised within logistical capacity.

The community survey protocol followed Malaria Indicator Survey procedures, mapping and randomly selecting 25 households per survey site [46], but with the primary sampling unit defined as primary school catchment area. Random selection of participating households was repeated for each of the eight survey iterations. A questionnaire was completed for each household and all individuals at the household were invited to provide a single finger prick blood sample for multi-species RDT (CareStart HRP2/panLDH, AccessBio, USA) and blood film. School surveys followed a standard methodology previously used in Ethiopia and Kenya [47, 48], with random selection of children was repeated at each survey iteration. Each child completed a questionnaire and was requested to provide a single finger-prick blood sample for multi-species RDT and blood film.

Attendance register data were extracted to calculate weekly absenteeism by class, defined as total child-days absence recorded, divided by the product of total children enrolled and number of days that attendance was recorded by the teacher. In addition, weekly malaria case data were collected from health centres and health posts serving the six study sites. Indicators included clinical and confirmed malaria cases and number tested by microscopy (at health centres) or RDT (at health posts).

Assigning sites to the two pilot systems (Phase 2)

Design of two surveillance systems was informed by Phase 1 findings, including feasibility of collecting various indicators at school-level, and the correlation between the indicator and number of malaria cases reported at health facilities. Indicators selected for piloting during Phase 2 were: weekly school absenteeism measured by attendance register, and the proportion of school-attending children reporting recent fever, recent absence from school or absence from school due to illness.

The two surveillance systems were piloted during the second school semester, from early October 2012 to the first week of January 2013 when the semester ended. All sites included in Phase 1 were retained for Phase 2. A further 14 sites (from 14 woredas) were purposively chosen using the same inclusion criteria as for Phase 1 sites. Woredas were assigned to participate in either the cluster A or B pilot without randomisation, according to location of woreda within higher administrative unit

Table 1 Selected syndromic surveillance systems reported in the literature: the setting, target diseases, indicators, system complexity and outcomes of their application. Reported studies are those which use school absenteeism as a key indicator, or systems applied in resource-limited settings for epidemic prone diseases including malaria

Setting	Target disease(s)	Indicators	Reporting frequency	Complexity of system	Surveillance system findings	Ref
Canada	H1N1 influenza	Elementary and high school absenteeism due to influenza-like illness exceeding the defined threshold of 10 % of total enrolment	Daily analysis of absenteeism, reporting if exceed threshold	Low – schools report data when indicator exceeds the threshold	Absenteeism was well correlated with hospitalisation rates for school age children and PCR positive tests for influenza. Peak absenteeism preceded peaks in hospitalisations by one week	[7]
United Kingdom	H1N1 influenza	School absenteeism in primary and secondary schools, comparing against telephone health hotline, general practitioner sentinel network & confirmed influenza data	Weekly mean percentage absenteeism	Low – collation of school % absenteeism data	Weekly school absenteeism peaked concomitantly with existing influenza alert systems, and would not have identified pandemic influenza earlier than other systems. Daily attendance data may have improved timeliness	[8]
Japan	Influenza	School influenza-related absenteeism, where child absent with confirmed diagnosis from physician	Daily school influenza-related absenteeism rate	Low – daily attendance routinely recorded and absent children require doctor's note	School influenza-related illness can be used to predict outbreaks and determine when a school should close to limit ongoing spread. Thresholds for influenza-related absenteeism proposed.	[9]
China (rural)	Respiratory infections, gastroenteritis	Symptoms reported at health clinics, over-the-counter drug sales at pharmacies and primary school absenteeism	Daily input to web-based system	High – collation and analysis of data at central level	Labour-intensive data entry to electronic system. Presentation of six months' pilot data, no validation of data from surveillance system against other sources	[11, 43]
Madagascar	Malaria, influenza, dengue, diarrhoeal disease	Malaria case confirmed by RDT, fever & respiratory symptoms, fever & 2 possible dengue symptoms, diarrhoea.	Daily report by encrypted SMS. Weekly summary paper report.	Moderate – SMS reports entered to database. Temporal & spatial analysis by syndrome	Ten cases of fever clusters occurred which weren't detected by the traditional surveillance system. Five outbreaks identified – two dengue, two influenza and one malaria.	[42]
French Guiana	Dengue	Dengue index: percentage of patients attending the emergency department who had thrombocytopenia but were negative for Plasmodium infection	Weekly generation of indicators	Low – plotting of simple indicators on weekly basis, minimal analysis	Dengue index was specific – increasing during what was confirmed to be a dengue epidemic, but showing no strong increase during two respiratory infection epidemics. Total emergency department attendance with thrombocytopenia but malaria negative was also a specific indicator.	[38]

Table 1 Selected syndromic surveillance systems reported in the literature: the setting, target diseases, indicators, system complexity and outcomes of their application. Reported studies are those which use school absenteeism as a key indicator, or systems applied in resource-limited settings for epidemic prone diseases including malaria (Continued)

Setting	Target diseases	Indicators	Reporting	System complexity	Outcomes / Application	Ref
Pacific island countries and territories	Measles, dengue, rubella, meningitis, leptospirosis, gastroenteritis, influenza, typhoid, malaria	Hospitals report total cases for four syndromes: acute fever & rash, diarrhoea, influenza-like illness, prolonged fever	Weekly reporting of data to national level	Moderate – data reported from national to WHO regional level for analysis	The system successfully identified an outbreak of diarrhoeal disease linked to breakdown of water disinfection, and two outbreaks of influenza. The system alert was timely and allowed fast implementation of control measures	[39]
India	Cholera, dysentery, malaria, measles, meningitis, typhoid fever, and 8 others	Suspected cases (clinical diagnosis) of target diseases from public and private health facilities, except malaria, where slide-confirmation required for reporting	As clinical cases identified (daily), using pre-formatted post cards with postage pre-paid	Low – doctors report cases on simple form to central level. Minimal analysis.	Several outbreaks were detected early and interventions applied, the most notable was cholera. Leptospirosis and acute dysentery also commonly reported. Monthly summary of reported diseases distributed to participating facilities for feedback and updates on the surveillance system.	[41]
Cambodia	Respiratory and diarrhoeal diseases	School absenteeism (aggregated daily by schools), compared against overall health facility attendance	Daily SMS report of school absenteeism due to illness, collated at weekly level for analysis	Low – daily data reported by schools to central level, compared against all cause health centre attendance	Illness-specific absenteeism identified two peaks in incidence of illness. Absenteeism data preceded peaks in health centre attendance by 0.5 weeks on average. Cross correlation analysis indicated moderate correlations between illness specific absenteeism and reference data.	[13]
Papua New Guinea	Influenza, cholera, typhoid, malaria, poliomyelitis, meningitis, measles, dengue	Syndromes relating to target diseases identified in patients presenting to health facilities.	Weekly report by mobile phone, transcription to database	Low – health facilities submit data for analysis at provincial/national level, and automatic generation of feedback reports	System was more sensitive than the reference system for measles, but low sensitivity for malaria, due to poor case definition. Data were more timely than the reference system (mean 2.4 weeks compared to 12 weeks lag)	[54]

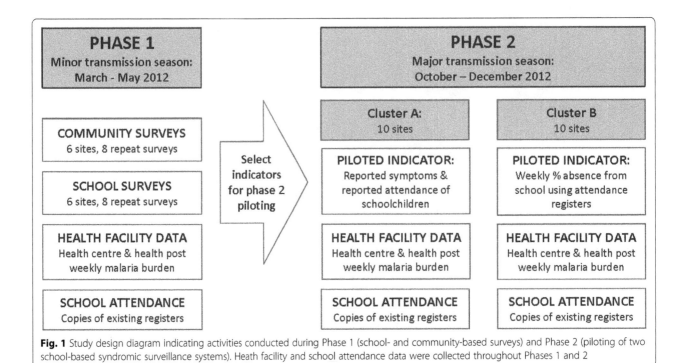

Fig. 1 Study design diagram indicating activities conducted during Phase 1 (school- and community-based surveys) and Phase 2 (piloting of two school-based syndromic surveillance systems). Heath facility and school attendance data were collected throughout Phases 1 and 2

(zones) (Fig. 2). This approach was used to reduce potential confusion between the two pilot methodologies by any zone health office staff supporting implementation. A one-day training event was held for three individuals from each site (the school director, a teacher and a representative from the woreda health office) on the relevant pilot methodology.

Piloted surveillance system methodology (Phase 2)

Cluster A sites used symptom questionnaires to investigate schoolchildren's reported recent fever, absenteeism due to illness and absenteeism for any reason. The symptom questionnaire was completed by a teacher every Monday, immediately after the attendance register. Each child was called in turn to the teacher's desk to respond to the questionnaire. The symptom questionnaire was restricted to grades two to four inclusive, since higher grades were unavailable due to exam preparations. Interviews were rotated weekly between grades to minimise disruption to normal teaching. The questionnaire included 10 symptoms (e.g. headache, cough, stomach ache), which were primarily included to mask fever as the symptom of interest; however, the additional symptoms could be of interest if the system was adopted with a remit including other epidemic-prone infectious diseases.

Cluster B sites were simply requested to use data recorded in their usual attendance registers to complete a weekly summary across all grades of the proportion absent, with total children enrolled multiplied by number of days attendance recorded as the denominator. At the end of the pilot period, copies of attendance registers were collected for validation purposes from a convenience sample of schools. Weekly health facility malaria data were also collected from 20 health centres and 20 health posts serving the Phase 2 study populations.

Data entry and analysis

Questionnaire data from Phase 1 surveys were entered into a customised Microsoft Access 2007 database with consistency and range checks. Microscopy results, health facility data and absenteeism extracted from attendance registers were entered into Microsoft Excel. Data were merged in Stata 12.0 (Stata Cooperation, College Station, Texas USA). Household coordinates for Phase 1 sites were imported into ArcMap 10.0 (Environmental Systems Research Institute Inc., Redlands, California USA) for display and calculation of Euclidean distance between household and school (at approximately 100 m resolution). Phase 2 data were entered into Excel spreadsheets and exported to Stata 12.0 for merging and analysis.

Analysis of Phase 1 data

The primary aim of Phase 1 analysis was to identify indicators which could be further piloted in Phase 2 school-based surveillance system, with secondary aims to determine the representativeness of the school-enrolled population compared to the wider community, and assess reported reasons for short-term absence from school.

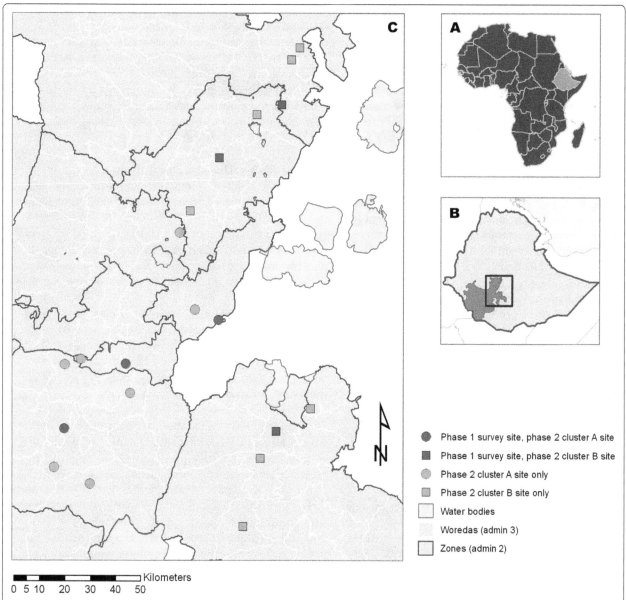

Fig. 2 Locator maps of Ethiopia (**a**) and SNNPRS (**b**), with a map of study kebele location (**c**) Six sites which were included in the Phase 1 school and community surveys as well as Phase 2 pilot are indicated by red markers, while the remaining 14 sites participating in Phase 2 pilots only are indicated by orange markers. Assignment to cluster A (symptom questionnaire) during Phase 2 is indicated by circular markers, assignment to cluster B (absenteeism estimated from attendance registers) is indicated by square markers

A wealth index was created using principal component analysis [49], at household level for community survey data and individual level for school survey data. Indicators associated with school enrolment reported during community surveys were assessed using binomial extension to generalised linear modelling at household level, with standard error estimates adjusted for clustering by study site. Mixed effects logistic regression was used to develop multivariate multilevel models describing risks of non-enrolment in school, with household-level and site-level random effects. A backward step-wise method was used to exclude the fixed effects in order of least

significance: a likelihood ratio test was used to re-test excluded variables for inclusion in the final model.

Analysis of Phase 2 data

Analysis of Phase 2 data focussed upon describing the characteristics of indicators collected at schools during the pilot. Box plots and logistic regression were used to describe absenteeism by grade over the study period. To explore dropout levels in these populations, mean absenteeism was evaluated by time. Accuracy of weekly summary absenteeism calculated by cluster B sites was determined by comparing teacher-generated summaries against the original registers.

Ethical considerations

Approval for this study was granted by the London School of Hygiene & Tropical Medicine ethical committee (6003) and the SNNPRS Health Research Ethics Review committee (P026-19/6157). Written, informed consent for participation of children in school surveys was collected from parents. Parents were free to withdraw consent at any time by informing the school director. Children were informed of the study procedures and their right to withdraw prior to random selection, and gave assent to take part. The head of household provided written consent for inclusion of household members in community survey, and verbal assent was sought from all household members before collection of blood samples.

A community health extension worker was present throughout school and community surveys. Participants with positive RDT were provided with treatment according to national guidelines: chloroquine for *P. vivax* and artemether-lumefantrine for *P. falciparum* or mixed infections.

Results

Population participating in Phase 1 school- and community-based surveys

RDT results were available from 4117 individuals participating in community surveys, aged from two months to 101 years (median 14 years). A total of 5189 school aged children participated in the school survey, with RDT results available from 5145 children (RDT data missing for 44 (0.8 %) of school children).

The prevalence of *Plasmodium* infection by RDT across all sites and survey iterations was 2.0 % (range

across site and survey iteration 0–12.3 %) for school surveys and 2.6 % (0–8.9 %) for community surveys. At any single site, the maximum difference in RDT prevalence over all survey visits was 7.6 %. Variation in both the prevalence of infection by RDT in school- and community-survey, as well as number of passively detected malaria cases at health facilities showed fluctuations during Phase 1, but no clear seasonal peak was observed (data not shown).

Reported primary school enrolment of school-aged children

School-aged children comprised 32.7 % of the population living in sampled households, and 54.0 % of these children (range by site 42–62 %) were reported by their head of household to be enrolled at the local primary school. From multivariate modelling, key risk factors for non-enrolment of school-aged children in school were the distance of the household from school, low household wealth, and the number of children of school age in the household (Table 2). Odds of enrolment also varied with education level of the head of household, with children from households where the head had attended any education having higher odds of school enrolment than those from households headed by an individual with no education.

Child-reported reasons for absence from school

Across all sites, 94 % of children reported usually attending school five days per week. Of all absences reported by children, 28 % were due to illness, while 67 % of absences were in order to assist in the home or with farming activities. Variations by site were seen, with two sites reporting the majority of absences being due to illness. Where children reported absence from school due to illness, fever was the most common symptom (88 %);

Table 2 Multivariate model of risk factors for non-enrolment of school-aged children (as reported by head of household during community survey)

	Odds ratio	95 % confidence interval	P
Age (increasing)	0.91	0.88, 0.95	<0.001
Number of children 7-16 years in household	1.20	1.08, 1.33	<0.001
Distance from school in km	1.57	1.30, 1.89	<0.001
Household wealth			
Poorest	1	-	-
Median	0.73	0.49, 1.10	0.132
Least poor	0.64	0.49, 0.84	0.001
Parental education			
None	1	-	-
Primary incomplete	0.66	0.51, 0.86	0.002
Primary complete or higher	0.64	0.42, 0.96	0.030

Fixed effects are presented, the multilevel model included random effects at household- and study-site level. Data were available from 1794 unique children and total 908 households, sampled from six sites in SNNPRS in 2012 however, only 50 % of those who reported fever as a reason for absence from school attended a health facility.

Phase 2 surveillance system pilot

Nine of the 10 cluster A schools submitted weekly summaries of the symptom and reported absence questionnaire. Schools collected the weekly indicators for a mean 11 weeks (range 6–14), overlapping with the peak transmission season from October to December. On average 68 children per school were interviewed each week (range 16–170). All ten cluster B schools submitted weekly estimates of absenteeism, calculated by summarising absent sessions recorded in attendance registers. Schools reported a mean 12 weeks of data (range 11–13). Schools summarised attendance for an average of 508 children each week (range 118 to 914).

In addition to the indicators collected from cluster A and B sites, available attendance registers were collected from a convenience sample of seven schools (five from cluster A and two from cluster B) for validation of weekly absenteeism in cluster B schools, and estimation of absenteeism in cluster A schools.

Absenteeism and drop-out recorded by school attendance registers

Weekly summary rates of absenteeism calculated from attendance registers were similar between classes within schools (data not shown). However, changes in proportion of enrolled children who are absent from school is expected to increase over the semester due to drop-out. Strong evidence for an increase in average weekly absenteeism was found when analysing grade total absenteeism

and allowing for clustering by school ($p = 0.008$). Absenteeism fluctuated on a weekly basis and varied by school, but showed an overall increase of 10 % during the study period.

Do syndromic surveillance indicators from schools correlate with health facility malaria trends?

Testing of the syndromic surveillance system was hampered by the lack of strong seasonal increase in malaria cases seen at the study sites during both Phases 1 and 2. Health facility data from all sites demonstrated weekly fluctuations in number of cases, but no clear peak in transmission and no epidemic during either the minor or major transmission seasons (Phase 1 and 2, respectively).

Few statistically significant correlations were seen between confirmed malaria at health facilities and the majority of the piloted indicators (i.e. child-reported fever, reported recent absence from school, absence from school due to illness, or teacher-summarised weekly absenteeism). There was evidence for an association between the proportion of child-days absent by week extracted from attendance registers collected for validation purposes and health facility total positive cases ($p = 0.002$) or RDT test positivity rate ($p = 0.028$). No evidence was found for an association between confirmed malaria at health facilities and teacher-summarised absenteeism from cluster B sites ($p = 0.197$, Fig. 3).

The difference in association with health facility data using absenteeism data from different sources may be a result of differences in malaria transmission levels between sites, with different locations contributing data to the attendance registers collected for validation purposes

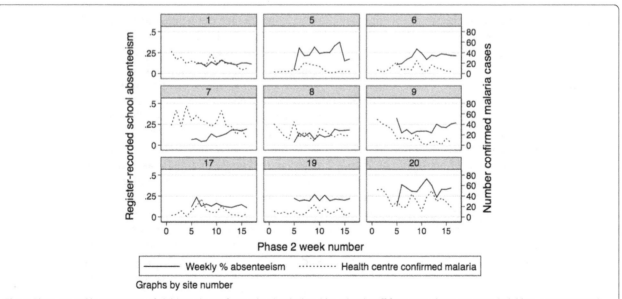

Fig. 3 Phase 2 weekly proportion of children absent from school, calculated by school staff from attendance registers (solid line, primary y-axis) and total confirmed malaria infections identified at local health centre by routine passive surveillance (dotted line, secondary y-axis)

from both clusters A and B, and the teacher-summarised data from cluster B sites only. There were insufficient data to conduct site-specific analysis to further investigate patterns associations between piloted indicators and health facility data at different transmission levels.

Discussion

This study is the first application of a surveillance system based on school absenteeism to the context of malaria epidemic early warning in a resource-poor setting. The study hypothesised that school attendance could act as a surrogate indicator of sudden increases in malaria burden or other infectious disease epidemics at community-level. However, during both the first and second phases of the study no seasonal peaks in malaria were observed from passive case detection at health facilities or cross-sectional survey RDT prevalence. Consequently, the majority of absences from school were reported to be not due to illness, and it was not possible to rigorously assess the study's primary hypothesis.

In Phase 1 of the study, enrolment of school aged children was found to be lower than expected, although those who were enrolled attended routinely. At schools, collection of daily attendance occurs routinely, and schools were able to generate accurate weekly summary indicators to describe absenteeism. An alternative approach where teachers interview their pupils to answer simple questions on recent illness and absence was also completed but it was found to be less feasible for scale-up due to the time required for interviews. While this study demonstrated that school absenteeism is a feasible indicator for weekly collection and could supplement existing health system surveillance, this approach is likely to be less representative in locations with low primary school enrolment, particularly if there are common risk factors for non-enrolment and exposure to malaria.

School enrolment

Our study found primary enrolment to be substantially lower than reported in national level data (42–62 % by site compared to 79 % national net enrolment in 2012 [24]). Our data concur with previous findings indicating that household wealth, education of household head and age of the child are associated with enrolment of children in primary school [50]. We found that the odds of enrolment were reduced with increasing number of school-aged children in the household, and increasing distance between household and school. Considering that universal enrolment and attendance at primary school has yet to be achieved in Ethiopia, it is likely that the sensitivity of a school-based syndromic surveillance system is reduced, since the whole community will not be captured at a school-level platform. Further piloting

of school-based syndromic surveillance approaches is recommended in areas of higher primary school enrolment, where sensitivity will be improved.

School absenteeism

Absence in schools can be classified as temporary or permanent (i.e. dropout). Illness was the second most commonly reported reason for temporary absence, but the most common reason was to assist with chores in the home or farm. Absence due to economic activities, attending market and lack of school materials were infrequently reported. Food insecurity has also been shown to be a determinant of school absenteeism and attainment in Ethiopia [51], and was a contributing factor to the severity of previous malaria epidemics in East Africa [20]. While the shift system used in many rural primary schools allows children to balance their schooling with farming, herding or domestic chores [52], it remains likely that school absenteeism will increase during periods of peak agricultural activity. Weekly absenteeism calculated from attendance registers was found to be similar across grades, and absenteeism could therefore be monitored from any grade as part of future implementation of the surveillance system.

While absence due to illness may be an intuitively more sensitive indicator for malaria surveillance, all-cause absenteeism is a more reliable indicator to collect on a daily basis. It is not feasible in this setting to trace a sibling, neighbour or parent to find out the reason for absence on their first missed day of school, unless a sibling attends the same class. It is not currently routine practice for schools in SNNPRS to record the reason for absence. This approach differs from school-based syndromic surveillance approaches in higher income countries, where reasons for absence can be rapidly determined by contacting parents by telephone.

The Ministry of Education target drop-out rate for the academic year 2010/11 of 8 %, but actual drop-out rate was 13 % [45]. Drop-out of approximately 10 % over the semester was observed at the study sites. While reasons for drop-out were not specifically investigated in the current study, drop-out can either be due to relatively stable factors such as number of children under five years in the household [53], as well as by economic shocks such as drought, crop failures, death and illness of family members [45].

Benefits and drawbacks of the piloted system

Identification of valid indicators for piloting was limited by inclusion of only six sites in Phase 1 and the low malaria transmission experienced in SNNPRS in 2012. The study was also limited by inability to provide a formal sample size calculation for the comparisons we sought to undertake, due to lack of data describing changes in these indicators during normal and abnormal transmissions seasons.

Of the two piloted syndromic surveillance systems, monitoring school absenteeism is a less time-intensive activity than weekly completion of symptom questionnaires. Consequently, we propose absenteeism to be a more feasible indicator for long-term implementation. Absenteeism is routinely recorded and generation of a weekly absenteeism total is a simple addition to existing responsibilities for school staff. Registers in use were found to often not be standardised, with limited validation of class registers by senior staff since registers are often stored in teachers' homes. For any future school absenteeism-based surveillance system, it is recommended to roll-out standard register formats and symbols for recording pupils' daily presence and absence, as well as regular checking and feedback on attendance register completion by senior staff.

Differences in "normal" absenteeism rates between schools would likely remain due to systematic differences in populations across epidemic-prone areas. The usefulness of the system would be dependent on motivation of the school director and teachers to collect and assess absenteeism data, and report to health extension workers when increases occur. No thresholds would be assigned to schools, but it would be the responsibility of the school director to determine when absenteeism becomes unusual and to alert the health extension workers.

Syndromic surveillance systems in high-income countries generally use electronic data capture or web-based systems to collate reported and existing data for analysis [7, 8, 30, 31]. While low- and middle-income countries are increasingly adopting web-based or SMS technology, the current pilot did not require data to be reported upwards, and therefore these technology solutions were not required. Instead of submitting data to a central level for analysis and then response, the aim was to create simple indicators which would allow an alert to be passed from school to community health extension worker of possible increases in illness in the community. This information would then act as a prompt for the health extension worker to review their recent case data, or to conduct active surveillance in targeted areas of the kebele. While this system has low specificity, it builds upon existing links at community level between the school and health extension workers, through the kebele committee's weekly meetings to discuss local issues, and may prove more sustainable in the long-term than any surveillance system requiring data to be reported upwards for analysis and feedback. The lack of strict thresholds to generate an alert from school data also allows flexibility to respond to rumours and local opinion, and could also capture non-malaria epidemics. Health extension workers routinely spend a proportion

of their time making home visits in the kebele, and it is credible that intelligence from the syndromic surveillance system may allow targeting of home visits at the sub-kebele level to areas of highest absenteeism.

Conclusions

In the current study, the lack of any malaria epidemic or strong seasonal peak in malaria transmission during the data collection period at the study sites prevented evaluation of the performance of a school-based syndromic surveillance system for malaria epidemic detection, resulting in inconclusive findings.

School-based surveillance approaches are limited by drop-out during the academic year and low rates of enrolment. Implementing a system without fixed thresholds for alert generation, and relying on subjective identification of "unusual" increases by school staff is one approach to avoid bias due to drop-out. Low school enrolment is a major limitation of the piloted surveillance system, and further investigation is required to assess if there are common risk factors for non-enrolment and malaria, and the extent to which this may reduce the sensitivity of school-based surveillance.

This syndromic surveillance approach could be further refined by piloting in malaria endemic or epidemic-risk settings with high primary school enrolment. Adapting the system to report absenteeism data by mobile phone to the local health facility or a central automated system combining syndromic and clinical data is an alternative approach to generate alerts. Mobile technology could also enable regular feedback to schools on the malaria situation in the wider area, or facilitate behaviour change communication messaging to pupils. Regardless of the data collation mechanism, piloting during a strong seasonal increase in malaria transmission or an epidemic would likely be required to demonstrate the sensitivity of a syndromic surveillance approach.

Competing interest
The authors declare that they have no competing interest.

Authors' contributions
The study was conceived and designed by RAA, TK, GT, SC, RR and SB. Data were collected by RA, TK, EB, TA, ZK and TM. Data were analysed by RA. RA and SB prepared the first draft of the manuscript. All authors reviewed and approved the final version of the manuscript.

Acknowledgements
The authors would like to thank the SNNPRS Regional Health Bureau, and woreda health offices for their collaboration on the study. We also wish to thank the school directors, teachers, parents and children, as well as the wider communities, for their time and participation. We thank the survey teams for their commitment to completing school and community surveys, often in challenging environmental conditions.
This work was funded by a Cooperative Agreement (663-A-00-09-00404-00) from the U.S. Agency for International Development under the President's Malaria Initiative to Malaria Consortium. Simon Brooker is supported by a Wellcome Trust Senior Fellowship in Basic Biomedical Science (098045). Ruth Ashton receives additional support from the John-Henry Memorial Foundation. The opinions expressed herein are those of the authors and do not necessarily reflect the views of the authors' employing organisations.

Author details

[1]Malaria Consortium, London, UK. [2]Faculty of Infectious and Tropical Diseases, London School of Hygiene & Tropical Medicine, London, UK. [3]Malaria Consortium Ethiopia, Addis Ababa, Ethiopia. [4]Malaria Consortium Southern Nations, Nationalities and People's Regional State sub-office, Hawassa, Ethiopia. [5]Southern Nations, Nationalities and People's Regional State Health Bureau, Hawassa, Ethiopia. [6]President's Malaria Initiative, U.S. Agency for International Development, Addis Ababa, Ethiopia. [7]RTI International, Washington, DC, USA.

References

1. Abeku T, Van Oortmarssen GJ, Borsboom G, De Vlas SJ, Habbema JDF. Spatial and temporal variations of malaria epidemic risk in Ethiopia: factors involved and implications. Acta Trop. 2003;87:331–40.

2. Mutonga D, Langat D, Mwangi D, Tonui J, Njeru M, Abade A, et al. National surveillance data on the epidemiology of cholera in Kenya, 1997-2010. J Infect Dis. 2013;208 Suppl 1:S55–61.

3. Halperin SA, Bettinger JA, Greenwood B, Harrison LH, Jelfs J, Ladhani SN, et al. The changing and dynamic epidemiology of meningococcal disease. Vaccine. 2012;30 Suppl 2:B26–36.

4. Racloz V, Ramsey R, Tong S, Hu W. Surveillance of dengue fever virus: a review of epidemiological models and early warning systems. PLoS Negl Trop Dis. 2012;6, e1648.

5. Last JM. A Dictionary of Epidemiology. 4th ed. New York: Oxford University Press; 2001.

6. Najera JA. Prevention and control of malaria epidemics. Parassitologia. 1999; 41:339–47.

7. Kom Mogto CA, De Serres G, Douville Fradet M, Lebel G, Toutant S, Gilca R, et al. School absenteeism as an adjunct surveillance indicator: experience during the second wave of the 2009 H1N1 pandemic in Quebec, Canada. PLoS One. 2012;7, e34084.

8. Kara EO, Elliot AJ, Bagnall H, Foord DG, Pnaiser R, Osman H, et al. Absenteeism in schools during the 2009 influenza A(H1N1) pandemic: a useful tool for early detection of influenza activity in the community? Epidemiol Infect. 2012;140:1328–36.

9. Sasaki A, Hoen AG, Ozonoff A, Suzuki H, Tanabe N, Seki N, et al. Evidence-based tool for triggering school closures during influenza outbreaks, Japan. Emerg Infect Dis. 2009;15:1841–3.

10. Besculides M, Heffernan R, Mostashari F, Weiss D. Evaluation of school absenteeism data for early outbreak detection, New York City. BMC Public Health. 2005;5:105.

11. Yan W, Palm L, Lu X, Nie S, Xu B, Zhao Q, et al. ISS–an electronic syndromic surveillance system for infectious disease in rural China. PLoS One. 2013;8:e62749.

12. Fan Y, Yang M, Jiang H, Wang Y, Yang W, Zhang Z, et al. Estimating the effectiveness of early control measures through school absenteeism surveillance in observed outbreaks at rural schools in Hubei, China. PLoS One. 2014;9:e106856.

13. Cheng CKY, Channarith H, Cowling BJ. Potential use of school absenteeism record for disease surveillance in developing countries, case study in Cambodia. PLoS One. 2013;8, e76859.

14. Some ES. Effects and control of highland malaria epidemic in Uasin Gishu District, Kenya. East Afr Med J. 1994;71:2–8.

15. Fontaine RE, Najjar AE, Prince JS. The 1958 malaria epidemic in Ethiopia. Am J Trop Med Hyg. 1961;10:795–803.

16. President's Malaria Initiative. Malaria Operational Plan for Ethiopia FY2015. In.; 2014.

17. World Health Organization. Systems for the early detection of malaria epidemics in Africa. An analysis of current practices and future priorities. In.; 2006: 108.

18. Federal Democratic Republic of Ethiopia MoH. Guidelines for malaria epidemic prevention and control in Ethiopia. 3rd edition: Addis Ababa, Ethiopia; 2009.

19. Jima D, Wondabeku M, Alemu A, Teferra A, Awel N, Deressa W, et al. Analysis of malaria surveillance data in Ethiopia: what can be learned from the integrated disease surveillance and response system? Malar J. 2012;11:330.

20. Checchi F, Cox J, Balkan S, Tamrat A, Priotto G, Alberti KP, et al. Malaria epidemics and interventions, Kenya, Burundi, southern Sudan, and Ethiopia, 1999-2004. Emerg Infect Dis. 2006;12:1477–85.

21. Brown V, Abdir Issak M, Rossi M, Barboza P, Paugam A. Epidemic of malaria in north-eastern Kenya. Lancet. 1998;352:1356–7.

22. Negash K, Kebede A, Medhin A, Argaw D, Babaniyi O, Guintran JO, et al. Malaria epidemics in the highlands of Ethiopia. East Afr Med J. 2005;82:186–92.

23. Tanner M, Greenwood B, Whitty CJ, Ansah EK, Price RN, Dondorp AM, et al. Malaria eradication and elimination: views on how to translate a vision into reality. BMC Med. 2015;13:167.

24. World Development Indicators: primary school enrollment [http://data.worldbank.org/indicator/SE.PRM.NENR] (2013). Accessed 30 Dec 2015.

25. Stevenson JC, Stresman GH, Gitonga CW, Gillig J, Owaga C, Marube E, et al. Reliability of school surveys in estimating geographic variation in malaria transmission in the western Kenyan highlands. PLoS One. 2013;8:e77641.

26. Baliraine FN, Afrane YA, Amenya DA, Bonizzoni M, Menge DM, Zhou G, et al. High prevalence of asymptomatic Plasmodium falciparum infections in a highland area of western Kenya: a cohort study. J Infect Dis. 2009;200:66–74.

27. Ogutu B, Tiono AB, Makanga M, Premji Z, Gbadoe AD, Ubben D, et al. Treatment of asymptomatic carriers with artemether-lumefantrine: an opportunity to reduce the burden of malaria? Malar J. 2010;9:30.

28. Okell LC, Bousema T, Griffin JT, Ouedraogo AL, Ghani AC, Drakeley CJ. Factors determining the occurrence of submicroscopic malaria infections and their relevance for control. Nat Commun. 2012;3:1237.

29. Henning KJ. What is syndromic surveillance? MMWR Morb Mortal Wkly Rep. 2004;53(Suppl):5–11.

30. Enserink R, Noel H, Friesema IH, de Jager CM, Kooistra-Smid AM, Kortbeek LM, et al. The KIzSS network, a sentinel surveillance system for infectious diseases in day care centers: study protocol. BMC Infect Dis. 2012;12:259.

31. Andersson T, Bjelkmar P, Hulth A, Lindh J, Stenmark S, Widerstrom M. Syndromic surveillance for local outbreak detection and awareness: evaluating outbreak signals of acute gastroenteritis in telephone triage, web-based queries and over-the-counter pharmacy sales. Epidemiol Infect. 2013;142:303-13.

32. Bounoure F, Beaudeau P, Mouly D, Skiba M, Lahiani-Skiba M. Syndromic surveillance of acute gastroenteritis based on drug consumption. Epidemiol Infect. 2011;139:1388–95.

33. Patwardhan A, Bilkovski R. Comparison: Flu prescription sales data from a retail pharmacy in the US with Google Flu trends and US ILINet (CDC) data as flu activity indicator. PLoS One. 2012;7:e43611.

34. Signorini A, Segre AM, Polgreen PM. The use of Twitter to track levels of disease activity and public concern in the U.S. during the influenza A H1N1 pandemic. PLoS One. 2011;6:e19467.

35. Chunara R, Andrews JR, Brownstein JS. Social and news media enable estimation of epidemiological patterns early in the 2010 Haitian cholera outbreak. Am J Trop Med Hyg. 2012;86:39–45.

36. Broniatowski DA, Paul MJ, Dredze M. National and local influenza surveillance through Twitter: An analysis of the 2012-2013 influenza epidemic. PLoS One. 2013;8, e83672.

37. Mook P, Joseph C, Gates P, Phin N. Pilot scheme for monitoring sickness absence in schools during the 2006/07 winter in England: can these data be used as a proxy for influenza activity? Euro Surveill. 2007;12:E11–2.

38. Carme B, Sobesky M, Biard MH, Cotellon P, Aznar C, Fontanella JM. Non-specific alert system for dengue epidemic outbreaks in areas of endemic malaria. A hospital-based evaluation in Cayenne (French Guiana). Epidemiol Infect. 2003;130:93–100.

39. Kool JL, Paterson B, Pavlin BI, Durrheim D, Musto J, Kolbe A. Pacific-wide simplified syndromic surveillance for early warning of outbreaks. Glob Public Health. 2012;7:670–81.

40. Durrheim DN, Harris BN, Speare R, Billinghurst K. The use of hospital-based nurses for the surveillance of potential disease outbreaks. Bull World Health Organ. 2001;79:22–7.

41. John TJ, Rajappan K, Arjunan KK. Communicable diseases monitored by disease surveillance in Kottayam district, Kerala state, India. Indian J Med Res. 2004;120:86–93.

42. Randrianasolo L, Raoelina Y, Ratsitorahina M, Ravolomanana L, Andriamandimby S, Heraud JM, et al. Sentinel surveillance system for early outbreak detection in Madagascar. BMC Public Health. 2010;10:31.

43. Yan WR, Nie SF, Xu B, Dong HJ, Palm L, Diwan VK. Establishing a web-based integrated surveillance system for early detection of infectious disease epidemic in rural China: a field experimental study. BMC Med Inform Decis Mak. 2012;12:4.

44. Federal Democratic Republic of Ethiopia MoH. Health Sector Development Program IV, 2010/11 - 2014/15. Final draft. In.; 2010.

45. Woldehanna T, Hagos A. Shocks and Primary School Drop-out Rates: A Study of 20 Sentinel Sites in Ethiopia. In.: Young Lives, Oxford Department of International Development, Oxford University; 2012.

46. Malaria Indicator Survey [http://www.malariasurveys.org/toolkit.cfm]. Accessed 30 Dec 2015.

47. Ashton RA, Kefyalew T, Tesfaye G, Pullan RL, Yadeta D, Reithinger R, et al. School-based surveys of malaria in Oromia Regional State, Ethiopia: a rapid survey method for malaria in low transmission settings. Malar J. 2011;10:25.

48. Gitonga CW, Karanja PN, Kihara J, Mwanje M, Juma E, Snow RW, et al. Implementing school malaria surveys in Kenya: towards a national surveillance system. Malar J. 2010;9:306.

49. Filmer D, Pritchett LH. Estimating wealth effects without expenditure data–or tears: an application to educational enrollments in states of India. Demography. 2001;38:115–32.

50. Admassu KA. Primary school enrollment and dropout in Ethiopia: Household and school factors. In: Population Association of America 2011 Annual Meeting. Washington D.C, USA; 2011.

51. Belachew T, Hadley C, Lindstrom D, Gebremariam A, Lachat C, Kolsteren P. Food insecurity, school absenteeism and educational attainment of adolescents in Jimma Zone Southwest Ethiopia: a longitudinal study. Nutr J. 2011;10:29.

52. Pereznieto P, Jones N. Young Lives Policy Brief 2. Educational Choices in Ethiopia: what determines whether poor children go to school? In: Young Lives. Oxford, UK; 2006: 12.

53. Woldehanna T, Jones N, Tefera B. Children's Educational Completion Rates and Achievement: Implications for Ethiopia's Second Poverty Reduction Strategy (2006-10). In: Young Lives Working Paper 18. Oxford: Young Lives; 2005.

54. Rosewell A, Ropa B, Randall H, Dagina R, Hurim S, Bieb S, et al. Mobile phone-based syndromic surveillance system, Papua New Guinea. Emerg Infect Dis. 2013;19:1811–8.

12

Complexity in simulation-based education: exploring the role of hindsight bias

Al Motavalli[1*] and Debra Nestel[2]

Abstract

Simulation-based education (SBE) has the potential to misrepresent clinical practice as relatively simplistic, and as being made safer through simplistic behavioural explanations. This review provides an overview of a well-documented and robust psychological construct - *hindsight bias* in the context of learning in healthcare simulations. Motivating this review are our observations that post-simulation debriefings may be oversimplified and *biased* by knowledge of scenario outcomes. Sometimes only limited consideration is given to issues that might be relevant to management in the complexity and uncertainty of real clinical practice. We use literature on *hindsight bias* to define the concept, inputs and implications. We offer examples from SBE where hindsight bias may occur and propose suggestions for mitigation. Influences of hindsight biases on SBE should be addressed by future studies.

Background

Hindsight bias can be defined as the tendency to overestimate the foreseeability, inevitability, or likelihood of outcomes after they become manifest and known [1, 2]. This can systematically influence perceptions of past events [1, 2], and therefore potentially the processes of reflection, debriefing, and learning. Debriefing that includes a deliberate re-examination of simulation experiences is established practice [3–6], and studies have investigated methods of promoting learners' reflections [7, 8]. However, the potential influences of hindsight bias on the nature of reflective processes in this context are unknown, as there is a gap in the literature exploring this issue [9]. The purpose of this commentary is to review hindsight bias in simulation-based education (SBE).

Using a vignette, the review explores our notion that debriefing is sometimes oversimplified and biased by outcome knowledge. We have observed that on occasion only limited consideration is given to potentially relevant issues related to the complexities of clinical practice. Often entailing multiple, dynamic, and sometimes conflicting demands and goals, clinical practice is complex. Such demands and goals are context-dependent, and exist under conditions of variable time pressure. We describe features of the hindsight bias literature,

* Correspondence: al@myanaesthetist.com.au
[1]Department of Anaesthesia, The Royal Victorian Eye & Ear Hospital, 32 Gisborne St, East Melbourne, VIC 3002, Australia
Full list of author information is available at the end of the article

including the broad empirical support base, and the types of populations and contexts where hindsight bias has been investigated. The potential relevance and implications of hindsight bias to SBE are then examined and strategies to mitigate their impact offered.

Simulation-based education for complex clinical practice

When conducting or observing debriefings, there are occasions where it might be suitable to explore a broad range of factors related to how and why learners managed a simulation scenario the way they did, in the face of uncertainty and complexity. After all, management in the context of uncertainty and complexity is surely an indisputable feature of clinical practice. However, it is our experience that when examining past simulation events (debriefing), there is a tendency for facilitators and learners to construct and accept very simplified explanations for actions and occurrences. These explanations seem to fail to account for the complexity encountered by participants in the simulation.

The vignette in Box 1 is used to illustrate relevant concepts. The situation is likely to resonate with many facilitators during debriefing. A timely call for assistance can have significant implications to patient morbidity and mortality, and may therefore be considered an important learning point [10]. As learners demonstrate this step in subsequent simulations, often immediately prompted by any sign of patient deterioration, it is reasonable to think that this learning point was successfully processed. The

Box 1 Vignette of an inter-professional simulation

An inter-professional high-fidelity crisis simulation session was conducted with a group of senior medical and nursing students.

The learning objectives were to:
- Demonstrate management of a deteriorating ward patient
- Demonstrate advanced life support
- Demonstrate crisis resource management skills

The scenario involved a ward patient who is complaining of nausea and dizziness, but with normal vital signs. This was initially conducted with one medical and one nursing student.

During the first few minutes of the simulation, the medical student carried out initial diagnostic and therapeutic interventions with the assistance of the nursing student.

When the patient's blood pressure dropped mildly, the students made intensive efforts to quickly establish intravenous access and set up intravenous fluids.

The medical student stated that he was unsure about the diagnosis and he re-examined the patient. The patient's blood pressure briefly improved, but then rapidly declined and he progressed to cardiac arrest.

After the cardiac arrest was diagnosed, the medical student requested that the nursing student leave to call for help.

Resuscitation activities initially appeared to be very challenging in the face of limited human resources.

During debriefing in a separate room with all students present and watching, the facilitator used video playback to replay the scenario up to and including the initial cardiac arrest management.

The facilitator asked the lead medical student participant to discuss their experience. The student stated that he should have requested for extra assistance much earlier, as this would have helped with the arrest resuscitation.

The facilitator agreed, and in the subsequent discussion, several of the other simulation participants stated that they would call for help early in future.

decision to call for help is likely to be embedded within a range of potential concerns faced by practitioners in the moment during a clinical situation. These may include assessing and managing the patient's immediate condition, resolving diagnostic dilemmas, prioritising tasks and deciding when and where to allocate scarce human resources. Further, they are to be accomplished when the trajectory of the patient's progress is uncertain and *unknown*.

In the face of such a situation, the judgement of when to relinquish immediately valuable and limited human resources to call for help is unlikely to be a clear and easy one. A learner who is overwhelmed with negotiating competing demands and goals might even overlook the decision-making step of seeking extra assistance for a prolonged period of time. This picture of context-specific complexity contrasts sharply with that of relative simplicity made with hindsight during the debriefing described in our vignette.

In light of knowledge that the patient progressed to cardiac arrest, it is possible to look back at the simulation and conclude that calling for help early was obvious and would have avoided challenges encountered with

the arrest resuscitation. It might also seem that this learning point is simply and easily transferable to the management of future situations in practice. These conclusions, however, fail to address the practical issue of how the participants are to go about recognising and resolving this decision-making step amongst a number of other potential issues, particularly when the patient's progress will *not* be readily foreseeable.

Debriefing discourse of learners and facilitators often simplifies the examination of past events, and in a way that is influenced by the knowledge of actual outcomes of the simulation. Specifically, this simplification leads to appraisals of actions made in light of simulation outcomes, even though these outcomes may not have necessarily eventuated from the same set of antecedent events, and could not have necessarily been foreseeable by learners within the simulation. In the vignette, the patient condition may not have progressed to cardiac arrest, and intense management efforts made by the two learners may have delayed or even prevented deterioration. From this perspective, which does not assume the inevitability of the patient progressing to cardiac arrest, the decision of when to call for help becomes less obvious. By calling for help early in future simulations, participants might be demonstrating that they have learned management for simulation rather than for clinical practice.

If simplification as described earlier might limit the learning that occurs for complex clinical practice, then this may have consequences for patient management and safety. *Why is it that simplification occurs and is evident in both facilitators and learners?* Fenwick and Dahlgren have recently noted limitations in SBE highlighting *complexity theory* as a means to "make visible important material dynamics, and their problematic consequences, that are not often *noticed* in simulated experiences..."(Fenwick & Dahlgren 2015, p. 359; emphasis added) [11]. That is, they acknowledge not only the interpersonal relationships of those involved in the simulation but confer at least equal power on the environment and other artefacts shaping behaviours. We propose *hindsight bias* as one possible answer to this question.

Review strategy

We searched the databases of PsychINFO, PubMed, ERIC, CINAHL plus, Web of Science, and SCOPUS using the terms: 'hindsight bias' AND 'simulation' – no articles dedicated to exploring hindsight bias in SBE were found. The same databases were searched with the terms: 'hindsight bias' AND 'reflection' – only one relevant empirical study was found. The same databases were then searched with the term: 'hindsight bias', which generated 763 unique articles. Of these, two recent articles had an explicit aim to review and synthesise the hindsight bias literature [2, 12]. These were selected for outlining definitions, inputs and implications of hindsight bias. Further details on selected topics were found by searching for articles with: 'specific term' (e.g., video) AND 'hindsight bias' in the same databases. Additionally, the references of articles were used to identify relevant articles. All databases were searched on September 1 2014. Cognitive psychology books were also used.

Cognitive biases and hindsight bias: definitions and consequences

Cognitive psychology describes cognitive biases as mental processes, that lead to systematic deviations in judgement from a norm [13]. A norm in this case, *"reflects what should be the outcome of a task carried out rationally or in a manner suitable to the situation at hand"* (Caverni et al. 1990, p.8) [13]. So using the vignette, an assertion could be made that a 'rational' and 'suitable' re-examination of the simulation includes an articulation and exploration of several factors and conditions related to management in the face of complexity and uncertainty as experienced by practitioners in the moment. This would contrast with a re-examination that offers a single cause and effect explanation or one that supports a potentially unforeseeable outcome.

Cognitive biases are considered to be unconscious, automatic, mental processing strategies, which have evolved as adaptive mechanisms to simplify complex information inputs, yet as a result, lead to biased judgements and inferences [14]. Additionally, individuals lack awareness for how these biases might impact their perception. That is, they do not realise that their judgements are biased [15]. Hindsight bias belongs to a group of biases where simplification involves a mental emphasis on factors that confirm or support a known outcome, while diminishing the significance of those identifiable factors that may favour potentially different or even contradictory outcomes [12]. Biases clearly do not prevent valuable reflective judgements and learning processes from occurring. The key issue is that with the tendency for *simplification* of this nature, the judgements and inferences are necessarily limited and biased. In SBE, this might have implications for what aspects of the simulation facilitators and learners *notice* and focus on, and hence possibly the scope and nature of learning opportunities that might be derived from reflecting.

In their review of the hindsight bias literature, Roese and Vohs summarised two important consequences of hindsight bias [2].

1. The first consequence is the construction and focus on unitary or limited causal narratives for explaining past events in relation to known outcomes, particularly with attribution of responsibility given to those most proximal to a particular outcome [2, 16, 17]. Thus hindsight bias leads to simple causal explanations that link to a manifest outcome, even though such explanations may be flawed [2]. Some empirical studies demonstrate hindsight bias occurrence depends on a plausible cause being identified and linked to an outcome [18, 19]. This feature of hindsight bias resonates with our experience of the explanations of simulation events found in debriefing discourse. In the vignette, the construction and acceptance of a simple causal link between a late call for help by the lead participant, and the difficult arrest resuscitation illustrates this point.

2. The second consequence is overconfidence in analysing and performing in similar future situations [2, 20]. This is thought due to hindsight bias minimising detailed scrutiny of past personal performances, leading to a false sense of heightened self-belief for future performance [2]. It may lead to a failure to appreciate and address the breadth and depth of factors at play when making similar future decisions – with potentially hazardous consequences. Using the vignette, the learners may be confident that they have learned to appropriately call for help early in future. However, they might fail to do so if they do not recognise the conditions that may or may not favour such an intervention in the clinical context. For example, a more explicit reflection upon conditions such as the concurrent presence of diagnostic uncertainty, vital sign changes and the limited number of novice practitioners, may support learners to quickly recognise similar conditions and act by calling for help early.

Hindsight bias empirical evidence and investigation in other contexts

In contrast with other potentially relevant cognitive bias constructs, an extensive literature base supports hindsight bias. A recent psychology review identified over 800 published articles on this bias [2]. Cognitive psychology researchers describe hindsight bias as a 'robust' phenomenon - that is, observable under a wide variety of experimental conditions [12, 21–23]. It has been measured and demonstrated across age groups [21, 24], and in different cultures [25, 26]. It has been investigated in a variety of domains, including legal decision-making [27], medical diagnosis and malpractice claims [28–30], forecasting in finance [31], elections [32], consumer satisfaction studies [33], and accident investigations [34]. Safety experts have frequently cited hindsight bias as a barrier to acknowledging complexity and foreseeability issues in relation to analysing accident investigations - this can lead to investigation reports that may not maximise learning to improve future safety [35–38]. In some of these contexts, implications also extend to consequences regarding the attribution of blame or negligence.

One article was found that studied the effect of hindsight bias in relation to nurses' reflective practices. Nurses were asked to read the same written clinical vignette describing a patient's clinical presentation, with or without a final physician statement offering a single likely patient diagnosis (either the correct diagnosis, or one from a limited set of incorrect differentials). This physician statement was considered to represent outcome knowledge. All nurses were then asked to select what they considered to be the most likely patient diagnosis from a list that included the correct diagnosis and the limited set of incorrect differentials. Although the study suggested that nurses who were provided with a final physician statement tended to exhibit hindsight bias for the offered diagnosis, whether it was correct or not, it was acknowledged that nurses might have actually supported that diagnosis because it was stated to have come from a physician.

Hindsight bias inputs and managing its influences

A greater understanding of hindsight bias might be gained through a brief exploration of its inputs, and this might also suggest potential targets for practice and research. Cognitive and metacognitive processes, rather than motivational ones, are considered to represent the most important factors in producing and modifying hindsight bias [2, 12]. Roese & Vohs [2] categorised three main cognitive memory inputs and described one metacognitive contributor:

1. *Recollection:* If memories cannot be clearly and accurately recalled, people tend to articulate distorted 'memories' that link closely with known outcomes. This is considered to be a minor effect in comparison to other inputs.
2. *Belief updating:* When presented with new information, there tends to be automatic integration with existing memory structures such that memories most consistent with this information are reinforced, and less congruous ones minimised [39, 40].
3. *Sense-making:* Simple, coherent, linear explanations of outcomes in relation to antecedent events provoke a sense of clear inevitability, and increase hindsight bias [41].
4. *Metacognitive contributions:* The apparent subjective ease with which we are able to form or process a particular explanation is found to strengthen its acceptability and increase hindsight bias. This is

thought to be one mechanism by which playing video representations of past events has been demonstrated to increase hindsight bias. This is thought to result from the depiction of past events in clear continuity with their outcomes.

Because it is considered an automatic and unconscious process, hindsight bias influences have proven to be extremely difficult to eliminate [42]. Simply having knowledge that hindsight bias exists has not been demonstrated to reduce it [43]. Currently, the only empirically supported strategy that has consistently demonstrated hindsight bias reduction is the use of *counterfactual explanations* [44–48]. 'Counterfactual' means contrary to facts [49]. This involves the deliberate formulation of explanations for how *potential* alternative outcomes could have eventuated from the same *actual* antecedent events. Conversely, it can also involve constructing explanations for how certain *actual* outcomes could have come about as a result of different *potential* antecedent events. Experts consider it effective to use at most two to three counterfactual explanations, as generating more could increase hindsight bias, by making it subjectively difficult from a metacognitive point of view [2, 50].

In the vignette, rather than simply being designated a consequence of oversight or error, the delayed call for assistance 'outcome' could be reformulated to be a function of diverted attention toward immediate diagnosis and management. These immediate and intense management efforts can also be articulated as having had the purpose and potential to minimise patient deterioration. This plausible counterfactual explanation offers a *potential* alternative outcome (of delaying or preventing deterioration) for the same *actual* antecedent events (initial management actions). After acknowledging this complexity and uncertainty, a discussion may then follow which includes an appraisal of the *conditions* that did or did not favour an earlier call for help, and how these might be recognised and acted upon in a timely manner in future.

Potential implications of hindsight bias to learning and simulation practices

Experiential learning theories share learner *reflection* of an experience as a key stage of the learning process, whereby a learner needs to "...recapture, notice and re-evaluate their experience, to work with their experience, to turn it into learning" (Boud et al. 1993, p. 9) [51]. A number of complex contextual factors might interact and influence the learner's reflective process, including, but not limited to those related to the learner, the facilitator, the simulation design and so forth. Clearly then, hindsight bias is only one such factor that might modify this process alongside others. However, despite the potential complexity related to reflective processes and judgement formation, hindsight bias does have a strong empirical basis and has been demonstrated to be *robust*. There is compelling reason to suggest that it also has relevance in SBE, even if these involve variable and unique contexts and conditions. As such, further investigation seems warranted. Additionally, unlike other disciplines, in SBE we have the opportunity to modify future simulation experiences that will then be re-examined in debriefings. This might mean that beyond introducing counterfactual explanations to the debriefing, reducing hindsight bias through elements of simulation design may be possible. Understanding hindsight bias might serve as a useful perspective to critically appraise various simulation and debriefing practices. Clearly, any modifications to practices would need to be contextualised and balanced with other goals and overriding concerns. Below we outline some considerations and theoretical strategies to mitigate the impact of hindsight bias in SBE.

Simulation design and debrief timing

- The *pause and discuss* method of debriefing, based Schön's *reflection-in-action* [52–54], may prove valuable. With pauses occurring prior to significant simulation outcomes manifesting, this may help with exploring and addressing immediate learner perceptions within a simulation experience by preventing belief updating and sense-making tied to particular outcomes.
- Ending a simulation scenario prior to a significant deterioration might be another useful strategy. In our vignette, designing and running subsequent simulations where patient arrest or progressive deterioration does not occur would be one way of shifting focus toward decision-making and management in conditions of uncertainty, and away from perceptions of inevitability.
- Simulations with less experienced learners may be more at risk of oversimplification during debriefing. This can be addressed in scenario design (not single cause and effect relationships), during briefing (alerting learners to multifactorial antecedents), during the simulation (a confederate may introduce complexity) and during debriefing (proposing *did you notice* questions with counterfactuals).

Video-assisted debriefing

- Through the clear depiction of events in continuity with outcomes, video-assisted debriefing might increase hindsight bias and this could challenge the intuitive assumption made by some simulation experts that video playback "…allow[s] participants to see

how they performed rather than how they thought they performed, and…help reduce hindsight bias in assessment of the scenario." (Fanning & Gaba 2007, p. 122) [3].
- Multiple visual perspectives (display clip from different camera angles) may interrupt the apparent simple linearity by which events may appear to be linked to one another when viewing from a single point [2].
- A facilitator could replay selected clips and direct learners focus to different physical locations, events or issues that were occurring simultaneously.
- To raise awareness and test hindsight bias, a facilitator could pause a video during playback and ask learners what happened next.

Facilitators

- Facilitators hold significant power during debriefing [55] and therefore influence what learners focus on and how they judge their performances.
- A facilitator's understanding of events borne of hindsight might help learners to focus on areas that yield valuable learning points. The potential pitfall is that from within this perspective, there may be an inadequate exploration of a variety of learner-centred concerns encountered in simulation. This concern also extends to facilitators debriefing one another.
- Facilitators may consider the potential influence of debriefing techniques that offer or ask for simple causal explanations linking learner actions and outcomes such as, in the *advocacy and inquiry* approach, where the facilitator promotes learner reflection by stating a combination of what is termed an *advocacy* statement – that is, an observation of learner action[s] and subjective judgment of this observation, with an *inquiry* statement [56]. Although this can prompt the learner to notice elements related to the complexity of a situation, the structure of the *advocacy* statement can sometimes be one that links a learner action with a specified outcome through a *single*, plausible, explanatory narrative. This might increase hindsight bias in participants. A potential strategy is to avoid *single* explanations and introduce at least one other counterfactual in the advocacy statement.

In seeking to notice and address issues of complexity and uncertainty, research might also be directed at defining a set of relevant contextual factors or conditions related to management in complex situations. This may lead to debriefings discussing issues experienced in the moment during complex clinical practice. This might include those factors that favoured or disfavoured certain actions being taken, whether these were intended or not. Potential debriefing topics could include issues and constructs such as: managing competing goals, task prioritisation, resource allocation strategies in time-critical and/or resource-poor situations, recognising and managing cognitive overload and fixation errors. Also, potentially relevant could be sociocultural barriers to making certain decision-making steps, including perceived consequences of decisions and issues surrounding power imbalances. Of course, these could not all be addressed in the same debriefing, but across a number of sessions, and according to specific learning objectives, simulation experiences, learner populations, and importantly, learner concerns. These conceptual distinctions could be focused on during reflection, and form the basis for articulations during debriefing discourse. Consequently, this might enable learning that is more aligned to complex, context-specific, clinical practice.

Conclusions
Clinical practice often involves complexity and uncertainty, and learning from SBE should address issues related to management in these contexts. Drawing on findings from published reviews of hindsight bias, the construct has an extensive empirical foundation, and is pervasive across a variety of contexts. During debriefings, hindsight bias might lead to oversimplification of explanations of simulation events, with a failure to acknowledge issues related to management in complex situations, as they are experienced in the moment by learners. This might influence facilitators and learners, leading to a failure to address learning opportunities that might be relevant to patient management in practice. Knowing that the bias exists has not been demonstrated to influence its effects. Given we do not know the impact of oversimplification during debriefing on subsequent practice, it is an important target for further inquiry and research, together with inputs and consequences of hindsight bias for all facets of SBE.

Competing interests
The authors declare that they have no competing interests.

Authors' contributions
AM developed the concept as an assignment in a post-graduate course. AM worked with DN as supervisor in this taught course to develop and apply the concept in simulation-based education. Both authors read and approved the final manuscript.

Author details
¹Department of Anaesthesia, The Royal Victorian Eye & Ear Hospital, 32 Gisborne St, East Melbourne, VIC 3002, Australia. ²HealthPEER, Faculty of Medicine, Nursing and Health Sciences, Monash University, Melbourne, VIC, Australia.

References
1. Blank H, Peters JH. Controllability and hindsight components: understanding opposite hindsight biases for self-relevant negative event outcomes. Mem Cognit. 2010;38(3):356–65.
2. Roese NJ, Vohs KD. Hindsight bias. Perspect Psychol Sci. 2012;7(5):411–26.
3. Fanning RM, Gaba DM. The role of debriefing in simulation-based learning. Simul Healthc. 2007;2(2):115–25.
4. Motola I, Devine LA, Chung HS, Sullivan JE, Issenberg SB. Simulation in healthcare education: a best evidence practical guide. AMEE Guide No. 82. Med Teach. 2013;35(10):e1511–e30.
5. Levett-Jones T, Lapkin S. A systematic review of the effectiveness of simulation debriefing in health professional education. Nurse Educ Today. 2014;34(6):e58–63.
6. McGaghie WC, Issenberg SB, Petrusa ER, Scalese RJ. A critical review of simulation-based medical education research: 2003–2009. Med Educ. 2010; 44(1):50–63.
7. Rudolph JW, Simon R, Dufresne RL, Raemer DB. There's no such thing as "nonjudgmental" debriefing: a theory and method for debriefing with good judgment. Simul Healthc. 2006;1(1):49–55.
8. Dreifuerst K. The essentials of debriefing in simulation learning: a concept analysis. Nurs Educ Perspect. 2009;30(2):109.
9. Jones PR. Hindsight bias in reflective practice: an empirical investigation. J Adv Nurs. 1995;21(4):783–8.
10. Chen J, Bellomo R, Flabouris A, Hillman K, Finfer S, Centre tMSIftS, et al. The relationship between early emergency team calls and serious adverse events. Crit Care Med. 2009;37(1):148–53.
11. Fenwick T, Dahlgren MA. Towards socio-material approaches in simulation-based education: lessons from complexity theory. Med Educ. 2015;49(4): 359–67.
12. Pezzo MV. Hindsight bias: a primer for motivational researchers. Soc Pers Psychol Compass. 2011;5(9):665–78.
13. Caverni JP, Fabre JM, Gonzalez M. Cognitive biases. North Holland: Amsterdam; 1990.
14. Heuer Jr RJ. Psychology of intelligence analysis. Washington DC: Center for the Study of Intelligence; 1999.
15. Fischhoff B, Gonzalez RM, Lerner JS, Small DA. Evolving judgments of terror risks: foresight, hindsight, and emotion: a reanalysis. J Exp Psychol. 2012; 18(2):e1–e16.
16. Shaklee H, Fischhoff B. Strategies of information search in causal analysis. Mem Cognit. 1982;10(6):520–30.
17. Shah AK, Oppenheimer DM. The path of least resistance using easy-to-access information. Curr Dir Psychol Sci. 2009;18(4):232–6.
18. Nestler S, Blank H, von Collani G. Hindsight bias and causal attribution: a causal model theory of creeping determinism. Soc Psychol. 2008;39(3):182–8.
19. Yopchick JE, Kim NS. Hindsight bias and causal reasoning: a minimalist approach. Cogn Process. 2012;13(1):63–72.
20. Granhag PA, Strömwall LA, Allwood CM. Effects of reiteration, hindsight bias, and memory on realism in eyewitness confidence. Appl Cogn Psychol. 2000;14(5):397–420.
21. Bernstein DM, Erdfelder E, Meltzoff AN, Peria W, Loftus GR. Hindsight bias from 3 to 95 years of age. J Exp Psychol. 2011;37(2):378–91.
22. Wu D-A, Shimojo S, Wang SW, Camerer CF. Shared visual attention reduces hindsight bias. Psychol Sci. 2012;23(12):1524–33.
23. Guilbault RL, Bryant FB, Brockway JH, Posavac EJ. A meta-analysis of research on hindsight bias. Basic Appl Soc Psychol. 2004;26(2–3):103–17.
24. Bayen UJ, Pohl RF, Erdfelder E, Auer T-S. Hindsight bias across the life span. Soc Cogn. 2007;25(1):83–97.
25. Pohl RF, Bender M, Lachmann G. Hindsight bias around the world. Exp Psychol. 2002;49(4):270–82.
26. Heine SJ, Lehman DR. Hindsight bias: a cross-cultural analysis. Jpn J Exp Soc Psychol. 1996;35:317–23.
27. Harley EM. Hindsight bias in legal decision making. Soc Cogn. 2007;25(1): 48–63.
28. Caplan RA, Posner KL, Cheney FW. Effect of outcome on physician judgments of appropriateness of care. JAMA. 1991;265(15):1957–60.
29. LaBine SJ, LaBine G. Determinations of negligence and the hindsight bias. Law Hum Behav. 1996;20(5):501–16.
30. Arkes HR. The consequences of the hindsight bias in medical decision making. Curr Dir Psychol Sci. 2013;22(5):356–60.
31. Biais B, Weber M. Hindsight bias, risk perception, and investment performance. Manage Sci. 2009;55(6):1018–29.

32. Blank H, Fischer V, Erdfelder E. Hindsight bias in political elections. Memory. 2003;11(4–5):491–504.

33. Zwick R, Pieters R, Baumgartner H. On the practical significance of hindsight bias: the case of the expectancy-disconfirmation model of consumer satisfaction. Organ Behav Hum Decis Process. 1995;64(1):103–17.

34. MacLean CL, Brimacombe C, Lindsay DS. Investigating industrial investigation: examining the impact of a priori knowledge and tunnel vision education. Law Hum Behav. 2013;37(6):441.

35. Dekker S. A field guide to understanding human error. 3rd ed. Burlington, VT: Ashgate Publishing Company; 2014

36. Cook RI, O'Connor MF. Thinking about accidents and systems. Medication safety: a guide for healthcare facilities. Bethesda: American Society of Health Systems Pharmacists; 2005. p. 73–88.

37. Leveson N. Engineering a safer world: Systems thinking applied to safety. Mit Press: Massachusetts; 2011.

38. Reason JT. Managing the risks of organizational accidents. Ashgate Aldershot: Hampshire; 1997.

39. Hoffrage U, Hertwig R, Gigerenzer G. Hindsight bias: a by-product of knowledge updating? J Exp Psychol. 2000;26(3):566.

40. Blank H, Nestler S. Cognitive process models of hindsight bias. Soc Cogn. 2007;25(1):132–46.

41. Wilson TD, Gilbert DT. Explaining away: a model of affective adaptation. Perspect Psychol Sci. 2008;3(5):370–86.

42. Arkes HR, Faust D, Guilmette TJ, Hart K. Eliminating the hindsight bias. J Appl Psychol. 1988;73(2):305.

43. Pohl RF, Hell W. No reduction in hindsight bias after complete information and repeated testing. Organ Behav Hum Decis Process. 1996;67(1):49–58.

44. Koriat A, Lichtenstein S, Fischhoff B. Reasons for confidence. J Exp Psychol. 1980;6(2):107.

45. Markman KD, Dyczewski EA. Mental Simulation: Looking Back in Order to Look Ahead. The Oxford Handbook of Social Cognition. 2013. p. 402.

46. Croskerry P. Cognitive forcing strategies in clinical decisionmaking. Ann Emerg Med. 2003;41(1):110–20.

47. Arkes HR. Costs and benefits of judgment errors: implications for debiasing. Psychol Bull. 1991;110(3):486.

48. Hirt ER, Markman KD. Multiple explanation: a consider-an-alternative strategy for debiasing judgments. J Pers Soc Psychol. 1995;69(6):1069.

49. Lewis D. Counterfactuals. 2nd ed. Malden, MA: Wiley-Blackwell; 2001.

50. Sanna LJ, Schwarz N, Stocker SL. When debiasing backfires: accessible content and accessibility experiences in debiasing hindsight. J Exp Psychol. 2002;28(3):497.

51. Boud D, Cohen R, Walker D. Using experience for learning: Society for Research into Higher Education and Open University Press. 1993.

52. Newby J, Keast J, Adam W. Simulation of medical emergencies in dental practice: development and evaluation of an undergraduate training programme. Aust Dent J. 2010;55(4):399–404.

53. Schön DA. Educating the reflective practitioner: Toward a new design for teaching and learning in the professions. San Francisco: Jossey-Bass; 1987.

54. Flanagan B. Debriefing: Theory and techniques. Manual of simulation in healthcare. Oxford: Oxford University Press; 2008. p. 155–70.

55. Stewart LP. Ethical issues in postexperimental and postexperiential debriefing. Simul Gaming. 1992;23(2):196–211.

56. Rudolph JW, Simon R, Rivard P, Dufresne RL, Raemer DB. Debriefing with good judgment: combining rigorous feedback with genuine inquiry. Anesthesiol Clin. 2007;25(2):361–76.

13

A systematic review: Children & Adolescents as simulated patients in health professional education

Andrée Gamble[1*], Margaret Bearman[2] and Debra Nestel[3,4]

Abstract

Simulated patients (SP) contribute to health professional education for communication, clinical skills teaching, and assessment. Although a significant body of literature exists on the involvement of adult SPs, limited research has been conducted on the contribution of children and adolescents. This systematic review, using narrative summary with thematic synthesis, aims to report findings related to children/adolescents as simulated patients in health professions education (undergraduate or post-graduate). A systematic review of qualitative and quantitative literature published between 1980 and September 2014 was undertaken using databases including CINAHL, Ovid Medline and Scopus. The lack of literature related to the employment of children and adolescents in nursing education dictated the expansion of the search to the wider health professions. Key search terms related to the employment of children and adolescents in health professional education programs. A total of 58 studies reduced to 36 following exclusion based on abstract review. Twenty-two studies reached full text review; following application of inclusion and exclusion criteria, 15 English language studies involving children and/or adolescents in simulation formed part of this systematic review. Five key themes emerged: Process related to recruitment, duration and content of training programs, support and debriefing practice, ethical considerations, and effects of participation for key stakeholders such as children and adolescents, parent and faculty, and learner outcomes. The results suggest that the involvement of children and adolescents in simulation for education and assessment purposes is valuable and feasible. The review identified the potential for harm to children/adolescents; however, rigorous selection, training and support strategies can mitigate negative outcomes. The ability of children to portray a role consistently across assessments, and deliver constructive feedback remains ambiguous.

Keywords: Simulation, Education, Simulated/standardized patient, Child, Adolescent, Nursing, Health professionals, Systematic review

Background

Learning through clinical practice has traditionally been the mainstay of practice-based health professional education programs. As an example, nursing education has reducing access to clinical placements and exposure to appropriate clinical learning environments is less certain. The inclusion of clinical practicum into the first year of many nursing undergraduate education programs, both nationally and internationally, has also necessitated

students are exposed to professional, psychomotor and developmentally appropriate communication skills earlier than was historically necessary. Holistic, realistic and safe approaches to learning professional and psychomotor skills prior to patient exposure are necessary. These approaches need to equip the student with useful and transferable skills they can apply in the complex clinical environment [1]. This is especially critical now that the National Council of State Boards of Nursing (NCSBN) study has identified the potential for replacing at least some proportion of clinical hours with simulation [2]. Results from this study of nursing students who had a proportion of their clinical hours replaced with simulation

* Correspondence: Andree.gamble@holmesglen.edu.au
[1]Health Science & Biotechnology Department, Holmesglen Institute, Chadstone, Victoria, Australia
Full list of author information is available at the end of the article

(10 %, 25 % or 50 %) indicates no statistically significant differences between the groups at the end of their nursing program in relation to clinical competency, comprehensive nursing knowledge assessments, and NCLEX pass rates. Six months into employment, no statistically significant differences were identified by their managers in relation to clinical competence or readiness for practice.

Paediatrics is a specialised field; the nuances and specific characteristics of children and adolescents must underpin all education approaches. However, learners with limited personal experience or exposure to children can find communication, interaction, assessment and the provision of developmentally appropriate care difficult [3]. Without the opportunity to apply, practise and evaluate these important skills prior to clinical placement, learners may find assimilation into the paediatric clinical environment difficult [1]. Simulation has been identified as a powerful active learning strategy, and an important part of health professional education. Learners are immersed in realistic situations where they have an opportunity to engage in skills-based scenarios in a 'patient-safe' environment. Simulation can offer learners exposure to professional domains such as teamwork, communication and time management and provide participants with almost all the essential components of a real situation. This exposure can then serve as a reference point to guide actions should the situation arise during clinical exposure [4].

Simulated patients (SPs) are defined as well people who have been trained to portray patients with a specific condition in a realistic way [5]. Adult SPs have contributed to clinical skills teaching since proposed by Barrows and Abrahamson in the late 1960s [6]. The benefits of SPs are numerous and widely researched in literature. Often employed in healthcare education programs to portray roles, SPs enable students to immerse more fully in the reality of a clinical situation [7, 8]. Working with SPs also reduces the haphazard nature of student/patient encounters in the clinical environment, resulting in standardization and fairness in exposure to learning opportunities and therefore also during assessment [9]. SPs can also communicate, interact and provide the learner with humanistic and developmentally appropriate responses that are difficult to replicate in a manikin-based program.

There is an obvious threat to patient safety with novice health professionals practising skills on real patients. By contrast, SPs are usually more widely accessible, able to portray a role multiple times and can work in situations where a real patient would be inappropriate. Consistent and standardized role portrayal also makes SPs suitable for clinical assessments where neither manikins nor real patients would be appropriate [10].

Paediatric education is most commonly introduced using a range of technologically diverse manikins. Although an excellent medium for teaching and learning in some areas, manikins can limit realism as their communication and behaviour is often unrealistic and may not reflect the developmental stage required by the simulation role [11]. In addition, manikins are unable to replicate the well child, or the child with a normal childhood illness, both of which are critical to adequate clinical preparation for practice. For these reasons, true learner engagement and immersion is often difficult to achieve.

Communication with children and adolescents is an essential element of health professional socialization, but is difficult to teach and/or assess in the educational setting. Clinical environments are often identified as a more appropriate setting for this learning to occur. However, a reducing number of placements, disparity in the quality and available learning experiences during placement and parental control over access to sick children has made learning more challenging [2]. An ever present patient safety agenda and ethical concerns associated with utilizing sick children for learning can also impact on student exposure to learning opportunities.

It is reasonable to suggest that children and adolescents should become a more important part of SP methodology. Simulation based education with children/adolescents has been used for many years to successfully engage students in various domains of learning. Across the physical examination and professional skills continuum, studies have demonstrated the value of adolescent SPs to education and assessment programs, particularly those related to communication [11].

In paediatrics, the use of children as employed SPs has long been questioned with regard to ethics and the examination of validity, reliability, and feasibility [12]. There are also inherent difficulties in employing real children. Ensuring children are adequately prepared, trained and supported using developmentally appropriate strategies can be challenging. The ethical considerations, particularly of employing children below the age of consent, must be considered when working with children and/or adolescents. Additionally, the age of the child, the role they play and the duration of engagement are crucial considerations.

Definition of terms

Child SPs (CSPs), for the purpose of this review, are aged between 5–12 years, while adolescent (ASPs) refers to participants aged 13–19 years. We use the Child and Adolescent SPs (CASPs) to include babies, CSPs and ASPs. In choosing to differentiate between children and adolescents, a developmental approach was considered appropriate due to the ambiguous nature of consent and Victorian (Australia) labour laws regarding employment of children. This review considers the employment of children for simulation as work in the entertainment industry;

as such, all ages from infancy through to adolescent can be employed for a variable duration dependent on age and employment guidelines [13].

Aim

The aim of this systematic review is to analyse the available literature and generate discussion and recommendations for future research related to the involvement of CASPs in health professional education.

Review question

This review aims to answer the following question: What is reported in the literature regarding children and adolescents who work as SPs in health professional education?

Methods

A systematic search was undertaken for qualitative, quantitative and mixed method papers related to employment of CASPs in all health professional education programs.

Search strategy

Between June – September 2014, seven databases were searched (CINAHL, Ovid Medline, PsychInfo, Google Scholar, Scopus, Cochrane database of systematic reviews, and Informit,). Reference lists from all papers and grey literature were also searched. The search solely focused on literature written in English; no date restrictions were applied. Search terms fell into three broad categories: Education, simulation and developmental stage, (Table 1). For example, a CINAHL search was conducted using the terms; simulated patient AND adolescent OR child AND education.

Table 1 Key Search Terms

Education	Simulation	Developmental Stage
Nursing	Simulated patient	Child
Nurs*	Simulation	Children
Medicine	Sim*	Adolescent
Health professions	Standardized patient	Paediatric
Medical students	SP	Toddler
Undergraduate		Pre-School*
Postgraduate		School Age
Education		Teen*
Role play		Teenager
Communication		
Patient simulation		
Scenario		
Nurse education		

Study selection

Initially, the involvement of children and/or adolescents as SPs in nursing education programs was the intended primary focus. However, limited numbers of papers dictated expansion to all health professional groups, undergraduate and post-graduate students and professional development programs. This review considers multiple research methods, including randomized control trials, control trials, qualitative studies, observation and exploratory studies. Studies written in English with reference to children and/or adolescents as SPs were included without application of date restriction. All peer-reviewed studies, including literature and systematic reviews, were included.

Data extraction

More than 1000 studies were identified in the initial search. This number was reduced to 60 through application of the exclusion criteria to the title alone. A large majority of the literature was further excluded based on review of title and abstract, resulting in 22 full text studies Table 2. Full review of these 22 studies resulted in extraction of data from the final fifteen papers presented in Table 3.

The PRISMA diagram has been utilised to represent the study inclusion and exclusion process underpinning this review (Fig. 1). PRISMA is an evidence-based set of terms used for reporting in systematic reviews [14]. Initial exclusion of studies occurred on abstract review; the lack of involvement of children and/or adolescents as SPs, and a primary focus on subjects not directly related to the review topic resulted in the greatest proportion of exclusions at this stage. Twenty-two studies progressed to full-text inclusion with 7 discarded following review. Four main reasons underpinned their exclusion; children/adolescents who although identified in the studies, were secondary in focus to adult SPs; lack of direct correlation between study content and research focus of this review; no explicit identification of research or review methodology and publication of study in a non-peer reviewed journal.

Table 2 Inclusion/Exclusion criteria

Inclusion Criteria	Exclusion Criteria
All studies focusing on children/adolescents as SPs	Content focused on adult SP rather than child/adolescent SP
	SPs not children or adolescents
Health education program	Non-health education program
Peer reviewed	Not peer reviewed
All study designs including reviews	Research or review not focused on topic
English	Manikin based programs

Table 3 Data Extraction Table

Reference	Study location	Sample	Study Purpose	Study design	SP Population	SP preparation
Austin et al. [17]	USA	Nursing students N = 263	Identify the impact on health professionals & children following their involvement in disaster preparedness simulation	Qualitative evaluation	16 children 6–15 years	Multiple sessions targeting different areas of preparation & role practice
Blake et al. [22]	Canada	Final year medical students N = 57 intervention groupN = 35 in control group	To determine if feedback from adolescent and mother leads to improvements in 4th year medical students' psychosocial interviewing To evaluate whether this skill persists in the long term (2–12 months post intervention, average 6.6 months)	Prospective randomized double blind study with 3 armsIntervention group received feedback from adolescent SP & SP mother after 2 interviews, 4 weeks apart. 2nd intervention group received feedback once after 2nd interview only. 3rd group did not participate in interview	9 SPs as mothers10 female adolescent SPs	Standardized feedback training Adolescents guided by SP mothers to give feedback Adolescent focus group
Blake et al. [23]	Canada	N = 54 final year medical students	To identify any adverse effects on adolescents who regularly undertake risk-taking roles; to capture the viewpoint of adolescents over time; to describe the training and monitoring process for adolescents as risk-taking SPs	Prospective study involving control groups	$n = 11$ female adolescents aged 13–15 Y Control $n = 6$ SPs of same age & grades completed	Information session
Bokken et al. [29]	Netherlands	2nd year medical students over 5 years	Evaluate the views of teachers, students & adolescent SPs regarding the SP program; Evaluate the extent to which all 3 felt the program had changed over 5 years; Evaluate the lessons learner 5 year experience of the SP program	Pre/post tst	$n = 16$ adolescent girls 13–19yn = 2 males	Introduction session & feedback training
Bokken et al. [30]	Netherlands	Medical students N = 341	Evaluation of effects on adolescent SP of performing a role, the quality of their role playing and feedback	Descriptiveevaluation	Adolescents aged 16–18N = 12	Role developed with adolescents based on their own experience. Role related & feedback training
Brown et al. [18]	USA	Medical students & Residents	Description of a pilot program to aid in training residents & medical students in complex interviewing skills addressing adolescent mental health issues	Qualitative	Children & adolescents aged 9–19 years	2 training sessions Not involved in case preparation
Feddock et al. [19]	USA	Medical students N = 95 intervention N = 91 control group	Determine effect of adolescent medicine workshop on knowledge & clinical skills	Randomised controlled trial Intervention: Medical students participating in adolescent medical workshop Control: Medical students in alternative workshop		

Table 3 Data Extraction Table (Continued)

Study	Country	Participants	Aim	Study design	SPs	Training
Hanson et al. [24]	Canada	2nd year medical students	Evaluation of adolescent selection methods & simulation effects for low & high stress roles in a psychiatry OSCE	Randomised controlled trial SP assigned to low stress/ high stress role or control group	Secondary school age adolescents	Information & training session Employment & psychological screening
Hanson et al. [25]	Canada		Evaluating safety of suicidality sim	Pre-post	N = 24 14–17 years	Information sessionScreening Group training
Hanson et al. [26]	Canada	N = 34 paediatric residents	Determine association between simulation discomfort & mental illness stigma	Randomised controlled trial	N = 2414–17 years Randomised to suicide/ depression or cough scenario	4 hours training & rehearsal
Lindsey-Lane et al. [20]	USA	Paediatric medical residents N = 56	Obtain qualitative data about the appropriateness, feasibility & responses of child SPs in CSA	Observational	n = 11 aged 7–16 n = 9 adults paired with children	Training sessions until consistency gained between history, PE & professional skills
Pullon et al. [27]	NZ	N = 69 medical students	Assess consultation skills teaching & risk of harm to involved adolescent SPs	Retrospective evaluation	Adolescent girls (14–18) n = 4n = 3 adult SPs	Discussion about suitability of case Training
Rowe et al. [28]	Africa	5 rural community & one city health service	To evaluate health care worker performance during consultations	Evaluation survey	6 children aged 6 m–59 m5 SP mothers	SP mothers: 3 training days 3 months prior and a 2 day refresher just prior to study. No child SP preparation identified
Tsai [12]	Taiwan	19 studies – English, searched via Medline	Review use of child SPs & difficulties in using children in assessment of competence	Systematic review	Children as SPs in clinical assessments	
Woodward, & Gliva-McConvey, [21]	USA	N = 7 Children 6-18	Identifying the effects of simulation on children	Qualitativeretrospective	N = 7 Children 6-18	Random selection from existing pool of child SPs

Table 3 Data Extraction Table

Reference	Outcome Measures	Learner Outcomes	SP Outcomes	SP related Considerations
Austin et al. [17]	Parental interview to gain understanding of child & parent experiences; Written evaluations from nursing students about nursing process, confidence & knowledge gain	Identified 3 main nursing roles during mass casualty; assessment, triage & interventions; work in multi-professional team to improve rapid assessment & decision making skills; improved confidence (52 % reported some confidence, 21 % very confident & 19 % slightly more confident); 42 % gained awareness of hectic nature of mass casualty	Parents reported children had an increased awareness of disaster-readiness;Children loved the experience;Parents felt education & preparation was excellent; Would allow child to participate again	Parental consent & presence; School support;Nurse dedicated to 1:1 support during Sim;Avoidance of critical events; 'Opt out' option
Blake et al. [22]	Pre-test review by psychologist using modified Calgary-Cambridge guide of interview with adolescent and mother SP;Post-test review of second interview 4 weeks after pre-test Evaluation of knowledge & psychosocial interviewing scores on 2 OSCE stations	Group who received feedback after 1st interview scored better on post-test;Both intervention groups had higher scores in psychosocial inquiry station in OSCE but not in knowledge;Adolescent interviewings kills can be taught & retained up to a year.		Time spent recruiting & training is important.
Blake et al. [23]	SP;Pre & post Interviews using Achenbach's youth self-report & Piers Harris Children's self-concept scale;Focus groups;Parental interview & questionnaire		PRE: SCS &YSR not in clinical range of concern for study or control groups; Focus groups: Develop attachment to SP mother; Wish to come out of character to give feedback;Benefitted from experience but SP work did lose glamour and become a job Parent interview: Saw as opportunity for adolescent empowerment & to better understand how difficult it is for doctors, no increased interest in risk-taking behaviours	Recruitment & screening important; Debrief; Exit strategy; Paid
Bokken et al. [29]	Students rated quality of SP role performance & feedback using Maastricht assessment of simulated patients (MaSP); Adolescent SP questionnaire about their experience; Faculty completed questionnaire about SP consultation, quality of feedback & role play & students reactions	Authenticity of encounter 7.5-8/10, adolescent SP fits role & stays in it; general performance of adolescent SP decreased over 5 years; Faculty saw encounter as authentic, able to address specific aspects of communication not able to be assessed in other ways, SPs able to give natural & spontaneous feedback	No personal disadvantage; Some difficulty with feedback; 8 role plays per day ideal; No differences in evaluation across 5 years	Parents advised by adolescent; Paid; Individualized role
Bokken et al. [30]	Students rated quality of SP role performance & feedback using MaSP; Adolescent questionnaire about effects of SP role; Faculty evaluation of, quality of feedback & role play	Learners indicated satisfaction with quality of role play & feedback; Student doctor & observer rated SP performance differently; Teachers noted a positive & authentic experience & acknowledged students may feel attracted to SP	Positive experience; Easier playing a role close to own experience; Need more feedback training	Given letter for parents but not mandatory to give it to them; Paid for their time
Brown et al. [18]	Resident & medical student questionnaire about the program & achievement of learning outcomes;Focus groups with child-parent SP dyads focused on preparation for roles, reactions to participation, ability to give feedback, reactions to roleplaying with biological/SP mother	Learning outcomes achieved & mostly positive program feedback – 2 learners preferred SP approach whilst 3 preferred lecture format	Child: Fun; empowering; contribute to learning for doctors; financial benefitSP & SP parent: Training was good preparation; Mixed reaction to providing feedback – some would prefer to give to faculty instead of directly to learner ; Varied opinion about biological/SP mother	No psychological follow up Children made links with personal experiences Don't need own parent present 'Opt out' clausePaid
Feddock et al. [19]				

Table 3 Data Extraction Table *(Continued)*

Study				
	End of year clerkship exam with adolescent SP encounters; 3rd year clinical exam; written exercise & questions specific to adolescent medicine on clerkship written exam	Performance of intervention group higher on clinical skills & written exam		Adolescent & parent consent
Hanson et al. [24]	Simulation impact questionnaire; Interview; Focus group; Adolescent self-perception profile; Achenbach behaviour questionnaires; Parental version of simulation impact questionnaire; 3 months after participation – interview; project role questionnaire to identify comfort enacting various roles		Identify good/bad doctors; Importance of training for SP work; Some adverse effects on relationships with peers, parents & school performance; No pre/post change in self-perception or Achenbach questionnaire; Discomfort with sexually explicit questions Parents reported no adverse effects, small increase in self-confidence, job skills & sense of responsibility	
Hanson et al. [25]	Suicidal ideation questionnaire; Reynolds adolescent depression scale; behavioural measures		No deterioration in mental health status; Suicidality role showed negative reaction with; 2 reports of brief depression	ConsentEthics approvalMH specialistStress relief methodsdebriefing
Hanson et al. [26]	Project role questionnaire		Discomfort with sex questions due to lack of knowledge; Adolescents experienced in mental illness roles anticipated greater comfort portraying subsequent stigma associated roles	ConsentEthics approval
Lindsey-Lane et al. [20]	Adult SP: Patient encounter checklists; Child SP gave overall patient satisfaction rating on checklist; SP focus groups with child/adolescents or SP and real parents; Residents completed questionnaires related to realism & challenge	Residents ratings low for fairness (2.9/5), but higher for enjoyment (3.1), realism (3.9) & challenge (4.1)	Child & adult SP satisfaction ratings concordant; Parent Focus Groups gave positive feedback about learning, working hard at a real job; SP parents noted child SP had negative reactions if ignored or talked down to Children found experience at times exciting, nerve wracking & boring, tiring by the end of 6 hours, but good to earn money	Careful selection, in-depth training and debriefing by individuals experienced in communication with children
Pullon et al. [27]	Student self-evaluation, video tape review of consultations by tutor; Interviews with adolescent SPs; Retrospective student evaluation via focus group	Increased confidence in consultation skills, however no clear effect on clinical performance	Adolescents positive about role, no negative effects but able to identify possible harm if supports not put in place	Parental & student consent Clear criteria of concern
Rowe et al. [28]	Survey result analysis – client survey & conspicuous observation		No serious problems for SPs	Ethics approval obtained
Tsai [12]			Children from infancy to adolescence can participate as SPs in clinical assessments; Children should have a substitute; Can provide feedback; More negative impacts for younger children; Use of	Only work with children for assessments that cannot be measured by other methods

Table 3 Data Extraction Table

Woodward, & Gliva-McConvey, [21]	Focus group	Important skills & information gained; Positive & negative outcomes for younger children; fun can disassociate from role; Mainly positive for older children; Help adults learn; Identify good & bad doctors	Mothers included if children <13 Role close to the child's personality & developmental age. Greater risk in younger children. Methods to monitor effects on children

children should be avoided for ethical reasons

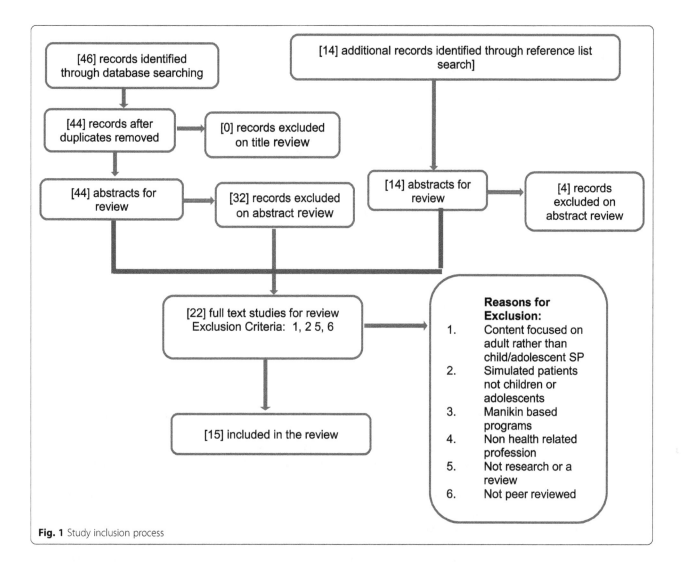

Fig. 1 Study inclusion process

Assessment of methodological quality

Studies underwent a quality analysis process relevant to their research methodology. Qualitative studies were analysed according to the Criteria for appraising qualitative research designed by Walsh and Downe [15]. This is an 8 item checklist, structured into three sections: stages, essential criteria and specific prompts which further delineate into sub-sections focusing on various criteria related to analysis of qualitative research studies. Quantitative literature was appraised using the Medical Education Research Study Quality Instrument (MERSQI). The MERSQI is a ten-item instrument designed to assess the methodological quality of experimental, quasi-experimental, and observational medical education research studies. The ten items reflect six domains of study quality: study design, sampling, data type (subjective or objective), validity of assessments, data analysis and outcomes [16]. Refer to Table 4 and Table 5 for study assessments.

Results

Description of Studies

There were 15 included studies; Tables 3, 4, 5 outline overviews of content and quality. Of these studies, 5 were conducted in the USA [17–21] or Canada [22–26] while one study was a systematic review from multiple countries [12]. The remaining four studies originated in New Zealand [27], Africa [28] and The Netherlands [29, 30].

Eleven studies identified the health professional group to which the learner belonged. Nursing students [17] were involved in one study, while 10 studies focused on medical students or physicians. Participant numbers ranged from 34 paediatric residents [26] to 341 medical students [30]. Two randomised control trials were included, and in both cases, baseline data of participants was comparable [19, 23].

In relation to the central focus of the intervention, two studies focused on Objective Structured Clinical Examination (OSCE) or Clinical skills assessment (CSA),

Table 4 Quality Analysis (Walsh & Downe, [15])

Author	Clear statement of purpose	Method consistent with research intent	Sampling strategy appropriate	Appropriate analytic approach	Interpretation	Data used to support interpretation	Researcher reflexivity demonstrated	Sensitivity to ethical concerns	Relevance & transferability
Austin et al. [17]	1	2	3	2	1	2	2	1	1
Bokken et al. [29]	1	2	2	2	1	1	2	2	1
Bokken et al. [30]	1	2	1	2	1	2	2	2	1
Brown et al. [18]	1	2	1	2	2	3	2	2	1
Lindsey-Lane et al. [20]	1	2	1	2	2	2	4	4	2
Pullon et al. [27]	1	1	1	2	1	1	1	1	1
Rowe et al. [28]	1	1	2	2	1	2	1	1	1
Tsai [12]	1	1	1	1	1	2	NA	NA	1
Woodward & Gliva-McConvey [21]	1	1	2	1	1	1	3	2	1

Key: 1 = Yes, 2 = Partially, 3 = No, 4 = Unknown

eleven related to simulation, while two studies addressed these in combination. Communication was the primary learning outcome for participants in ten studies and four studies related to a combination of communication and physical examination skills.

All studies discussed the experience of children or adolescents as SPs with varying degrees of focus on participant numbers, gender, ages and recruitment strategies. SP participant numbers ranged from four to twenty-four. Ten studies either did not specifically identify gender of the children or adolescent SPs or employed both males and females [12, 17–21, 24–26, 28], three studies focused solely on females [22, 23, 27] and two studies included a small number of males through convenience rather than planning [29, 30]. SPs were recruited from an existing database, following contact with a local community theatre or drama group or from faculty willing to involve their own children. Seven studies focused solely on adolescents whilst five expanded

their CASP involvement to children aged 6–7 years [17, 18, 20, 21, 28].

For qualitative studies, the experience of children and adolescents was captured in post simulation interviews and focus groups. Perspectives of CASPs, biological parents and SP parents were sought at variable points after CASP involvement although Austin [17] chose to focus solely on evaluation data collected from parents. In contrast, a selection of studies used a multi-layered approach to analyse effects of participation on adolescent SPs. Tools employed to gather data included pre and post administration of behavioural type questionnaires and specific project surveys designed to assess the impact of role playing on CASP participants [23–26].

In two studies, CASP evaluated the performance of students. Feddock et al. [19] provided SPs with case-specific checklists designed to assess adolescent medicine knowledge and general interviewing/counselling skills. While not completing a specific checklist, Lindsey-Lane et al.

Table 5 Quality Analysis (MERSQI)

	Study Design	Sampling	Type of data	Validity of evaluation instrument	Data Analysis	Outcomes
Blake et al. [22]	3	2	3	2	2	1.5
Blake et al. [23]	2	2	3	3	3	3
Feddock et al. [19]	3	2	3	1	2	1.5
Hanson et al. [24]	2	0.5	1	1	3	3
Hanson et al. [25]	1.5	2	1	2	2	3
Hanson et al. [26]	3	2	1	2	2	3

[20] allowed children as young as 7 years to give an overall satisfaction rating on the simulated encounter. Students were also involved in direct assessment of CASP performance. Bokken *et al.* [29] applied the Maastricht assessment of SP (MaSP) to evaluate role performance and quality of feedback provided by adolescent SPs.

The type of outcome measures and associated data collection tools varied widely. A variety of data was captured through the use of questionnaires, interviews, focus groups, assessment results and validated screening instruments. Of note was the repeated focus on the specific outcomes for the child and their ability to give feedback. However, even within these diverse data collection methods, the impetus for many studies appeared to be the identification of risk or adverse outcomes for the child or adolescent.

Whilst diversity in outcome is apparent, most studies chose to refine their focus to specific aspects of learning, most prominent being the choice between clinical skills or knowledge. Limited studies chose to evaluate both of these domains despite their obvious need to inter-link in clinical practice. When both domains were assessed in end of clerkship written and clinical exams, a higher score was attained by those learners receiving SP based education in comparison to those who did not.

In most cases, SP views were included in data collection in those situations where an adolescent rather than a child had fulfilled the SP role. Additionally, those studies that did involve younger children chose to focus more on the evaluation provided by either the child's biological parent, or the adult role playing their parent within the simulation activity. Perhaps an opportunity exists in this situation for the incorporation of developmentally appropriate evaluation tools as a means to ensure the valuable feedback of children is not omitted.

Longitudinal application and retention of knowledge were not common outcome measures, despite the potential for these to reinforce the value of child and adolescent SPs to educational outcomes. Two studies included these measurements with variation in the result apparent. Although one study indicated the retention of knowledge for up to one year [22], a second paper provided contrast by identifying that even in the short term there was no appreciable positive impact on clinical performance [27].

Synthesis

All studies were read and reread numerous times to obtain an overall sense of the data. Content that stood out as meaningful was identified and utilised as the basis for theme formation. Studies were initially analysed by the primary researcher, with some further checking for themes undertaken by secondary authors [31].

Analysis of the 15 studies identified five critical considerations that may impact on the inclusion of children

and/or adolescents in simulation based education or assessment programs. These are: recruitment, training, participation and support, ethical issues and the impact of CASP involvement on the learner. Two key additional themes emerged from the analysis: parental and child perspectives.

Critical considerations
Recruitment

The recruitment and screening processes for children and adolescents are clearly important [20–24, 27]. Ensuring adolescents are able to cope with the simulation content, are mature and have a sense of reality about the role, particularly if it involves risk-taking, is vital. Careful selection appears to correlate with more successful and realistic role portrayal [23] as does matching developmental age and personality with the content and expectations of the role [12, 21].

Studies that identify source of recruitment indicate that local schools and community theatre groups in close proximity to the simulation location, and employing children of faculty and their friends were the most effective in finding suitable participants [17, 18, 20, 21, 22, 24, 27, 29, 30]. Collaborating with schools is considered important during selection processes. Teachers are ideally situated to identify suitable students, such as those who have interest in drama, or conversely, those who cannot afford to miss time from school [18, 23].

Recruitment processes ranged from a convenience sampling approach to implementation of strict pre-selection testing using a various assessment tools. Brown *et al.* [18] only employed children with no personal experience of the condition they were to simulate. In contrast, Hanson *et al.* [23–25] and Blake *et al.* [23] used a more rigid approach to selection with a combination of validated tools investigating constructs such as suicidal ideation and adolescent depression [25].

CASP training

Detail about preparatory training time and content was difficult to gauge. The number of hours in training, if specified, ranged between 2, 4 and 8 hours [20, 23, 25]. The content of training also varied within the studies with options encompassing the core role of an SP, specific case training [20, 25], tips to remember the role and multiple practice opportunities. In studies related to adolescent mental health or risk-taking behaviours, the need to engage specialists in training was acknowledged [25, 26].

The duration, level and content of preparatory programs appears to be depend on the age of the child and the role content. Where there is critical content and CASPs are involved in delivery of feedback, their preparation is more time intensive and detailed. In contrast, studies where feedback is not given directly by the child, or the content is less psychologically stressful, the time dedicated to training decreases.

The ability to give effective feedback to participants was identified as a key component of the CASP role [18, 22, 29, 30]. However, this was not always recognized or acted on during training. Studies indicate that CASP feedback is powerful, but there are mixed reactions from both children and adolescents [18, 29, 30]. Brown et al. [18] identified that whilst one adolescent felt uncomfortable giving direct feedback to a student, another reported that the protective mantle of the role and the perceived importance of the information enabled them to feel more comfortable.

Bokken et al. [30] suggest that a role developed in consultation with, and based largely on, the child's personal experience is easier to play, and thus potentially increases perceived realism. In contrast, Brown et al. [18] suggest that collaboration with children/adolescents in role creation is inappropriate given the personal and potentially painful nature of past experience. Training young children for consistent role portrayal could be problematic, so distancing the role from their own personal experience may not necessarily be a protective mechanism, rather one that leads to an increased need for training. Closely aligning the role to their developmental stage and personality, or enhancing engagement through inclusion of personal belongings, could perhaps be the ideal method for accurate, consistent and realistic role depiction. Level of SP engagement is critical, but it is not feasible to involve them every time in scenario design.

Participation and support

CASPs' actual participation in the simulation was difficult to ascertain. Only two studies identified the duration of active participation as 90 minutes and an average of 10.1 60–70 minute interviews [17, 23]. An additional 3 studies [27, 29, 30] indicated that CASPs were involved in 4 to 8 consultations per day. Regardless of the actual active participation time, it is clear that in some instances it is ethically inappropriate to repeatedly expose children, especially younger children, to repeated examinations.

A variety of support measures were implemented prior to, during and after the simulation. Austin et al. [17] implemented a number of these during the preparation and active phase, including parental presence and nursing support for younger children. A number of studies suggested that the presence of an adult SP is an effective support mechanism [22, 23, 27, 28]. Particularly in risk-taking scenarios, Blake et al. [23] identified that developing a relationship with the SP mother can be protective and enabling, thus mitigating the negative impact of involvement. Involving mental health or child communication specialists pre and post simulation was also particularly critical for young children, risk-taking or psychologically stressful roles [25]. In two studies [17, 18], children were also given a method by which they could indicate their desire to end scenario participation. Several studies also recognised the critical need for follow up using either independent interview or focus group methods [18, 20, 21, 23, 24, 25, 27].

Despite the successful involvement of children as young as 6 years of age in simulation (Austin et al. [17]), the majority of studies focused on adolescents aged between 11–19 years. This could be attributed to the focus and content of the simulation; however, Tsai [12] suggests that young children are not reliably able to reproduce a role with enough credibility to create realism or consistency.

Ethical Issues relating to children as SPs

Given the legal age and developmental stage of children and adolescents, their engagement in SP work raises ethical concerns. Gaining consent from children, adolescents and/or parents is one critical ethical issue. The participation of young children was consented to by parents, although one study (12) does suggest that as young children are unable to understand their role or effects of involvement, consent should not be given particularly where there is no observable benefit for the child. In the absence of benefit, the impetus for safeguarding child participants rests in negating harm. Multiple studies raised the notion that adolescents 16 years or above need not gain parental consent prior to involvement as their cognitive level suggests ability to comprehend the requirements and potential adverse consequences of involvement. However, in most cases, information was provided to adolescents should they wish to inform their parents.

The principles of autonomy, beneficence, and non-maleficence are critical ethical considerations when employing vulnerable populations such as children or adolescents. Respecting the autonomy of children is somewhat difficult, given their developmental inability to make decisions based on informed choices. It presumably then falls to the parents of younger children to determine whether participation as an SP truly reflects the child's best interests. In the situation where a young child is to be engaged in SP work, the principle of beneficence emerges. Health professionals must make a critical decision regarding their involvement, balancing benefits to the child with the potential for risk or harm to either the child or the learner.

The principle of non-maleficence dictates that harm should be limited and importantly not disproportionate to the benefits of involvement [32]. Younger children are more at risk of adverse outcomes related to underdeveloped psychological and psychosocial defence mechanisms. ASPs involved in risk-taking, sexuality or mental health scenarios acknowledge a transient negative or discomfort reaction, however there is no evidence to support the presence of long-term adverse effects. The addition of appropriate selection, training, support and debriefing strategies can also serve to ameliorate any deleterious effects (18, 24, 25, 26, 30]. In the decision making process, the risk/harm to benefit ratio must be carefully balanced to ensure the possibility of harm does not outweigh the benefits of involvement.

The potential for harm can be mitigated by reducing the number of examinations, duration of involvement and regular substitution of children to avoid long periods of involvement. There is need to ensure appropriate safeguards are in place prior to, during and post simulation including identification of an 'exit' clause for children, whereby if distressed, unsure or anxious, a child can remove themselves from the scenario. Debriefing, including developmentally aware and content specialists, is clearly supportive whilst adequate follow up is also necessary for monitoring potential medium and long-term consequences.

Because ASPs felt they could be could be viewed as risk-takers outside of the research context, coming 'out of character' to give feedback was implemented as a psychological safeguard. One study [27] identified that as a result of the vulnerability of adolescents, there is potential they adopt risk-taking behaviours. Whilst this is possible, adolescents in another study reported that the enactment of a substance abuse role actually had a preventive rather than incentive effect [24].

The impact of CASP involvement on the learner

Overwhelmingly, the literature suggests that key areas of professionalism, such as communication, are well suited to CASP based simulation. CASP inclusive education and assessment can provide experiential learning opportunities capable of impacting on the preparation of health professionals for clinical work. However, whilst the involvement of CASPs can be beneficial, there is limited evidence that it is actually the child or adolescent who is responsible for positive learning outcomes. In some circumstances, the performance of participants in OSCE who were prepared with an educational program involving ASP simulation surpassed that of others educated using an alternative teaching method. It is difficult to accurately confirm that it was the adolescent, rather than the entire preparatory program, that resulted in better outcomes.

Six studies addressed participant involvement and evaluation as their primary focus, with the majority indicating the positive impact of education programs involving CASP. Austin et al. [17] identify the positive impact

on learner knowledge and confidence, whilst multiple other studies (18, 20, 23, 28, 30] indicate beneficial aspects of CASP involvement including the achievement of realism and the addition of high level challenge. Despite the myriad of beneficial outcomes, the most powerful one appears to be adolescent feedback. Regardless of whether feedback was given to participants in their role playing persona, or as themselves, adolescent evaluation of the learner's performance was incredibly powerful [22]. Blake et al. [22] in their research involving simulation based education and subsequent OSCE based assessment, further emphasize the powerful nature of feedback indicating that performance improved in an OSCE if the participant received feedback after simulation.

There is distinct variability within the studies regarding outcomes for the learner. Blake et al. [22] indicate that interviewing skills can be retained for up to one year if adolescents are involved, whilst in contrast Pullon et al. [27] suggest that although a positive experience, education programs involving CASP has little, if any, direct impact on learner clinical performance. The question therefore remains as to whether it is the program alone, or the involvement of children and/or adolescents that results in positive learner outcomes.

Children and adolescents are included in simulation for different purposes including: application and expansion of knowledge, repetitive practice and assessment. This variability in purpose could actually be the factor that impacts on learning to a far greater extent than that which could be attributed solely to CASP involvement. The implementation and management of CASP based programs can be challenging on many levels. There is a fundamental need therefore to carefully consider if their involvement is the critical element of student learning, or the same outcomes would have been achieved with an alternative modality [12].

Parents' perspectives

Parents across all studies identified positive outcomes for children, with the most common responses categorised as the development of knowledge and empowerment, particularly in regards to the preventative nature of risk-taking scenarios, and the opportunity for financial gain. Blake et al. [23] identify expanding knowledge in regard to empowerment as a consumer, along with an increased understanding of difficulties associated with being a doctor and importantly, no elevated interest in risk-taking behaviours. Parents also noted positive effects in relation to self-confidence, job skills and sense of responsibility. Lindsey-Lane et al. [20] conducted parental focus groups that identified positive outcomes including development of knowledge related to interpersonal dynamics. Parents in this study felt that their child's participation was a privilege and they were proud of 'having a real job and earning money'.

Although primarily positive, some parents suggested that SP work was not suitable for all adolescents; rather they emphasized the need for CASP to be self-aware and understand boundaries [23]. In addition, the propensity for training to be scheduled at night, rather than during school hours, impacted on further participation for the adolescent of one parent [24]. Parental feedback garnered by Lindsey-Lane et al. [20] indicated that at times children found their involvement boring and tiring. In addition, the need to accompany their child to simulation had financial implications in relation to missing paid employment, travel costs and costs of alternate care provision for other children [12].

Child perspectives

The experience for children and adolescents involved in SP work can be positive or negative. Positive impacts include development of knowledge, contributing to the education of future health professionals and financial gain. For adolescents particularly, the preventative nature of risk-taking scenarios is also emphasized as a positive outcome.

Blake et al. [23] identified that gaining medical knowledge for adolescents was interesting. However and perhaps more importantly, the ASPs developed empathy for peers with medical problems. The emergence of assertiveness when interacting with their own GP and an elevated understanding of the difference between 'good and bad doctors' also proved beneficial. Satisfaction in making an important contribution to the training of future health professionals, having fun, making new friends, and gaining important skills for future employment were considered positive outcomes for CASP [24] as were helping adults learn and knowing those adults valued their input into medical training programs [21]. Younger children particularly felt they were having fun by play-acting, and that their involvement was a good excuse to miss school [21]. Financial gain was repeatedly recognized as a beneficial outcome of involvement [18, 20, 21, 23, 24, 30]. Although in direct contrast, adolescents in one study revealed that money was not a major motivator for participation [24].

Two studies found that enactment of a substance abuse or risk-taking role actually had a preventative, rather than encouraging, effect on adolescents [23, 24]. Involvement in high-risk and mental health simulations also had limited negative effects, with only transient rather than long-term depressive reactions experienced.

Adolescents identified that giving feedback was troublesome, and at times anxiety provoking (18, 30]. Adolescents expressed worry that exhibiting risk-taking behaviour within the scenario would follow them to an external context, and they clearly expressed a desire for feedback to be given in their real persona, rather than in 'role' [23]. Losing its glamour and becoming a real job that required commitment was cited as negative (Blake et al., [23]) whilst the impact on social plans because of travel and training schedules was problematic. Missing school and declining school performance, anxiety and tiredness were also identified as significant issues, particularly for younger children [17, 20, 24].

Some adolescents expressed discomfort with the content of some roles. Hanson et al. [24] found that sexually explicit questions caused some discomfort for participants who often reacted with anxiety and shock. Roles could also be seen as increasing the adolescents' worries about their own health or mortality, particularly when they overheard statements about the possible death [21, 24].

Discussion

This systematic review analysed the literature related to children and adolescents who work as SPs in health professional education. It has indicated that the inclusion of CASPs in education and assessment programs is a viable option for health professions. Fifteen studies arising from various sources and involving different health professions, developmental age groups and focus clearly suggest that CASP involvement is feasible as both a learning and assessment strategy. The review demonstrates that children of various age groups can be involved in simulated case scenarios, short objective structured clinical examinations (OSCE) and clinical skills assessment (CSA).

Several studies did indicate that the content of scenarios should be based on real experience [12, 30]. In addition, research does suggest that matching the developmental age and personality of the child to the required role is also a means to improve performance [12, 21]. This is particularly important for younger children who can find it difficult to portray an actual patient well enough to convince of realism. Overall, studies indicated that even risk taking roles are appropriate if sufficient support is available. However, the literature does clearly inform that scenarios involving death are inappropriate, particularly for younger children [17, 21].

In comparing studies where SPs provided learner feedback, the literature agreed that it results in powerful learning outcomes for participants [18, 23, 24, 30]. Children may not be able to complete long feedback reports, however their ability to deliver concrete and direct feedback is equally as powerful as the adolescent whose feedback tends to be more abstract and reflective [18, 27]. Although children and adolescents may find the provision of feedback difficult [30], the addition of an SP mother to the dyad can guide the process [23].

Outcomes for SPs must be positive if their inclusion in health professional simulation is viable. Interestingly, the power of financial gain is not paramount for SPs. What is of importance is that SPs are able to identify more with their own medical care, and make changes if necessary. SPs became more assertive when assessing the quality of their own medical care, and declared an increased ability to discriminate between good and bad doctors [18, 21, 23, 24]. Even young children, who perhaps are less able to clearly articulate their thoughts regarding medical care, exhibited a strong reaction to poor interpersonal communication [20].

Dissent within the literature is apparent around key areas including: preparation of children and adolescents for the SP role, ethical considerations when employing children, and the impact of the child or adolescent on tangible participant learning outcomes. Inability to realistically portray a role consistently for long periods can affect fairness and reliability of assessment whilst it may also be inappropriate for a child to simulate particular conditions or consent to interventions where there is no benefit. Much of the literature does identify strategies that can be employed to address possible harm Careful selection, preparation, support and debriefing are critical, whilst the inclusion of an SP parent is an addition deemed both supportive and encouraging.

Children and adolescents should only be involved in simulation where benefit clearly outweighs any possible negative outcomes. Where children can either provide assent or consent, there should be clear and developmentally appropriate explanation of the role. In situations where younger children are involved, the literature agrees that parents must be provided with adequate information to enable provision of informed consent prior to their child's participation.

Although children and adolescents have been involved in simulation for teaching and assessment for many years, they remain under-utilised in health professional education. The reducing nature of clinical placement availability and appropriateness, in conjunction with the patient safety agenda, demands educators adopt a more realistic and feasible strategy to adequately prepare students and professionals for practice.

Review limitations

Although an extensive search strategy was utilised, the total number of papers included is low. This number may have been reduced due to exclusion of papers written in languages other than English. Although the process and tools utilised for data collection were mostly robust and validated, the inclusion of self-evaluation processes may not be as reliable in capturing learning outcomes. The sample size of studies focusing on child and adolescent SPs rather than the learner was also quite

low. Given this, the ability to extrapolate data to different age groups, health professional groups or clinical practice environments could be limited. Despite these limitations, the review suggests that employment of children and adolescents in health professional education is feasible and there are demonstrable positive outcomes for both learners and child/adolescent SPs.

Conclusion

The findings of this systematic review suggest that simulation based education and assessment programs involving children and adolescents are feasible and capable of producing positive outcomes for both CASPs and participants. There remains inherent variability in recruitment and preparation, developmental stage of CASPs and type of role they portray. The collective studies indicate that CASP involvement in paediatric simulation endeavours can enhance realism and preparation of health professional students for work, although further research is required to isolate the specific benefit of interacting with children and adolescents. The literature clearly suggests that consideration of ethical principles including autonomy, beneficence and non-maleficence, is a critical element of CASP programs. While there is recognition of the potential for negative outcomes, these can be managed.

Recommendations for future research

There is a lack of research regarding CASP based programs in nursing education despite a clear need for objective analysis of their impact on learning outcomes and assessment results. The significance of this could be seen as contentious given the ability to extrapolate from other health professional domains. However, it would however be fruitful for nursing education to have credible research on which to base and expand nursing specific simulation. The impact on longer term outcomes such as retention of knowledge and skill learning is also critical as the demand to produce simulation capable of exerting an impact, rather than just being enjoyable, grows.

A gender bias is obvious throughout the studies, with the majority of literature focused on adolescent females with the dyad of clinician and mother/daughter presentation also dominant. Expansion of studies to include younger children may be of benefit to future education endeavours, as would the involvement of males. These are particularly important given the potential for both these groups to need health care. Within a multicultural society where cultural and linguistic diversity exists, adequate exposure of the learning group to CASPs and families with English as a second language and varying cultural mores and values would be beneficial.

Although feedback is gained from CASPs, there are multiple studies where their voice in evaluation and assessment is absent. Incorporating developmentally appropriate strategies to enable provision of feedback from all age groups is one option for ensuring a breadth of feedback is received.

If health professional education programs continue to ponder replacing at least some proportion of clinical hours with simulation, the need to ensure experience and learning is equitable with placement outcomes is essential. Incorporating children and adolescents in simulation is one way of fostering this outcome.

Competing interests
The authors declare they have no competing interest.

Funding
This research received no specific grant from any funding agency in the public, commercial or not-for-profit sectors.

Author details
[1]Health Science & Biotechnology Department, Holmesglen Institute, Chadstone, Victoria, Australia. [2]HealthPEER - Health Professions Education and Educational Research, Monash University, Melbourne, Victoria, Australia. [3]Simulation Education in Healthcare, School of Rural Health, HealthPEER, Faculty of Medicine, Nursing and Health Sciences, Monash University, Melbourne, Victoria, Australia. [4]Graduate Programs in Surgical Education, University of Melbourne, Parkville, Victoria, Australia.

References
1. Davies J, Nathan M, Clarke D. An evaluation of a complex simulated scenario with final year undergraduate children's nursing students. Collegian. 2012;19:131–8.
2. Hayden JK, Smiley RA, Alexander M, Kardong-Edgren S, Jeffries P. The NCSBN National Simulation Study: A Longitudinal, Randomized, Controlled Study Replacing Clinical Hours with Simulation in Prelicensure Nursing Education. Journal of Nursing Regulation. 2014;5:S3–S64.
3. Jones DC, Sheridan ME. A case study approach: Developing critical thinking skills in novice pediatric nurses. The Journal of Continuing Education in Nursing. 1999;30:75–8.
4. Hovancsek M. Using simulation in nurse education. In: Jeffries PR, editor. Simulation in Nursing Education: From conceptualization to evaluation. New York: National league for Nursing; 2007.
5. Wind LA, Dalen JV, Muijtjens AM, Rethans J. Assessing simulated patients in an educational setting: the MaSP (Maastricht Assessment of Simulated Patients). Med Educ. 2004;38:39–44.
6. Barrows HS. Simulated patients in medical teaching. Can Med Assoc J. 1968;98:674–6.
7. Bornais JAK, Raiger JE, Krahn RE, El-Masri MM. Evaluating Undergraduate Nursing Students' Learning Using Standardized Patients. J Prof Nurs. 2012;28:291–6.
8. Ker JS, Dowie A, Dowell J, Dewar G, Dent JA, Ramsay J, et al. Twelve tips for developing and maintaining a simulated patient bank. Med Teach. 2005;27:4–9.
9. Webster D. Using standardized patients to teach therapeutic communication in psychiatric nursing. Clinical Simulation in Nursing. 2014;10:e81–6.
10. Cleland JA, Abe K, Rethans JJ. The use of simulated patients in medical education: AMEE Guide No 42. Med Teach. 2009;31:477–86.
11. Haddington N, Hanning L, Weiss M, Taylor D. The use of a high-fidelity simulation manikin in teaching clinical skills to fourth year undergraduate pharmacy students. Pharm Educ. 2013;13:54–60.
12. Tsai T. Using children as standardised patients for assessing clinical competence in paediatrics. Arch Dis Child. 2004;89:1117–20.
13. Child employment laws and requirements. State Government of Victoria, Melbourne. 2015. http://www.business.vic.gov.au/hiring-and-managing-staff/employing-children/laws-and-act. Accessed 16th October 2015.
14. Liberati A, Altman DG, Tetzlaff J, Mulrow C, Gøtzsche PC, Ioannidis JPA, et al. The PRISMA statement for reporting systematic reviews and meta-analyses of studies that evaluate healthcare interventions: explanation and elaboration. BMJ. 2009;339:b2700.
15. Walsh D, Downe S. Appraising the quality of qualitative research. Midwifery. 2006;22:108–19.
16. Reed DA, Beckman TJ, Wright SM, Levine RB, Kern DE, Cook DA. Predictive validity evidence for medical education research study quality instrument scores: Quality of submissions to JGIMs medical education special issues. JGIM: Journal of General Internal Medicine. 2008;23:903–7.
17. Austin EN, Hannafin NM, Nelson H. Pediatric disaster simulation in graduate and undergraduate nursing education. J Pediatr Nurs. 2013;28:393–9.
18. Brown R, Doonan S, Shellenberger S. Using children as simulated patients in communication training for residents and medical students: A pilot program. Acad Med. 2005;80:1114–20.
19. Feddock CA, Hoellein AR, Griffith CH, Wilson JF, Lineberry MJ, Haist SA. Enhancing knowledge and skills through an adolescent medicine workshop. Archives Of Pediatrics & Adolescent Medicine. 2009;163:256–60.
20. Lindsey-Lane J, Ziv A, Boulet J. A pediatric clinical skills assessment using children as standardized patients. Archives of Pediatric Adolescent Medicine. 1999;153:637–44.
21. Woodward CA, Gliva-McConvey G. Children as standardized patients: Initial assessment of effects. Teach Learn Med. 1995;7:188–91.
22. Blake K, Mann KV, Kaufman DM, Kappelman M. Learning adolescent psychosocial interviewing using simulated patients. Acad Med. 2000;75:S56–8 [12].
23. Blake KD, Gusella J, Greaven S, Wakefield S. The risks and benefits of being a young female adolescent standardised patient. Med Educ. 2006;40:26–35.
24. Hanson M, Tiberius R, Hodges B, Mackay S, McNaughton N, Dickens S, et al. Adolescent standardized patients: Method of selection and assessment of benefits and risks. Teaching and Learning in Medicine: An International journal. 2002;14:104–13.
25. Hanson M, Niec A, Pietrantonio AM, Johnson S, Young M, High B, et al. Effects Associated with Adolescent Standardized Patient Simulation of Depression and Suicidal Ideation. Acad Med. 2007;82:S61–4.
26. Hanson M, Niec A, Pietrantonio AM, Johnson S, Young M, High B, et al. Does Mental Illness Stigma Contribute to Adolescent Standardized Patients' Discomfort With Simulations of Mental Illness and Adverse Psychosocial Experiences? Acad Psychiatry. 2008;32:98–103.
27. Pullon S, McKinlay E, Wynn-Thomas S. Teaching complex consultation skills using adolescent and parent simulated patients. Focus on Health Professional Education: A Multi-disciplinary journal. 2003;5:48–60.
28. Rowe AK, Onikpo F, Lama M, Deming MS. Evaluating health worker performance in Benin using the simulated client method with real children. Implement Sci. 2012;7:1–11.
29. Bokken L, Van Dalen J, Scherpbier A, Van Der Vleuten C, Rethans J. Lessons learned from an adolescent simulated patient educational program: five years of experience. Med Teach. 2009;31:605–12.
30. Bokken L, Van Dalen J, Rethans J. The case of "Miss Jacobs": Adolescent simulated patients and the quality of their role playing, feedback, and personal impact. Simul Healthc. 2010;5:315–9.
31. Braun V, Clarke V. Using thematic analysis in psychology. Qual Res Psychol. 2006;3:77–101.
32. Beauchamp TL, Childress JF. Principles of Biomedical Ethics. New York: Oxford University Press; 2009.

14

Magnitude and factors associated with appropriate complementary feeding among children 6–23 months in Northern Ghana

Mahama Saaka[1*], Asamoah Larbi[2], Sofo Mutaru[3] and Irmgard Hoeschle-Zeledon[4]

Abstract

Background: Inappropriate complementary feeding is a major contributor to child malnutrition. Previous studies have described complementary feeding practice using single indicators but a combination of indicators is needed to better explain the role of complementary feeding practices in child growth. To adequately quantify appropriate complementary feeding, we used a composite indicator comprising three of the World Health Organization (WHO) core infant and young child feeding (IYCF) indicators that relate closely to complementary feeding.

Methods: A community-based cross sectional cluster survey was carried out in November 2013. The study population comprised mothers/primary caregivers and their children selected using a two-stage cluster sampling procedure. A total of 778 children aged 6–23 months were involved.

Results: Of the children aged 6–23 months; 57.3 % met the minimum meal frequency, 35.3 % received minimum dietary diversity (≥4 food groups), 25.2 % had received minimum acceptable diet and only 14.3 % received appropriate complementary feeding.

Multivariable logistic regression adjusted for cluster sampling showed that children aged 12–23 months were 26.6 times more likely [AOR 26.57; 95 % CI (3.66–193.12)] to receive appropriate complementary feeding compared to children aged 6–8 months. Children who were not bottled-fed were 2.5 times more likely to have been appropriately fed [AOR 2.51; 95 % CI (1.98–6.42)] compared to children who were bottle-fed in the last 24 h prior to study.

Conclusions: Findings from this study demonstrate appropriate complementary feeding and caring practices by caregivers remain a challenge for most households in Northern Ghana.

Keywords: Appropriate complementary feeding, Dietary diversity, Meal frequency, Acceptable diet, Northern Ghana

Background

Childhood malnutrition remains one of the most intractable public health problems throughout the developing world including Ghana. The estimated prevalence of chronic malnutrition for example, in Northern Region is 33.1 % compared with a national average of 19 % [1]. Variation in the prevalence of acute malnutrition among children across regions exists, ranging from a low of 3 to 9 %. Similarly, according to the survey, 66 % of children aged 6–59 months in Ghana have some level of anaemia (Hb < 11 g/dL) but anaemia in children is most common in Northern region with a prevalence of 82 %.

There are several determinants of under-nutrition, including poor dietary practices, non-availability of food and high rates of infection but these factors vary depending on geographic, social, and cultural settings. Mostly however, a major drawback on being fed an adequate diet is lack of access to diversified foods and insufficient meal frequency after 6 months of age [2, 3]. About 6 % of under-five deaths can be prevented particularly in the developing world if optimal complementary feeding is ensured, thereby contributing towards the

* Correspondence: mmsaaka@gmail.com
[1]University for Development Studies, School of Allied Health Sciences, P O Box 1883, Tamale, Ghana
Full list of author information is available at the end of the article

realization of the Millennium Development Goal four [4–6]. Complementary feeding is defined as giving children other foods or fluids in addition to the breast milk at six months age of child [7].

The World Health Organization (WHO) has developed eight core infant and young child feeding indicators to monitor and to guide the feeding practices of young children [8, 9] including the following: (1) early initiation of breastfeeding; (2) exclusive breastfeeding under six months; (3) continued breastfeeding for one year; (4) the introduction of solid, semi-solid or soft foods; (5) minimum dietary diversity; (6) minimum meal frequency; (7) minimum acceptable diet; and (8) consumption of iron rich or iron fortified foods.

The development of successful interventions to improve child-feeding practices, in particular, requires appropriate instruments that can adequately assess current feeding practices and monitor the impact of programmes designed to improve them [10]. Therefore, knowledge of the magnitude and predictors of appropriate complementary feeding practices is an important step in designing and evaluating appropriate interventions that seek to address poor infant and young child feeding practices. However, there is little information on the extent mothers adhere to the WHO recommended infant and young child feeding practices in Northern Ghana. Furthermore, given the strong links between diet diversity and nutritional outcomes [11–14], this study sought to assess the prevalence of appropriate complementary feeding practices and its determinants among children aged 6–23 months who reside in rural areas of Northern Ghana where child malnutrition is a serious concern.

Methods
Study area
The nutrition survey covered five programme districts of Northern Ghana comprising the Northern Region (NR), Upper East Region (UER) and Upper West Region (UWR). The five districts where International Institute of Tropical Agriculture (IITA) project is currently operating are Nadowli, Wa West, Tolon, Savelugu and Kassena-Nankana.

Majority of the people in the study area have agriculture as their main occupation while some are involved in trading. The main staple foods including maize, sorghum, millet and yam are usually harvested from October through December. Although the food security situation is usually good during the harvesting time, child care tends to suffer because of lack of time on the part of rural mothers. A high proportion of rural women work daily away from home, and therefore frequently face challenges to the care of children.

The rainfall pattern is unimodal and the period is usually short and lasts from May to August, followed by a long dry season (September – April) with dry harmattan winds.

Survey design, population and sampling
This paper is based on re-analysis of data which was collected in a base-line cross-sectional survey in November 2013. The overall aim of the community based cross-sectional study was to collect information on knowledge and practices related to infant and young child feeding (IYCF) practices which will serve as a baseline for future comparison after the implementation of IITA sponsored nutrition project.

A sample size of 288 was required to ensure that the estimated prevalence of the main outcome variable was within plus or minus 5 % of the true prevalence at 95 % confidence level. Assuming a correction factor of 2 (the "design effect") for cluster sampling, the sample size was increased to 576. A non response rate of 5 % and other unexpected events (e.g., damaged/incomplete questionnaire) was factored in the sample size determination and so the sample size is adjusted to 600 for 25 intervention communities that were already selected. The same number of children was selected from comparison communities using probability proportionate to size (PPS).

The basic primary sampling unit was the household and these were selected using a two-stage cluster sampling technique. PPS was used to select the comparison communities in adjacent districts given the lack of a comprehensive sampling frame and the geographic distribution of the population. Each comparison district was considered a stratum, from which clusters were selected based on stratified probability proportional to population size (PPS) sampling. The sampling frame of communities for each district was constructed using projected population figures based on 2010 Ghana population census. The Emergency Nutrition Assessment (ENA) software was used to randomly select the required number of clusters.

In each selected cluster, a complete list of all households was compiled, and systematic random sampling was used to select eligible households.

Data collection
Data were collected using face-to-face interview during house-to-house visit from mothers who had 6–36 months age children using structured questionnaire. The mother of the child or other caretaker provided information on the child's age, gender, morbidity in the past week and child feeding practices. Information on the household's composition, household wealth index (socio-economic), crop and poultry/livestock production practices and child anthropometry indicators were also collected.

Independent and dependent variables

The main outcome variable for this study was the prevalence of appropriate complementary feeding and its components. The independent variables were maternal, child and household characteristics. A brief description of main independent and dependent variables is as follows:

Assessment of infant and young child feeding (IYCF) practices

Infant and young child feeding indicators including minimum meal frequency, minimum dietary diversity and minimum acceptable diet were estimated by recall of food and liquid consumption during the previous day of the survey as per WHO/UNICEF guidelines [15].

A child was judged to have taken 'adequate number of meals if he/she received the minimum frequency for appropriate complementary feeding (that is, 2 times for 6–8 months and 3 times for 9–11 months, 3 times for children aged 12–23 months) in last 24 h. For non breast feeding children, the minimum meal frequency was 4. Adequacy of meal frequency was ranked by assigning a score of 1.

The WHO defined minimum dietary diversity as the proportion of children aged 6–23 months who received foods from at least four out of seven food groups [8, 9]. The 7 foods groups used for calculation of WHO minimum dietary diversity indicator are:

(i) grains, roots and tubers; (ii) legumes and nuts; (iii) dairy products; (iv) flesh foods; (v) eggs; (vi) vitamin A rich fruits and vegetables; and (vii) other fruits and vegetables.

From the dietary diversity score, the minimum dietary diversity indicator was constructed using the WHO recommended cut-off point with a value of "1" if the child had consumed four or more groups of foods and "0" if less. Minimum dietary diversity is the proportion of children who ate at least 4 or more varieties of foods from the seven food groups in a 24 h time period [8, 9]. Minimum acceptable diet is a composite indicator of minimum dietary diversity and minimum meal frequency. Breastfed children who meets both the minimum diversity and the minimum meal frequency are considered to have met the WHO recommended minimum acceptable diet.

Previous studies have described complementary feeding practices using single indicators but a combination of indicators is needed to better explain the role of complementary feeding practices in child growth. To adequately quantify appropriate complementary feeding, we used a composite indicator comprising three of the WHO core IYCF indicators that relate closely to complementary feeding. These are timely introduction of solid, semi-solid or soft foods at 6 months, minimum meal frequency, and minimum dietary diversity. In this study, a child was classified as having received appropriate complementary feeding if the child met all the following three criteria:

i. Complementary feeding commenced at 6th month of birth
ii. Minimum dietary diversity score was at least 4
iii. Minimum meal frequency was adequate for age of child

Complementary feeding was inappropriate if any of the three criteria was not fulfilled

Malnutrition classification

For the present study, we defined positive deviant children as having both height - for -age Z-score (HAZ) and weight – for height Z-score (WHZ) ≥ –2 (best nutritional status). A negative deviant child was defined as having both HAZ and WHZ < –2. Median deviant child was defined as having either HAZ or WHZ < –2.

Statistical data analyses

Both bivariate and multivariate analyses were done to identify the determinants of appropriate feeding practices and minimum dietary diversity (MDD). Firstly, bivariate analyses for all the various risk factors were performed using X^2 tests. Child, maternal and household characteristics that were significantly associated with the outcome variable were included in the logistic regression (LR) models. Multiple logistic regression analyses using appropriate measures to account for the complex survey design were applied to examine the associations between dependent variable (that is, appropriate complementary feeding) and potential predictors. Stepwise backward LR was used for multiple logistic regressions. Odds ratio with 95 % confidence interval to ascertain association between independent and dependent variable was used.

Ethics consideration

The study protocol was approved by the Ethical Committee of the School of Allied Health Sciences, University for Development Studies. Community leaders in the study communities were briefed about the study and permission sought to proceed. Informed consent was also obtained verbally after needed information and explanation. Participation was voluntary and each woman signed (or provided a thumb print if she was illiterate) a statement of an informed consent after which she was interviewed.

Results
Sample characteristics

Table 1 presents the summary statistics on key characteristics of mother - child pairs in our sample. The study sample comprised a total of 778 children aged 6–23 months with the majority of their mothers (69.8 %) had

Table 1 Sample characteristics

Characteristics	Frequency (n)	Percentage (%)
Religion of respondent		
Christianity	360	46.3
Islam	375	48.2
African traditional religion (ATR)	35	4.5
Other	8	1.0
Marital status		
Single	11	1.4
Married	762	97.9
Widow	3	0.4
Separated	2	0.3
Educational level of mothers		
None	543	69.8
Primary	115	14.8
Junior High School (JHS)	101	13.0
Senior High School (SHS)	18	2.3
Tertiary	1	0.1
Age Groups of mothers (years)		
Under 18	11	1.4
18–35	664	85.3
More than 35	103	13.2

Table 2 Nutritional status and dietary intake of children aged 6–23 months

Characteristics	Mean ± SD	Frequency (n)	Percentage (%)
Nutritional status			
WAZ	−1.13 ± 1.1		
HAZ	−0.88 ± 1.35		
WHZ	−0.91 ± 1.13		
Stunted (HAZ < −2)		130	16.8
Wasted (WHZ < −2)		116	15.0
Underweight (WAZ < −2)		163	21.0
Diarrhoeal infection the past 14 days		284	36.5
Currently breastfeeding		759	97.6
Prevalence of bottle feeding		87	11.2
Met minimum meal frequency		431	57.3
Met minimum dietary diversity		276	35.6
Met minimum acceptable diet		193	24.9
Appropriate complementary feeding rate		107	13.8

no formal education. The mean age of the respondents was 28.3 ± 6.5 years with the minimum and maximum ages of 15 and 52 years respectively. The sample comprised 63.6 % of children aged 12–23 months.

Nutritional status and dietary intake of children aged 6–23 months

With respect to nutritional status of children aged 6–23 months, 16.1 % (CI: 13.5 to 19.2), 19.2 % (CI: 15.5 to 23.6) and 23.1 % (CI: 19.2 to 27.5) of the study population were wasted, stunted, and underweight respectively. The proportion of children 6–23 months who met the minimum dietary diversity (≥4 food groups) was 35.6 and 57.3 % had adequate meal frequency. Only 24.9 % of the children aged 6–23 months met the minimum acceptable diet. Children who met the acceptable diet and started complementary feeding at six months were considered to have appropriate complementary feeding. Therefore the overall appropriate complementary prevalence was only 13.8 % (Table 2).

Factors found associated with appropriate complementary feeding practice

In bivariate analysis, place of residence, age of the child, religion of mother, avoidance of bottle feeding, timely initiation of breast feeding and absence of diarrhoeal infection were positively associate with appropriate complementary (Tables 3 and 4).

Multiple logistic regressions analysis showed three variables were significantly associated with appropriate complementary feeding practice. These were child's age, absence of illness and whether the child was classified as positive, median or negative deviants.

Compared with positive deviants, negative deviants were 2.7 times more likely to be fed appropriately [AOR 2.74; 95 % CI (1.12–6.71)]. In terms of appropriate complementary feeding, there was no difference between positive deviants and median growers. Younger children were less likely to be fed appropriately, compared with older children. Compared to children aged 6–8 months, older children aged 9–23 months were 14 times more likely to meet recommended complementary feeding practices [AOR 14.09; 95 % CI (1.87–106.30)].

Compared to children who were reported sick from diarrhoea at any time in the last two weeks, children who were well were 1.8 times more likely to receive appropriate complementary feeding [AOR 14.09; 95 % CI (1.87–106.30)] (Table 5).

Discussion

This study sought to quantify appropriate complementary feeding using a composite indicator comprising three of the WHO recommended core IYCF indicators. It also investigated factors that are associated with appropriate complementary feeding.

Table 3 Factors associated with appropriate complementary feeding practice among children aged 6–23 months (Bivariate analysis)

Characteristic	N	Complementary feeding practice		Test statistic
		Inappropriate n (%)	Appropriate n (%)	
Region of residence				
Northern	311	280 (90.0)	31 (10.0)	$\chi^2 = 6.9\ p = 0.03$
Upper East	156	133 (85.3)	23 (14.7)	
Upper West	308	255 (82.8)	53 (17.2)	
Age of child (months)				
6–11	285	265 (93.0)	20 (7.0)	$\chi^2 = 19.9\ p < 0.001$
12–17	242	205 (84.7)	37 (15.3)	
18–23	248	198 (79.8)	50 (20.2)	
Religion of mother				
Christianity	360	298 (82.8)	62 (17.2)	Fisher's exact test = 6.4 $p = 0.04$
Islam	372	331 (89.0)	41 (11.0)	
African Traditional Religion (ATR)	43	39 (90.7)	4 (9.3)	

Due to the multidimensional nature of feeding practices, which is also age-specific [16], an appropriate tool to determine the overall child-feeding practices is yet to be determined. Minimum dietary diversity, adequacy of meal frequency and timely initiation of complementary feeding were the WHO indicators factors used in building the composite index and this study is the first of its kind in which important WHO IYCF indicators were combined to quantify appropriate complementary feeding in Northern Ghana. This composite index reflects key components of child feeding, namely appropriate timing of introduction of complementary foods, dietary density and adequacy of meal frequency.

The results revealed that the prevalence of appropriate complementary feeding was only 13.8 % which is similar

Table 4 Factors associated with appropriate complementary feeding practice among children aged 6–23 months (Bivariate analysis)

Characteristic	N	Complementary feeding practice		Test statistic
		Inappropriate	Appropriate	
Timely initiation of breast feeding				
No	414	366 (88.4)	48 (11.6)	$\chi^2 = 3.6, p = 0.06$
Yes	361	302 (83.7)	59 (16.3)	
Child had diarrhoea in the last two weeks?				
Yes	283	253 (89.4)	30 (10.6)	$\chi^2 = 3.8, p = 0.05$
No	492	415 (84.3)	77 (15.7)	
Bottle feeding				
Yes	86	81 (94.2)	5 (5.8)	$\chi^2 = 5.2, p = 0.02$
No	689	587 (85.2)	102 (14.8)	
Currently breastfeeding?				
No	19	13 (68.4)	6 (31.6)	$\chi^2 = 5.2, p = 0.02$
Yes	756	655 (86.6)	101 (13.4)	

to what was reported from Northern Ethiopia, Sri Lanka, Nepal and Tanzania Bangladesh, Zambia, and [17–20]. This indicates the general low level of appropriate complementary feeding practices in many countries including Ghana.

The three consistent variables that were found to be significantly associated with appropriate complementary feeding practice in this study were increasing child's age, freedom from illness and whether the child was classified as positive, median or negative deviants. Other variables that were significant in bivariate analysis but failed to reach significance level in the multivariate analysis were region of residence, bottle feeding, religion of mother, timely initiation of breast feeding and absence of diarrhoeal infection.

Children within the age group 9–23 months were 14 times more likely to be appropriately fed as compared to infants in the age group 6–8 months. This finding is congruent with the findings in many countries including Ethiopia, Zambia Nepal, Indonesia and Tanzania where older children are more likely to be fed on complementary foods optimally [17, 20–22]. Education on complementary feeding should therefore target mothers of young children to give such children diversified diets that also meet adequate meal frequency. The 6–8 months age period is known to coincide with the period of the fastest growth faltering [23]. Poor complementary feeding practices in this age group should therefore be addressed effectively in order to greatly reduce the risk of growth faltering.

One would expect that positive deviant children will receive better appropriate feeding. Surprisingly, more of the negative deviant children (29.6 %) received appropriate complementary feeding compared to median growers (13.5 %) and positive deviants (13.2 %). The inverse

Table 5 Determinants of appropriate complementary feeding practices

Variable	Wald	Sig.)	Adjusted odds ratio (AOR)	95 % confidence Interval (CI) Lower	Upper
Free from diarrhoea in the past two weeks	6.78	0.009	1.83	1.16	2.90
Height of the child	10.11	0.001	1.07	1.03	1.12
Deviance (reference: positive deviants)	4.88	0.09			
Median growers	0.07	0.79	1.071	.649	1.768
Negative deviants	4.87	0.03	2.74	1.12	6.71
Age group (9–23 months)	6.59	0.01	14.09	1.87	106.30
Constant	30.39	<0.001	.000		

relationship was more pronounced with respect to acceptable diet whereby 51.9 % of negative deviants, 26.6 % of median growers and 23.2 % met the criterion for acceptable diet. The issue of reverse causality may be applicable here whereby the sick child is given better care with regards to appropriate complementary feeding. This means, the undernutrition gives the mother the opportunity to provide appropriate complementary feeding.

Our data also showed that children with diarrhoeal infection were less likely to be fed appropriately. The negative association between sickness and appropriate complementary feeding is for the fact that some mothers would avoid feeding or reduce the meal frequency during diarrhoeal episode of the child and this will be detrimental to appropriate complementary feeding as defined in this study. Mothers should be educated and encouraged to continue to feed their children even when they have diarrhoea.

This study revealed that there was no association between frequency of antenatal care (ANC) visits and appropriate complementary feeding practice and same was reported in Northern Ethiopia [17] but that disagrees with other studies in Nepal, India and Sri Lanka [18, 19, 24] where inadequate antenatal care was associated with inappropriate complementary feeding. The finding in our study could imply that appropriate complementary feeding messages were either not being given to mothers by health professionals during antenatal or there was little variation in ANC attendance among the mothers. Most of the mothers (84.2 %) actually made at least four visits during the last pregnancy. Similarly, maternal educational level and socio-economic status as measured by household wealth index were also not associated with complementary feeding practices in this study. The lack of association may be attributed to the little variation of these variables in our study sample. In other studies, higher maternal education attainment is reported to associate positively with appropriate complementary feeding [19, 20]

Geographic location was also an important determinant of appropriate complementary feeding. Children from the Upper West and Upper East Regions were more likely to receive appropriate complementary feeding when compared to the children from Northern Region. The regional differentials in complementary feeding practices strongly suggest the importance of ensuring that interventions to improve complementary feeding are evidence-based and are informed by context specific formative research.

As expected, higher household wealth significantly increases diet diversity. Household wealth index positively associated with a higher dietary diversity score (DDS). Rich families are more likely to be able to afford and provide a variety of foods to their children more frequently. The positive association between higher household wealth and increased diet diversity has been consistently reported in earlier studies in different countries including Bangladesh, India, Nepal, Pakistan and Sri Lanka [25–27]. The fact that household wealth is a predictor of minimum dietary diversity underlines the important role of household resources in determining optimal complementary feeding practices.

Families that reported keeping chickens, ducks, or other birds for the meat/sale were more likely to provide children with diversified foods. Initial studies show a strong positive relationship between biodiversity in agricultural production and improved diversified diets [28]. Therefore, an appropriate mix of behaviour change communication and production of local food varieties and poultry resources could be a feasible option to increase recommended infant feeding practices and reduce under nutrition. Educational interventions can be implemented through existing mother's group meetings, community health volunteers, and outreach clinics including primary health care outreach clinics will help promote good child feeding practices.

Conclusion

In conclusion, the overall prevalence of appropriate complementary feeding practices was very low, an indication that appropriate complementary feeding by caregivers remains a challenge for most households in

Northern Ghana. Focused behaviour change communication strategies should therefore target care-givers to provide diversified complementary foods timely to their children at six months of age.

The results presented in this study highlight the fact that both the magnitude and determinants of appropriate complementary feeding vary depending on what indicator or set of indicators are used. Furthermore, the findings underscore the need to always have context specific information in designing and evaluating appropriate interventions that seek to address poor infant and young child feeding practices. This is because factors that determine feeding practices are never the same in every environment and especially so when different indicators are used in measuring them.

Study limitations

Like any other observational studies, this study has some limitations. The cross sectional nature of the study prevents it from making causal inference. The information collected was mainly through interviews. There is possibility that some of the responses might suffer from recall bias and this may affect prevalence estimates. Also the complex nature of complementary feeding makes some aspects of it more difficult to capture and accurately assess.

Competing interests
The authors declare that they have no competing interests.

Authors' contributions
MS and SM designed the study, analyzed and interpreted the data. MS drafted the manuscript. AL and I H revised it critically for important intellectual content. SM assisted with the development of the questionnaire and data collection from the field. All authors read and approved the final manuscript.

Acknowledgements
The authors would like to gratefully acknowledge funding received from IITA Africa RISING Project under the USAID Feed the Future Nutrition. We are thankful to the data collection team members from the Ghana Health Service (GHS) for their hard work and commitment. The data could not have been obtained without the co-operation and support of the programme communities, especially the mothers and caregivers who took time off from their busy schedules to respond to the interviewers. Their involvement and cooperation is highly appreciated.

Funding
The study was funded by IITA Africa RISING Project under the USAID Feed the Future Nutrition.

Author details
[1]University for Development Studies, School of Allied Health Sciences, P O Box 1883, Tamale, Ghana. [2]International Institute of Tropical Agriculture (IITA), P O Box 6, Tamale, Ghana. [3]Ghana Health Service, Tamale, Northern Region, Ghana. [4]International Institute of Tropical Agriculture (IITA), PMB 5320, Oyo Road, Ibadan, Nigeria.

References
1. Ghana Statistical Service (GSS), Ghana Health Service (GHS), ICF International. Ghana Demographic and Health Survey 2014. Rockville: GSS, GHS, and ICF International; 2015.
2. Pan American Health Organization, World Health Organization. Guiding Principles for Complementary Feeding of the Breastfed Child. Geneva: World Health Organization; 2003.
3. Black RE, Allen LH, Bhutta ZA, Caulfield LE, de Onis M, Ezzati M, et al. Maternal and child undernutrition: global and regional exposures and health consequences. Lancet. 2008;371:243–60.
4. Black RE, Morris SS, Bryce J. Where and why are 10 million children dying every year? Lancet. 2003;361(9376):2226–34.
5. Jones G, Steketee RW, Black RE, Bhutta ZA, Morris SS, Bellagio Child Survival Study Group. How many child deaths can we prevent this year? Lancet. 2003;362:65–7.
6. Lutter C. Meeting the challenges to improve complementary feeding. Stand Committee Nutr News. 2003;27:4–9.
7. World Health Organization. Complementary Feeding: Summary of Guiding Principles. Report of the Global Consultation in 2001. Geneva: World Health Organization; 2002.
8. World Health Organization. Indicators for assessing infant and young child feeding practices Part 1 Definitions. Washington DC: World Health Organization, Dept. of Child and Adolescent Health and Development; 2007.
9. WHO, UNICEF, USAID, FANTA, AED, UC DAVIS, IFPRI. Indicators for assessing infant and young child feeding practices part 2: measurement. Geneva: The World Health Organization; 2010.
10. Ruel MT, Brown KH, Caulfield LE. Moving Forward with Complementary Feeding: Indicators and Research Priorities. In: FCND Discussion Paper No 146. Washington, D.C: Food Consumption and Nutrition Division, International Food Policy Research Institute; 2003.
11. Ruel MT, Menon P. Child feeding practices are associated with child nutritional status in Latin America: innovative uses of the demographic and health surveys. J Nutr. 2002;132:1180–7.
12. Rah JH, Akhter N, Semba RD, de Pee S, Bloem MW, Campbell AA, et al. Low dietary diversity is a predictor of child stunting in rural Bangladesh. Eur J Clin Nutr. 2010;64(12):1393–8.
13. Zongrone A, Winskell K, P M. Infant and Young Child Feeding (IYCF) Practices and Child Undernutrition in Bangladesh: Insights from Nationally Representative. Data Pub Health Nutr. 2012, doi:10.1017/ S1368980012001073
14. Arimond M, Ruel MT. Dietary diversity is associated with child nutritional status: evidence from 11 demographic and health surveys. J Nutr. 2004;134:2579–85.
15. WHO/UNICEF/IFPRI/UCDavis/FANTA/AED/USAID. Indicators for assessing infant and young child feeding practices. Part 1: Definitions. Geneva: World Health Organization; 2008.
16. Moursi MM, Arimond M, Dewey KG, Treche S, Ruel MT, Delpeuch F. Dietary diversity is a good predictor of the micronutrient density of the diet of 6- to 23-month-old children in Madagascar. J Nutr. 2008;138(12):2448–53.
17. Mekbib E, Shumey A, Ferede S, Haile F. Magnitude and factors associated with appropriate complementary feeding among mothers having children 6–23 months-of-age in Northern Ethiopia; A Community-Based Cross-Sectional Study. J Food Nutr Sci. 2014;2(2):36.
18. Senarath U, Godakandage SS, Jayawickrama H, Siriwardena I, Dibley MJ. Determinants of inappropriate complementary feeding practices in young children in Sri Lanka: secondary data analysis of demographic and health survey 2006–2007. Matern Child Nutr. 2012;8 Suppl 1:60–77.
19. Joshi N, Agho KE, Dibley MJ, Senarath U, Tiwari K. Determinants of inappropriate complementary feeding practices in young children in Nepal: secondary data analysis of demographic and health survey 2006. Matern Child Nutr. 2012;8 Suppl 1:45–59.
20. Rose V, Baines SK, Agho KE, Dibley MJ. Factors associated with inappropriate complementary feeding practices among children aged 6–23 months in Tanzania. Matern Child Nutr. 2012;23:22925557.
21. Disha AD, Rawat R, Subandoro A, Menon P. Infant and Young Child Feeding (IYCF) Practices in Ethiopia and Zambia and their association with child nutrition: analysis of demographic and health survey data. AJFAND. 2012;12(2):5895–913.
22. Charmaine SN, Dibley MJ, Agho KE. Complementary feeding indicators and determinants of poor feeding practices in Indonesia: a secondary analysis of 2007 demographic and health survey data. Food Nutr Bull. 2010;31(2):366–75.

23. Victora CG, De OM, Hallal PC, Blossner M, Shrimpton R. Worldwide timing of growth faltering: revisiting implications for interventions. Pediatrics. 2010;125:e473–80.

24. Aggrawal A, Verma S, Feridi MA, Chand D. Complementary feeding–reasons for inappropriateness in timing, quality and consistency. Indian J Pediatr. 2008;75:49–56.

25. Bhagowalia P, Menon P, Quisumbing AR, Soundararajan V: What Dimensions of Women's Empowerment Matter Most for Child Nutrition? Evidence Using Nationally Representative Data from Bangladesh. In: IFPRI Discussion Paper 01192. IFPRI, Washington D.C; 2012.

26. Senarath U, Agho KE, Dur-e-Samin A, Godakandage SSP, Hazir T, Jayawickrama H, et al. Comparisons of complementary feeding indicators and associated factors in children aged 6–23 months across five South Asian countries. Matern Child Nutr. 2012;8 Suppl 1:89–106.

27. Senarath U, Dibley MJ. Complementary feeding practices in South Asia: analyses of recent national survey data by the South Asia infant feeding research network. Matern Child Nutr. 2011;8 Suppl 1:5–10.

28. Bhagowalia P, Headey D, Kadiyala S. Agriculture, Income and Nutrition Linkages in India: Insights from a Nationally Representative Survey IFPRI Discussion Paper 01195. Washington DC: International Food Policy Research Institute; 2012. p. 31.

15

Observer roles that optimise learning in healthcare simulation education: a systematic review

Stephanie O'Regan[1*], Elizabeth Molloy[2], Leonie Watterson[1] and Debra Nestel[2]

Abstract

Background: Simulation is widely used in health professional education. The convention that learners are actively involved may limit access to this educational method. The aim of this paper is to review the evidence for learning methods that employ directed observation as an alternative to hands-on participation in scenario-based simulation training. We sought studies that included either direct comparison of the learning outcomes of observers with those of active participants or identified factors important for the engagement of observers in simulation. We systematically searched health and education databases and reviewed journals and bibliographies for studies investigating or referring to observer roles in simulation using mannequins, simulated patients or role play simulations. A quality framework was used to rate the studies.

Methods: We sought studies that included either direct comparison of the learning outcomes of observers with those of active participants or identified factors important for the engagement of observers in simulation. We systematically searched health and education databases and reviewed journals and bibliographies for studies investigating or referring to observer roles in simulation using mannequins, simulated patients or role play simulations. A quality framework was used to rate the studies.

Results: Nine studies met the inclusion criteria. Five studies suggest learning outcomes in observer roles are as good or better than hands-on roles in simulation. Four studies document learner satisfaction in observer roles. Five studies used a tool to guide observers. Eight studies involved observers in the debrief. Learning and satisfaction in observer roles is closely associated with observer tools, learner engagement, role clarity and contribution to the debrief. Learners that valued observer roles described them as affording an overarching view, examination of details from a distance, and meaningful feedback during the debrief. Learners who did not value observer roles described them as passive, or boring when compared to hands-on engagement in the simulation encounter.

Conclusions: Learning outcomes and role satisfaction for observers is improved through learner engagement and the use of observer tools. The value that students attach to observer roles appear contingent on role clarity, use of observer tools, and inclusion of observers' perspectives in the debrief.

Keywords: Simulation, Observer, Observer role, Directed observer, Vicarious learning

* Correspondence: saoregan@msn.com
[1]Sydney Clinical Skills and Simulation Centre, Royal North Shore Hospital, Level 6 Kolling Building, Reserve Rd, St Leonards, NSW 2065, Australia
Full list of author information is available at the end of the article

Background

There has not been a systematic review of the factors that promote learning in the observer roles in simulation. As more learners are allocated to observer roles there is an imperative to ensure that learning in this role is optimised. This review seeks to synthesise the factors that focus the observers' learning and satisfaction in the role and provide educators with guidance to employing observer roles within their simulations.

Simulation is an effective healthcare teaching strategy [1] and can improve knowledge, skills and behaviours when compared to traditional or no teaching [2]. Simulation conventionally enables learners to physically participate in realistic scenarios replicating real world practice and has been reported as an effective replacement for clinical hours for nursing students [3]. Increasing demand, cohort numbers and access limitations, particularly in professional entry programs has resulted in innovative approaches for learners using simulation. These approaches include role modelling [4, 5], peer and near-peer assisted learning [6–8], and alternative instructional design methods whereby learners are actively directed to observe without hands-on participation [9–11]. We refer to this as the directed observer. When simulation is used appropriately, it improves learning outcomes [2, 12]. However, the evidence supporting learning by observation is less clear.

This review presents evidence supporting directed observation as an educational method and features of this method that lead to positive educational outcomes.

The literature is not always clear on what constitutes observer roles. Here, observer roles are defined as two broad types. First, roles where the learner is external to the simulation. For example, the learner will be watching but not participating in the simulation, either within the simulation area or from an area removed from the simulation. Second, roles where the learner is given a role in the simulation that is not congruent with their professional one. For example, a nursing student could realistically be expected to perform the roles of medication nurse, bedside nurse or documentation nurse in their professional activities. However, they would not be a doctor, social worker or patient relative. In this paper, we describe these roles as 'in-scenario' observer roles. Further, observers are described as having a 'directed observer' role or a 'non-directed' role. A directed observer role would include a specific instructional briefing or use of an observer tool. A non-directed observer watches without specific guidance or objectives. The instructional briefing or observer tool contains information for the directed observer on specific learning objectives, behaviours or activities to consider, points for peer feedback or a checklist to measure against. These specifics would then form part of the debrief.

Methods

The search was conducted over five databases (Medline, Cinahl, PsycINFO, EmBase and ERIC) within a publication period of 1980 – July 2015 using 45 search terms and restricted to the English language. Hand searching of grey literature, journal contents and reference lists was also undertaken. The study population included any healthcare professional or student who participated in mannequin, simulated patient (actor) or role-play based simulations that included a specific observer role (Table 1). Studies selected included either direct comparison of the learning outcomes of observers with those of active participants following the simulation or identified the factors important for the engagement of observers in simulations and needed to identify their outcome measures and include changes in knowledge, skills, attitudes or behaviours of participants (Table 2) Specific exclusions included computer or virtual reality based simulations as the observer role was difficult to define, and specific task or skill training as the teaching methodology is different than case based scenarios. Video based learning and expert role

Table 1 Search terms

Population	Intervention	Outcome
Nurs* or	Simulation or	Learn* or
midwif* or	Patient simulation or	Knowledge or
Medic* or	Manikin* or	Skill* or
doctor or	Mannequin* or	Attitude* or
surgery or	Simulated patient* or	Behav*
Allied health or	Standardised patient* or	
Physiotherap* or	Standardized patient* or	
Occupational therap* or	Role play or	
Dental or	Actor or	
Dentist* or	Acting or	
Social work* or	theatre	
Respiratory therap* or		
Dietet* or	AND	
Paramedic* or	Observ* or	
Aboriginal torres strait	Observ* role or	
islander health or	Observational learn* or	
Indigen* or	Vicarious learn* or	
Inter professional or	Watching	
Interprofessional or		
Intra professional or		
Intraprofessional or		
Multi disciplin* or		
Multidisciplin* or		
Multi profession* or		
Multiprofession*		

Table 2 Inclusion and exclusion criteria

Inclusion/Exclusion Criteria		
Criterion	Inclusion	Exclusion
Population	Clinicians and students of any health profession	Non health professionals
Intervention	Undergoing a mannequin or simulated patient based learning experience *and*	Computer based, skill or part-task trainers, virtual reality, or cadaveric simulation/simulators.
	• Examines the role of the observer • Has an observer role defined as a learner within a scenario not in a clinically congruent role *or* • Has an observer role external to scenario participant roles	• Studies which do not explicitly examine the observer role. • Observers who are not participating in the learning, for example observers for the purpose of research study. • Expert modelling for learning
Outcome measures	• A direct or indirect change in knowledge, skills, attitudes or behaviours	• Description of behaviours without consideration of any changes in learner behaviour
Citations	Peer reviewed papers in the english language from 1980 to October 4th 2014.	• Non peer reviewed publications e.g thesis or reports • Descriptive papers • Published texts or books

modelling were also excluded, as there is no comparison of hands-on and observer roles (Table 2).

Results

Nine studies were selected from the 5469 potential papers identified using the PRISMA process [13] (Fig. 1). The studies are summarised in Table 3. The included studies used quantitative, qualitative and mixed methods. A modified version of Buckley's quality indicators, devised for assessment of quantitative, qualitative and mixed methods studies was selected as the quality assessment tool [14]. These 11 quality indicators relate to the appropriateness of study design, conduct, results analysis and conclusions and are not biased towards any particular research methodology (Table 4).

Two reviewers (SO, EM) rated the quality of the studies with an inter-rater agreement of 0.94 across 99 data points. Seven studies meeting seven or more criteria as specified by Buckley, were considered high quality studies [14]. There was a wide range of quality with scores from 3 to 11 out of a possible 11. Most common problems encountered were with data completeness, control for confounders, study replicability and addressing ethical issues. Two studies, Stegmann [15] and Thidemann, [16] met all 11 criteria. Two studies, Lau [17] and Stiefel, [18] met six or less criteria. Rater differences are shown in the table as two scores, with the lowest total score reported where there was a discrepancy (Table 4).

To provide composite data the nine included studies were examined using categories adapted from Cook et al [2]. There were a total of 1203 participants across the nine studies with the majority of studies focusing on undergraduate students in nursing (*n* = 527) and medicine (*n* = 484). There was one interprofessional study involving practising clinicians across four disciplines [19]. Five studies used mannequin-based simulations [11, 16, 20–22], two employed simulated patients [15, 18], one

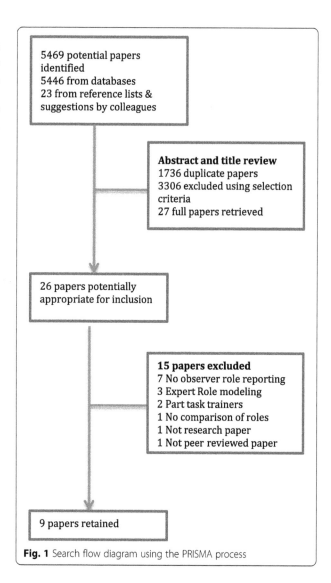

Fig. 1 Search flow diagram using the PRISMA process

Table 3 Summary of selected studies

Reference	Research paradigm, design & sampling[a]	Participants	Intervention	Learner Observation Style	Results
Bell, Pascucci, Fancy, Coleman, Zurakowski and Meyer [24]	Mixed methods Post-simulation survey design with qualitative and quantitative analysis Convenience sample	Health professionals from four disciplines (n = 192) Teaching faculty (n = 33) Actors (SP) (n = 10) Hands on participants (47 %) Observers (53 %)	Use of improvisational actors in difficult conversations to teach communication and relational skills to practicing health professional	Non-directed role: no use of observational tool or verbal guidance reported	No difference between observers and hands on learners in: perceived realism; usefulness of actors; usefulness of scenarios; and, opinions on non-actor role play
Harder, Ross and Paul [25]	Ethnographic stud Observational design with focused interview and journal review of selected participants Volunteer sample	Bachelor of Nursing students year 3 (n = 84) Participant/observation (n = 84) interview (n = 12) journal review (n = 4)	Role assignment within regular simulation session with analysis of experience and perceptions of learning within different role All participants experienced both roles	Non-directed role: no use of observer tool or verbal guidance reported	Students preferred assignment to nursing roles rather than observer or non nursing role Structured role descriptions positively affected learning outcomes
Hober and Bonnel [11]	Qualitative Survey and interview design Convenience sample	Bachelor of Nursing "senior" students (n = 50) Observers (n = 23) hands on learners (n = 27)	Immersive simulation scenarios with students randomly assigned to active or observer roles All completed survey Observers interviewed	Directed observer role: observer tool – educator provided activity guidelines	Observer role beneficial, less stressful Use of a guided observer tool useful Able to reflect in action and on action
Kaplan, Abraham and Gary [27]	Quantitative Randomised groups Convenience sample	Bachelor of Nursing "junior" students (n = 92) Observers (n = 46) Scenario participants (n = 46)	Immersive simulation scenarios - participants self selected roles Unclear whether observers self selected or were assigned Post scenario knowledge test and satisfaction survey	Directed observer role: observer tool -checklist	No difference in knowledge Limited as aggregated post satisfaction survey data
Lau, Stewart and Fielding [22]	Quasi experimental randomised to roles Convenience sample	Medical students (bilingual) year 1 (n = 160)	Student role plays with comparison of learning between interpreter role play and observer role Self rated pre & post knowledge	Directed observer role: observer tool -checklist	Observers rated post knowledge higher than learners in interpreter role-play

Table 3 Summary of selected studies (Continued)

Smith, Klaassen, Zimmerman and Cheng [26]	Mixed methods with increasing variables over three years Convenience sample	Bachelor of Nursing "junior" students year 1 (n = 67) year 2 (n = 72) year 3 (n = 85) Note only the year 2 and 3 data were included in review	Introduction of simulation year 1 Introduction non nursing participatory roles year Introduction non participatory observer roles year 3	Non-directed role: no use of observational tool or verbal guidance reported	No significant difference in learning outcomes, student perceptions or peer evaluations
Stegmann, Pilz, Siebeck and Fischer [20]	Quantitative Crossover design 2x2x2 pre-test post-test	Medical students (n = 200)	Comparison of participatory role and observer role in simulated patient scenario with and without observation tool	Non-directed and directed observer roles compared: checklists and feedback scripts used	Observational learning (especially if supported by observer script) more effective than learning by doing
Stiefel, Bourquin, Layat, Vadot, Bonvin and Berney [23]	Quantitative Randomised into 2 group Evaluation using instructor rating scale and student questionnaire Convenience sample	Medical students (masters level) (n = 124) Individual training (n = 49) Group training (n = 75) -participated in simulation (n = 14) observed (n = 61)	Individual training with simulated patient encounter Group training with simulated patient encounter Group training with observation of simulated encounter	Non-directed observer role: no use of observer tool or verbal guidance reported	Measured outcomes no difference Those who observed but did not participate felt they did not meet their learning objectives as well compared to the other 2 groups
Thidemann and Soderhamn [21]	Quasi experimental Pre - and post-simulation knowledge test and student questionnaire Convenience sample over two consecutive years	Bachelor of Nursing student year 2 (n = 144)	Immersive mannequin simulation with random allocation to groups Four volunteers within each group allocated to participatory and in scenario observer roles – remainder observers (n = 72)	Directed observer role: observer tool with specific task focus	Post-test scores higher in all groups independent of rol More satisfaction with nurse role

[a] as attributed by author where available

Table 4 Study ratings using Buckley's (modified) criteria

Criteria (Yes, No, Unclear) Note: rater disagreement shown as two scores	Bell	Harder	Hober	Kaplan	Lau	Smith	Stegmann	Stiefel	Thidemann
Clear research question	U	Y	Y	Y	U	Y	Y	U	Y
Subject group appropriate for study	Y	Y	Y	Y	Y	Y	Y	Y	Y
Reliable and valid methods (qualitative or quantitative) used	Y	Y	Y	Y	Y/U	Y	Y	Y	Y
Completeness of data (drop out, questionnaire response rate >60 %, attrition rate <50 %)	Y	Y	Y	Y	N	N	Y	N	Y
Controlled for confounders or acknowledged if non RCT design	N	U/N	N	U/N	U	N	Y	U	Y
Statistical and other analysis methods appropriate	Y	Y	Y	Y	Y	Y	Y	Y	Y
Data justifies the conclusions drawn	Y	Y	Y	Y	N	Y	Y	U/N	Y
Study could be replicated	Y/U	Y	Y	Y	U	N/U	Y	Y	Y
Prospective study	Y	Y	Y	Y	Y	Y	Y	Y	Y
Relevant ethical issues addressed	U	Y	Y	N	U	Y	Y	U	Y
Triangulation of data	Y	Y	Y	Y	N	Y	Y	N	Y
Total Score/11 (lowest score reported)	7	10	10	9	3	8	11	5	11

an actor [19], and one study involved role-play by the participant group [17] (Table 5).

Eight of the nine studies compared knowledge, skills, attitudes or behaviours between the hands-on role and the observer role [11, 15, 17, 18, 20–22]. Six studies used a pre and post-test design, three of which were self-assessment of improvement in knowledge and/or skills [17–19] and three studies tested knowledge [15, 16, 21]. Two studies examined knowledge in a post-test only design [22] one of which was a self-assessment [20]. Outcomes included knowledge (six), 'non-technical skills' (eight), technical skills (three), attitudes (two) and behaviours (one).

Four studies found no difference in outcomes between the hands-on learners and the observers [11, 16, 19, 22]. Two studies reported superior outcomes in the hands-on group [18, 20] and one study reported better outcomes in the observer group [15]. The study that found superior outcomes for the observer group and three of the four studies that found no difference in outcomes between the hands-on and observer groups [15–17, 22] incorporated an observer tool to guide the observer group. Neither study that demonstrated superior outcomes by the hands-on learners employed an observer tool [18, 20].

Six studies considered the perceived value of the hands-on learner and observer roles to the participants. Two studies reported that participants valued the hands-on roles more than the observer role [18, 20], one study highly valued the observer role [16] and three studies reported no difference in the value of the roles [11, 19, 22]. Two of the three studies with no value difference in roles [11, 22], and the study that valued the observer role highly [16] used an observer tool. The study that

valued the hands-on roles higher did not employ an observer tool for the observer group [18]. The observer tools included performance checklists [15, 17, 22], feedback or observation guides [11, 15], or observer role instructional briefing [16]. All studies except Bell [23] documented including observers in the post simulation debrief or feedback.

Discussion

We sought reported factors that contribute to the optimisation of learning in the observer role. It is clear from this review that the use of observer tools to focus the observer and role clarity are strongly associated with role satisfaction and learning outcomes in observer roles. This finding is supported by Bandura's social learning theory and Kolb's experiential learning cycle and we propose that these form the basis of the directed observer role.

One of the outstanding findings from this review is the association of observer tools with both satisfaction and equal if not better, learning outcomes in observer roles. The use of these tools may move observers from simply watching to actively observing. The activation of observers allows those in that role to experience the satisfaction and learning normally associated with hands-on experience. Simulation is described by Dieckmann et al as a social practice where people interact with each other in a goal orientated fashion [24]. The observer tool provides this necessary goal orientation for observer roles. Directed observers are focused on the learning objectives of the simulation.

This is explained by Bandura's social learning theory, which proposes that virtually all learning acquired experientially could also be acquired on "*a vicarious basis*

Table 5 Characteristics of included studies

Study Characteristics	Number of Studies	Number of Participants
All studies	9	1203
Study participants		
Medical students	3	484
Nursing students	5	527
Practicing clinicians	1	
Physician		43
Nurse		114
"Psychosocial clinicians"		20
Medical interpreter		14
Study settings		
Mannequin based simulation (high fidelity simulation - HFS)	5	527
Simulated patient (SP)	2	324
Actor (improvisation rather than scripted SP)	1	192
Role play by participant group	1	160
Study design		
Post test only (Knowledge)	1	92
Pre-test/post-test 1 group	1	157
Pre-test/post-test 2 groups	2	344
Self-assessment pre-test and post-test	3	476
Self-assessment post-test only	1	84
Observer role allocation		
Randomised	5	643
Self allocation	1	84
Unclear	2	284
Outcome		
Knowledge	6	869
Skills - technical	3	441
Skills - non technical	8	1059
Attitudes	2	134
Behaviours	1	84
Learning outcomes by role		
Participatory role better than observer	2	208
Observer role better than participatory	1	200
No difference	4	588
Satisfaction by role		
Participatory role more valued than observer	2	208
Observer role more valued than participatory	1	144
No difference in value	3	334
Observational tool used	6	803
Debriefing/feedback		
Observer led pairs	1	200
Faculty led group debrief	7	811
Feedback guide	1	200

through observation of other people's behaviour and its consequences for them [25]. Through observation learners can build behaviours without trial and error, experience emotions by watching others and resolve fears through other's experience. Bandura describes this as a process of attention, retention, reproduction and motivation [25]. Bethards reports on a program where *"simulation experiences are designed around the observer role using the four component processes of Bandura's observational learning construct"* [26]. They postulate that this provides all their learners, regardless of role, the same opportunities to achieve the learning objectives [26].

Vicarious learning requires active listening, reflective thinking and situational engagement [27]. Nehls describes this in the context of narratives; lived experiences shared for the purpose of learning [27]. The addition of "active watching" to Nehls' definition fits well in the simulation context. In a review of vicarious learning, Roberts concludes that vicarious learning occurs during story telling and discourse, and may require a teacher to help find meaning [28]. In the context of scenario-based simulation the story is the scenario or case; active listening and watching is engaged with the use of tools or tasks and the reflective facilitated discussion is the debriefing. It seems important that for optimal learning to occur, observers be engaged in all aspects including the debrief.

Experiential learning is viewed as fundamental to simulation and clinical practice [29, 30] and the theoretical foundations of simulation are commonly described in terms of Kolb's experiential learning cycle [29]. Kolb proposes a cycle of concrete experiences which on reflection are distilled into abstract concepts that can then provide the basis for future actions and further testing [31]. Kolb stresses that this is an unending cycle and educators need to be aware that learners have a preference for, and may enter at different stages of the experiential learning cycle, but need to be moved through the entire process. A dangerous presumption for educators and learners alike is that concrete experience requires hands-on participation. Vicarious learning theory and Kolb's experiential learning cycle form the theoretical basis for directed observation.

It seems that observers with the appropriate tools can benefit vicariously from the experience of the hands-on learners. Simulation is a facsimile of the clinical environment so the findings here may also translate to observation in similar clinical practice situations. This directed observer role is different to indirect workplace learning described by Le Clus, where the emphasis is on observers seeking learning to meet their personal needs [32]. However, the concept of observer learning as a social practice aligns with both [24, 32].

Stegmann reports better outcomes from observers preparing to provide feedback than those completing a checklist or in a hands-on role [15]. The impending 'debrief' where observers have an expectation that they will be asked to contribute their opinions about the encounter may sharpen the focus of their observations. Bandura describes this as an external motivator [25]. This 'heightened state' may mean observers are more likely to engage in standards of practice required for the simulation (for example, measures of good communication) and consider how the simulation participant's performance measures up to this standard. Thidemann used reporting on standards of practice in her directed observer role guidelines [16].

The learners who did not value observer roles as highly as a hands-on role described observer roles as passive, or boring [20]. They were not fully engaged in the learning process. Emotional engagement in simulation is connected to the feeling of relevance of the scenario to the goals of the session [24]. Lack of goal direction may have prevented observer engagement. It is not clear whether there is an optimal level of activation for learning in observer roles or whether it differs between learners. Learners that valued observer roles described it as being less stressful and providing them the opportunity to see the big picture, examine details from a distance, and provide meaningful feedback to the team [11]. Stress decompression, a feature of debriefing frameworks, is necessary for reflection [30, 33].

The ability to reflect is important in the provision of feedback. An understanding of performance requirements and a judgement regarding the observed performance and its relationship to the standard is required before bridging strategies can be formulated [34]. In directed observer roles, information was provided in the form of the observer tool (e.g. checklist) defining the standards and/or objectives for the learners. The directed observers were able to use these tools to observe, reflect upon and formulate their peer feedback for the debrief.

In-scenario observers, that is non-clinical or other professional roles within the scenario, reported that lack of scripts or clear direction detracted from the act of observation because of anxiety regarding role performance requirements [20]. These aspects of role fidelity have been identified as a barrier to student satisfaction with role play [35]. The other studies that used non-clinical or other non-congruent professional roles viewed these learners as hands-on participants and did not include specific findings for these in-scenario observer roles [17, 20, 21]. Thidemann commented that the nursing roles in their scenarios were the most preferred roles [16]. The lack of clarity in the separation between professionally congruent and incongruent hand-on roles in these studies prevents drawing any real conclusions from the data. In a report of a large study for the National League of Nurses Jefferies and Rizzola [1] concluded that whilst knowledge and self-confidence were unrelated to role allocation, there was a perceived lack of collaboration in the observer role and there was a responsibility for educators to provide structure for this to occur [9].

While learners have assessed the value of observer roles, there has not been a published assessment of the value placed upon observer roles in simulation by educators or facilitators. Use of observer tools or activities and the active involvement of observers in the post-scenario debrief could be considered an indirect indication of the value educators place on learning in observer roles.

It is also unclear as to whether there is a group of learners better suited to learning through observation than learning through hands-on participation in the simulation. Whilst most of the studies used role allocation, one study [20] had a portion of study participants who either self allocated or worked through the case as a group without assigned roles. There was confusion amongst the students in this study as to which roles were considered to be observers; for example some students viewed the documentation nurse as an observer role while others viewed it as a hands-on role. No studies examined whether self-allocation to roles would result in better learning outcomes. The reasons behind self-allocation were also not examined and may be worthy of further study.

An important area for further study includes establishing educator perceived value of observational roles, and the potential impact of these perceptions on simulation education design and orientation of learners to roles within the scenarios. Activation and emotional engagement in the observer role has also not been explored, and provides future research potential.

Limitations

This review examines one small area of observational learning within scenario-based simulation. Skills training, which is often taught in groups was not included. Also excluded were non peer-reviewed reports, including a major study of more than 400 nurses [9]. This report did however inform the discussion. We also narrowly defined simulation modalities excluding virtual reality simulations where there is even more blurring of boundaries between hands-on participants and observer roles. In some studies it was unclear how the authors defined the in-scenario roles. Reporting of observer roles was in some cases a secondary finding. Lack of clarity may have biased findings. The small number of included papers also limits the conclusions.

Conclusion

Learning outcomes for participants and observers in simulation can have value if all roles involve active learning either through hands-on roles within the simulation, or through use of tools to facilitate active observer learning. The value that students attach to observer roles seems to be related to the value educators place on them as evidenced through role briefing, use of observer tools to hone judgement of performance compared to standards, and inclusion of observers' perspectives in debriefing.

Endnotes

[1]This study was not included, as it did not meet the inclusion criteria of peer-reviewed publication however the findings are important and inform the discussion (see study limitations).

Competing interests

Stephanie O'Regan declares she has no competing financial or other interests.
Elizabeth Molloy declares she has no competing financial or other interests
Leonie Watterson declares she has no competing financial or other interests
Debra Nestel is the Editor in Chief of Advances in Simulation. She has no other competing interests.

Authors' contributions

SO conceived the study, drafted the study design, search protocol, conducted the search, selected the included studies, participated in the study ratings and drafted the manuscript. EM refined the study design and search protocol, participated in the study rating, helped draft the manuscript and contributed to the background literature. LW helped draft the manuscript and contributed to the background literature. DN refined the study design and search protocol, helped draft the manuscript and contributed to the background literature. All authors read an approved the final manuscript.

Acknowledgements

There are no other acknowledgments to be made for this manuscript. The authors received no external funding for the data collection or preparation of this manuscript.

Author details

[1]Sydney Clinical Skills and Simulation Centre, Royal North Shore Hospital, Level 6 Kolling Building, Reserve Rd, St Leonards, NSW 2065, Australia. [2]Health Professions Education and Educational Research (HealthPEER), Faculty of Medicine, Nursing and Health Sciences, Monash University, Building 13C, Office G09, Clayton Campus, Victoria 3800, Australia.

References

1. Issenberg BS, McGaghie WC, Petrusa ER, Lee Gordon D, Scalese RJ. Features and uses of high-fidelity medical simulations that lead to effective learning: a BEME systematic review. Med Teach. 2005;27(1):10–28.
2. Cook DA, Hatala R, Brydges R, Zendejas B, Szostek JH, Wang AT, et al. Technology-enhanced simulation for health professions education: a systematic review and meta-analysis. JAMA. 2011;306(9):978–88.
3. Hayden JK, Smiley RA, Alexander M, Kardong-Edgren S, Jeffries PR. The NCSBN National Simulation Study: a longitudinal, randomized, controlled study replacing clinical hours with simulation in prelicensure nursing education. J Nur Reg. 2014;5(S2):s4–s41.
4. LeFlore JL, Anderson M, Michael JL, Engle WD, Anderson J. Comparison of self-directed learning versus instructor-modeled learning during a simulated clinical experience. Sim Healthcare. 2007;2(3):170–7.
5. LeFlore JL, Anderson M. Effectiveness of 2 methods to teach and evaluate new content to neonatal transport personnel using high-fidelity simulation. J Perinat Neonat Nurs. 2008;22(4):319–28.
6. Nestel D, Kidd J. Peer assisted learning in patient-centred interviewing: the impact on student tutors. Med Teach. 2005;27(5):439–44.
7. Field M, Burke JM, McAllister D, Lloyd DM. Peer-assisted learning: a novel approach to clinical skills learning for medical students. Med Educ. 2007;41(4):411–8.
8. Ladyshewsky R. Building competency in the novice allied health professional through peer coaching. J Allied Health. 2010;39(2):e77–82.
9. Jeffries P, Rizzola MA. Designing and implementing models for the innovative use of simulation to teach nursing care of ill adults and children: a national, multi-Site, multi-method study. 2006. National League for Nursing.
10. Ertmer PA, Strobel J, Cheng X, Chen X, Kim H, Olesova L, et al. Expressions of critical thinking in role-playing simulations: comparisons across roles. J Comput in High Educ. 2010;22(2):73–94.
11. Hober C, Bonnel W. Student perceptions of the observer role in high-fidelity simulation. Clin Sim Nurs. 2014;10(10):507–14.
12. McGaghie WC, Issenberg SB, Petrusa ER, Scalese RJ. A critical review of simulation-based medical education research: 2003-2009. Med Educ. 2010;44(1):50–63.
13. Moher D, Liberati A, Tetzlaff J, Altman D. Preferred reporting Items for systematic reviews and meta-analyses: the PRISMA statement. PLoS Med. 2009;6(6):e1000097.
14. Buckley S, Coleman J, Davison I, Khan KS, Zamora J, Malick S, et al. The educational effects of portfolios on undergraduate student learning: A Best Evidence Medical Education (BEME) systematic review. BEME Guide No. 11. Med Teach. 2009;31(4):302.
15. Stegmann K, Pilz F, Siebeck M, Fischer F. Vicarious learning during simulations: is it more effective than hands-on training? Med Educ. 2012;46(10):1001–8.
16. Thidemann IJ, Soderhamn O. High-fidelity simulation among bachelor students in simulation groups and use of different roles. Nurs Educ Today. 2013;33(12):1599–604.
17. Lau KC, Stewart SM, Fielding R. Preliminary evaluation of "interpreter" role plays in teaching communication skills to medical undergraduates. Med Educ. 2001;35(3):217–21.
18. Stiefel F, Bourquin C, Layat C, Vadot S, Bonvin R, Berney A. Medical students' skills and needs for training in breaking bad news. J Cancer Educ. 2013;28(1):187–91.
19. Bell SK, Pascucci R, Fancy K, Coleman K, Zurakowski D, Meyer EC. The educational value of improvisational actors to teach communication and relational skills: perspectives of interprofessional learners, faculty, and actors. Patient Educ Counsel. 2014;96(3):381–8.
20. Harder N, Ross CJM, Paul P. Student perspective of role assignment in high-fidelity simulation: an ethnographic study. Clin Sim Nurs. 2013;9(9):e329–e34.
21. Smith KV, Klaassen J, Zimmerman C, Cheng AL. The evolution of a high-fidelity patient simulation learning experience to teach legal and ethical issues. J Prof Nurs. 2013;29(3):168–73.
22. Kaplan BG, Abraham C, Gary R. Effects of participation vs. observation of a simulation experience on testing outcomes: implications for logistical planning for a school of nursing. Int J Nurs Educ Scholarsh. 2012;9(1) doi:10.1515/1548-923X.2398.
23. Sanders A, Bellefeuille P, van Schaik S. Emotional impact of active versus observational roles during simulation learning. Sim Healthcare; 2013;8(6) p. 589.
24. Dieckmann P, Gaba D, Rall M. Deepening the theoretical foundations of patient simulation as social practice. Sim Healthcare. 2007;2(3):183–93.
25. Bandura A. Social Learning Theory. New York City: General Learning Press; 1971.
26. Bethards ML. Applying social learning theory to the observer role in simulation. Clin Sim Nurs. 2014;10(2):e65–e9.
27. Nehls N. Narrative Pedagogy: Rethinking nursing education. J Nurs Educ. 1995;35(5):204–10.
28. Roberts D. Vicarious learning: a review of the literature. Nurs Educ Pract. 2010;10(1):13–6.
29. Stocker M, Burmester M, Allen M. Optimisation of simulated team training through the application of learning theories: a debate for a conceptual framework. BMC Med Educ. 2014;14:69.
30. Rudolph JW, Simon R, Raemer DB, Eppich WJ. Debriefing as formative assessment: closing performance gaps in medical education. Acad Emerg Med. 2008;15(11):1010–6.

31. Kolb DA. Experiential Learning: Experience as the source of learning and development. 2nd ed. Pearson Education Inc: New Jersay; 2015.

32. Le Clus M. Informal learning in the workplace: a review of the literature. Aust J Adult Learn. 2011;51:355–73.

33. Husebo S, O'Regan S, Nestel D. Reflective practice and its role in simulation. Clin Sim Nurs. 2015;11:368–75.

34. Sadler DR. Formative assessment and the design of instructional systems. Instr Sci. 1989;18:119–44.

35. Nestel D, Tierney T. Role-play for medical students learning about communication: Guidelines for maximising benefits. BMC Med Educ. 2007;7:3.

Prehospital paths and hospital arrival time of patients with acute coronary syndrome or stroke, a prospective observational study

Carine J. M. Doggen[1*], Marlies Zwerink[1], Hanneke M. Droste[2], Paul J. A. M. Brouwers[2], Gert K. van Houwelingen[3], Fred L. van Eenennaam[4] and Rolf E. Egberink[1,5]

Abstract

Background: Patients with a presumed diagnosis of acute coronary syndrome (ACS) or stroke may have had contact with several healthcare providers prior to hospital arrival. The aim of this study was to describe the various prehospital paths and the effect on time delays of patients with ACS or stroke.

Methods: This prospective observational study included patients with presumed ACS or stroke who may choose to contact four different types of health care providers. Questionnaires were completed by patients, general practitioners (GP), GP cooperatives, ambulance services and emergency departments (ED). Additional data were retrieved from hospital registries.

Results: Two hundred two ACS patients arrived at the hospital by 15 different paths and 243 stroke patients by ten different paths. Often several healthcare providers were involved (60.8 % ACS, 95.1 % stroke). Almost half of all patients first contacted their GP (47.5 % ACS, 49.4 % stroke). Some prehospital paths were more frequently used, e.g. GP (cooperative) and ambulance in ACS, and GP or ambulance and ED in stroke. In 65 % of all events an ambulance was involved. Median time between start of symptoms and hospital arrival for ACS patients was over 6 h and for stroke patients 4 h. Of ACS patients 47.7 % waited more than 4 h before seeking medical advice compared to 31.6 % of stroke patients. Median time between seeking medical advice to arrival at hospital was shortest in paths involving the ambulance only (60 min ACS, 54 min stroke) or in combination with another healthcare provider (80 to 100 min ACS, 99 to 106 min stroke).

Conclusions: Prehospital paths through which patients arrived in hospital are numerous and often complex, and various time delays occurred. Delays depend on the entry point of the health care system, and dialing the emergency number seems to be the best choice. Since reducing patient delay is difficult and noticeable differences exist between various prehospital paths, further research into reasons for these different entry choices may yield possibilities to optimize paths and reduce overall time delay.

Keywords: Acute stroke, Prehospital paths, Delay, Acute coronary syndrome

* Correspondence: c.j.m.doggen@utwente.nl
[1]Department of Health Technology and Services Research (HTSR), MIRA institute for Biomedical Technology and Technical Medicine, University of Twente, RA 5252, PO Box 217, 7500 AE, Enschede, The Netherlands
Full list of author information is available at the end of the article

Background

In myocardial infarction (MI), percutaneous coronary intervention (PCI) is the treatment of choice usually followed by stent implantation. Treatment of ischemic stroke consists of intravenous thrombolysis with recombinant tissue plasminogen activator (rt-PA). In both cases treatment should start as soon as possible after first symptoms to prevent further tissue damage. According to guidelines, primary PCI should preferably start within 90 min after first medical contact for patients with ST-elevated myocardial infarction [1]. Most stroke guidelines recommend treatment with rt-PA within 4.5 h after first symptoms [2, 3]. In line with these guidelines, sets of quality indicators have been developed. Door-to-balloon time indicates the timeframe between arrival of the patient with myocardial infarction at the hospital and start of PCI. Door-to-needle time indicates the time between arrival of patient with ischemic stroke at the hospital and start of thrombolysis. However, mainly because of prehospital delay, many patients arrive too late for treatment, and in clinical reality across the entire stroke population this treatment can be given to only a minority (1–8 %) of such patients [4]. Improving these disappointing numbers seems to be very difficult.

Prior to arrival at the hospital patients may have had contact with several healthcare providers. In the Netherlands most patients contact their general practitioner (GP), and outside office hours most patients contact a GP cooperative. Alternatively, patients dial the national emergency number, and the dispatch center will send an ambulance if requested and warranted according to a standard protocol. Others will directly visit the Emergency Department (ED) of the hospital. This points out that several healthcare providers, and thus various prehospital paths may be involved.

Information about various prehospital paths and associated time delays is scarce [5, 6]. Therefore, the aim of this study was to describe the prehospital paths of patients with a presumed diagnosis of acute coronary syndrome or stroke and measure time to hospital treatment. Additionally, door-to-balloon time of patients with ST-elevated myocardial infarction and door-to-needle time of patients with ischemic stroke were assessed.

Methods

Study design and study population

This is a prospective observational study. Patients with a provisional diagnosis of Acute Coronary Syndrome (ACS) or stroke, suggested by the health care provider who was contacted by the patient in the prehospital phase, were included between May 2012 and July 2012 and between September 2012 and October 2012. Patients were 18 years or older and living in the region of Twente and Oost Achterhoek, the Netherlands. About 750,000 inhabitants live in this area of 2093 km^2 where three hospitals, four GP cooperatives and two ambulance emergency medical services are active. No other in- or exclusion criteria were used.

Patients with a provisional diagnosis of ACS were hospitalized at a coronary care unit (CCU) in one of the three hospitals. One of these hospitals has the facilities to perform percutaneous coronary interventions (PCI). If a ST-elevated myocardial infarction was suspected based on the electrocardiogram (ECG) made in the ambulance, patients were transported to the hospital with PCI facilities; otherwise the patient was transported to the nearest hospital. Patients with a provisional diagnosis of stroke were transported to the nearest hospital. All three hospitals have a fully equipped stroke unit with facilities to provide thrombolysis.

Data collection

Nurses(specialists) at the CCU or stroke unit informed (both orally and written) and asked admitted patients to participate in the study within 24 h of arrival. Each participating patient provided written informed consent and filled in a questionnaire, sometimes with some help of a relative. This structured questionnaire included questions regarding date, time, circumstances of the ACS or stroke, date and time of seeking medical advice, and the healthcare provider(s) the patient had contact with. The ambulance emergency medical services, EDs of the three hospitals, individual GPs and GP Cooperatives received an electronic questionnaire, focusing on date, time of telephone call from the patient or others, and date and time of visit when applicable. Data on arrival date and time at CCU or stroke unit, time of PCI or thrombolysis, and final diagnoses at hospital discharge were retrieved from hospital registries. In the few cases where similar data was asked for but different answers were obtained, data from health care providers and hospital registries were used. The study was submitted to the accredited medical ethical committee Twente and was deemed to be non-intrusive and therefore did not fall under the Dutch law governing scientific research with humans.

Patient delay is defined as the difference between the time of onset of symptoms according to the patient and the time the patient, family member, friend or bystander decided to call or visit a healthcare provider (first medical contact where medical advice is given). Furthermore, time between first medical contact and arrival at CCU (ACS patients) or ED (stroke patients) is calculated. Additionally, time between onset of symptoms and arrival at hospital is calculated. No upper time limits were used. Door-to-balloon time for patients receiving PCI is defined as the difference between time at arrival in hospital and starting time of the PCI procedure. Since most patients in need for PCI are transported directly to the CCU, door-time of CCU is used. For those patients who arrived at the ED, arrival time at ED is used as door-time. Door-to-needle time for stroke patients receiving thrombolysis is defined as the difference between arrival time at the ED and start of thrombolysis.

Data analyses

For continuous variables means and standard deviations (SD) were calculated for normally distributed data. Median values with interquartile ranges (IQR 25-75th percentiles) were calculated for non-parametric continuous data. Categorical variables are presented as absolute values and percentages.

Results

Included in the study were 202 patients with a provisional diagnosis of acute coronary syndrome and 243 patients with a provisional diagnosis of stroke. Most patients with acute coronary syndrome were men (65.8 %) and the mean age was 63.3 years (Table 1). Final diagnoses of these 202 patients were: 19.3 % ST-elevated myocardial infarction, 20.8 % non ST-elevated myocardial infarction, 22.8 % unstable angina pectoris, 27.7 % aspecific thoracic complaints and 9.4 % other diagnoses, such as intercostal myalgia or atrial fibrillation. Half of the 243 patients with presumed stroke were men (50.2 %) and mean age was 69.4 years. Four patients were hospitalized twice during the inclusion period. Overall 74.9 % of the patients were finally diagnosed with acute ischemic stroke, 7.4 % transient ischemic attack, 7.8 % hemorrhagic stroke and 9.9 % with other diagnoses, such as peripheral vertigo or epileptic seizure.

About three-quarter of the patients were at home when symptoms started and in half of the events their partner was present. In the ACS group 57.4 %, and in the stroke group 28.4 % sought medical advice themselves.

Prehospital paths

The 202 patients of the ACS group arrived at the CCU by 15 different paths (Fig. 1). In the prehospital phase 39.2 % had contact with one healthcare provider and 60.8 % with two or more health care providers. The four most frequently used prehospital paths were 'GP cooperative and ambulance', 'GP and ambulance', 'GP only' and 'ambulance only' (Table 2). Of the 202 patients 96 (47.5 %) had first medical contact with their GP and 69 (34.2 %) with the GP cooperative. Only 27 (13.4 %) patients immediately called the national emergency number. Of the 96 patients who first had contact with their GP, 50 (52.1 %) were transported by ambulance, and 27 (28.1 %) arrived at the CCU using private transportation. Of the 69 patients who first had contact with a GP cooperative, 51 (73.9 %) were transported by ambulance, and 12 (17.4 %) arrived at the CCU by private transportation.

Overall, ambulances transported 140 out of 202 (69.0 %) patients with ACS of whom 133 directly to the CCU.

Patients in the stroke group arrived at the stroke unit through 10 different paths (Fig. 2). Almost five percent (4.9 %) of the 243 patients had contact with only one healthcare provider and 95.1 % with two or more health care providers before arriving at the stroke unit. The four most frequently used prehospital paths were 'ambulance and ED', 'GP and ED', 'GP, ambulance and ED' and 'GP cooperative, ambulance and ED' (Table 3). Of the 243 patients 120 (49.4 %) first sought medical advice from their GP, 55 (22.6 %) patients contacted the GP cooperative first, and 59 (24.3 %) patients immediately called the national emergency number. Almost half of the patients who first had contact with their GP were transported by ambulance (45.8 %) and others arrived at the ED using private transportation (45.8 %). Of the 55 patients who first contacted the GP cooperative 35 (63.6 %) were transported by ambulance and 20 (36.4 %) arrived at the ED by their own means. Overall, the ambulances transported 156 out of 243 patients (64.0 %) with a stroke.

Time delays

Median time between onset of symptoms and time to arrival at CCU in the ACS group was 385 min. Median patient delay was 180 min and 47.7 % of all the patients

Table 1 Characteristics and circumstances of 202 patients with ACS and 243 patients with stroke

	ACS (N = 202)	Stroke (N = 243)
	N (%)[b]	N (%)[b]
Men	133 (65.8)	122 (50.2)
Age, mean (SD)	63.3 (13.1)	69.4 (12.9)
Location when having symptoms[a]		
At home	146 (72.3)	188 (77.7)
Public place	47 (23.3)	39 (16.1)
Other	9 (4.5)	15 (6.2)
Other person present when having symptoms[a]		
Nobody	59 (29.2)	69 (28.6)
Partner	110 (54.5)	116 (48.1)
Family, friends or acquaintances	23 (11.4)	35 (14.5)
Other	10 (5.0)	21 (8.7)
Person who sought medical advice[a]		
Patient	112 (57.4)	69 (28.4)
Partner	47 (24.1)	80 (32.9)
Family, friends or acquaintances	17 (8.7)	57 (23.5)
Other	19 (9.7)	37 (15.2)

[a] ≤ two missings
[b] Number and percentage, unless otherwise stated

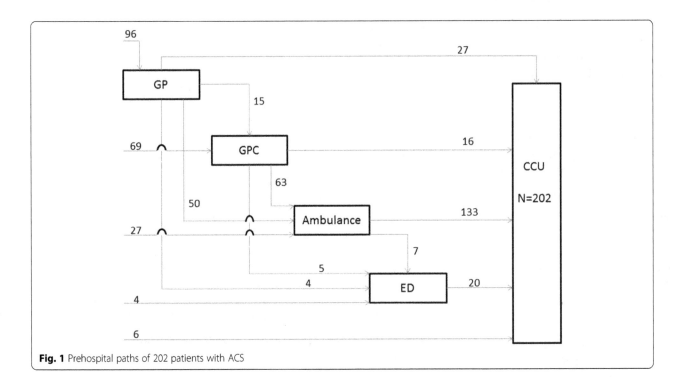

Fig. 1 Prehospital paths of 202 patients with ACS

Table 2 Time (minutes) between onset of symptoms, seeking medical advice and arrival at CCU for patients with ACS overall and by most common prehospital paths

	Overall	Most common prehospital path			
		GP cooperative – ambulance	GP – ambulance	GP only	Ambulance only
	$N = 202$	$N = 51$ (25.2 %)	$N = 49$ (24.3 %)	$N = 27$ (13.4 %)	$N = 25$ (12.4 %)
	N (%)[a]	N (%)[b]	N (%)[b]	N (%)[b]	N (%)[b]
Symptom - arrival					
Median (25-75th)	385 (130–2859)	172 (99–608)	582 (155–4285)	4333 (416–13,184)	120 (82–405)
< 90	24 (12.1)	7 (13.7)	3 (6.3)	2 (7.7)	6 (26.1)
90-239	61 (30.8)	23 (45.1)	15 (31.3)	3 (11.5)	10 (43.5)
240-359	8 (4.0)	3 (5.9)	3 (6.3)	1 (3.8)	0 (0.0)
> = 360	105 (53.0)	18 (35.3)	27 (56.3)	20 (76.9)	7 (30.4)
Symptom - medical advice[c]					
Median (25-75th)	180 (30–1425)	95 (20–360)	495 (60–4085)	1290 (53–13,020)	60 (30–353)
< 90	82 (41.2)	24 (47.1)	16 (34.0)	7 (26.9)	16 (64.0)
90-239	22 (11.1)	10 (19.6)	4 (8.5)	0 (0.0)	2 (8.0)
240-359	14 (7.0)	4 (7.8)	2 (4.2)	1 (3.8)	1 (4.0)
> = 360	81 (40.7)	13 (25.5)	25 (53.2)	18 (69.2)	6 (24.0)
Medical advice - arrival					
Median (25-75th)	95 (60–196)	80 (60–113)	100 (71–167)	197 (100–1678)	60 (45–74)
< 90	91 (46.0)	29 (56.9)	19 (39.6)	6 (23.1)	20 (87.0)
90–239	65 (32.8)	15 (29.4)	20 (41.7)	9 (34.6)	3 (13.0)
240–359	6 (3.0)	1 (2.0)	1 (2.1)	1 (3.8)	0 (0.0)
> = 360	36 (18.2)	6 (11.8)	8 (16.7)	10 (38.5)	0 (0.0)

[a] ≤ four missings
[b] ≤ two missings
[c] Is patient delay

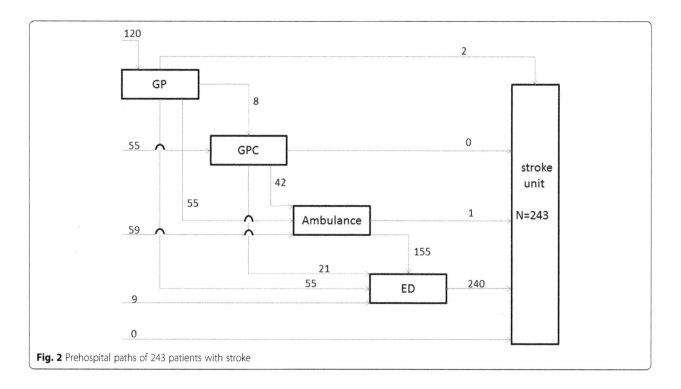

Fig. 2 Prehospital paths of 243 patients with stroke

Table 3 Time (minutes) between onset of symptoms, seeking medical advice and arrival at ED for patients with stroke overall and by most common prehospital paths

	Overall	Most common prehospital path			
		Ambulance – ED	GP – ED	GP – ambulance – ED	GP cooperative – ambulance – ED
	N = 243	N = 58 (23.9 %)	N = 55 (22.6 %)	N = 55 (22.6 %)	N = 35 (14.4 %)
	N (%)[a]	N (%)[b]	N (%)[b]	N (%)[b]	N (%)[b]
Symptom – arrival					
Median (25-75th)	240 (90–1031)	83 (49–288)	781 (291–1929)	209 (98–1031)	183 (83–1206)
< 60	34 (14.6)	21 (38.2)	1 (1.9)	6 (11.5)	5 (14.3)
60–239	82 (35.3)	17 (31.0)	9 (17.1)	23 (44.2)	18 (51.4)
240–359	24 (10.3)	6 (10.9)	8 (15.1)	5 (9.6)	2 (5.8)
> = 360	92 (39.7)	11 (20.0)	35 (66.0)	18 (34.6)	10 (28.6)
Symptom – medical advice[c]					
Median (25-75th)	60 (10–450)	15 (5–60)	195 (60–1140)	60 (15–315)	23 (5–300)
< 60	117 (48.8)	42 (73.7)	13 (23.6)	25 (46.3)	22 (64.7)
60–239	47 (19.7)	6 (10.5)	16 (29.1)	13 (24.1)	4 (11.8)
240–359	7 (2.9)	2 (3.5)	2 (3.6)	2 (3.7)	0 (0)
> = 360	69 (28.7)	7 (12.3)	24 (43.6)	14 (25.9)	8 (23.5)
Medical advice – arrival					
Median (25-75th)	98 (54–217)	54 (35–93)	238 (111–402)	106 (59–266)	99 (64–174)
< 60	62 (27.7)	28 (51.9)	4 (8.0)	12 (24.0)	7 (20.6)
60–239	111 (49.5)	21 (38.9)	22 (44.0)	25 (50.0)	23 (67.6)
240–359	18 (8.1)	1 (1.9)	9 (18.0)	6 (12.0)	1 (2.9)
> = 360	33 (14.7)	4 (7.4)	15 (30.0)	7 (14.0)	3 (8.8)

[a] ≤ 19 missings
[b] ≤ five missings
[c] Is patient delay

waited more than 4 h before seeking medical advice (Table 2). After first medical contact, 46 % of the patients arrived within 90 min at the CCU. Of the most common prehospital paths, median time between seeking medical advice and arrival at the CCU was shortest for 'ambulance only' (60 min). In line with this, the percentage of patients arriving at CCU within 90 min after first medical contact was highest for 'ambulance only' (87.0 %) and lowest for 'GP only' (23.1 %).

Median time between onset of symptoms and time to arrival at ED in the stroke group was 240 min. Median patient delay was 60 min and 31.6 % waited longer than 4 h before seeking medical advice (Table 3). After first medical symptoms, 49.9 % of the patients arrived within 4 h at the ED. Median time between seeking medical advice and arrival at ED was shortest for 'ambulance and ED' (54 min). Of patients using the path 'ambulance and ED' 69.2 % arrived within 4 h at ED after onset of symptoms and only 19.0 % of those using 'GP and ED'.

Door-to-balloon time and door-to-needle time

Overall 39 patients had a ST-elevated myocardial infarction. Six patients called or visited a healthcare provider more than 12 h after the first symptoms. ECG and clinical criteria of two patients were insufficient to perform PCI. One patient received a PCI in another hospital outside the region and details of the PCI were unknown. Median time between first medical contact and PCI for the remaining 30 patients with ST-elevated myocardial infarction was 132 min. Only one patient received a PCI within 90 min after first medical contact and 12 within 120 min (Table 4). Median door-to-balloon time was 50 min and 63.0 % received a PCI within a door-to-balloon time of 90 min.

Out of 182 patients with ischemic stroke, 31 (17.0 %) received thrombolysis. Median time between first medical contact and thrombolysis was 92 min. Almost all patients (93.5 %) received thrombolysis within 270 min (4.5 h) after symptoms (Table 4). Median door-to-needle time was 43 min, and 89.6 % received thrombolysis within 60 min after arrival in hospital. Of the 151 patients not receiving thrombolysis 89 (58.9 %) arrived at the ED more than 4 h after the start of the symptoms and were therefore too late for thrombolysis. Although 62 (41.1 %) patients arrived within 4 h after the symptoms were first noticed, 24 of these patients could not receive thrombolytic treatment because the symptoms were first noticed on awakening, and therefore the precise starting time of stroke was unknown. The other 38 patients had contra-indications for thrombolysis such as the use of oral anticoagulants, recent surgery, minor neurological deficit and loss of consciousness.

Table 4 Time between onset of symptoms, seeking medical advice, PCI and door-to-balloon time for 30 patients with ST-elevated MI, thrombolysis and door-to-needle time for 31 patients with ischemic stroke

30 patients with ST-elevated MI who received percutaneous coronary intervention (PCI)			
Time (minutes)	Symptom – medical advice[a,b]	Medical advice – PCI	Symptom – PCI	Door-to-balloon[b]
	N (%)	N (%)	N (%)	N (%)
Median (25–75th)	30 (15–180)	132 (108–209)	222 (139–416)	50 (33–150)
< 60	17 (63.0)	0 (0.0)	0 (0.0)	14 (51.9)
60–89	2 (7.4)	1 (3.3)	0 (0.0)	3 (11.1)
90–119	0 (0.0)	11 (36.7)	4 (13.3)	2 (7.4)
120–239	2 (7.4)	12 (40.0)	14 (46.7)	6 (22.2)
240–359	2 (7.4)	4 (13.3)	2 (6.7)	1 (3.7)
>= 360	4 (14.8)	2 (6.7)	10 (33.3)	1 (3.7)
31 patients with ischemic stroke who received thrombolysis			
Time (minutes)	Symptom – medical advice[a,b]	Medical advice – thrombolysis[b]	Symptom – thrombolysis	Door-to-needle[b]
	N (%)	N (%)	N (%)	N (%)
Median (25–75th)	10 (5–30)	92 (64–120)	110 (77–150)	43 (33–53)
< 60	26 (86.7)	7 (23.3)	3 (9.7)	26 (89.6)
60–89	3 (10.0)	7 (23.3)	9 (29.0)	1 (3.4)
90–119	0 (0.0)	8 (26.7)	6 (19.3)	0 (0.0)
120–269	1 (3.3)	7 (23.3)	11 (35.5)	1 (3.4)
270–359	0 (0.0)	1 (3.3)	2 (6.5)	0 (0.0)
>= 360	0 (0.0)	0 (0.0)	0 (0.0)	1 (3.4)

[a]Patient delay
[b]≤ three missings

Discussion

Patients in the ACS group arrived at the CCU through 15 different paths, and patients in the stroke group arrived at the stroke unit through 10 different paths. In these paths often two or more healthcare providers were involved (60.8 % ACS, 95.1 % stroke). Almost half of all patients first contacted their GP (47.5 % ACS, 49.4 % stroke). Some prehospital paths were more frequently used, and in 65 % of all events an ambulance was involved, which is much higher compared to other countries [7]. For paths involving the ambulance either alone or in combination with one other healthcare provider, time intervals were short. Time intervals of other paths without ambulances were longer and differed considerably in duration. The major part of the overall prehospital delay was caused by patients themselves, as they waited a long time before seeking medical advice.

Prehospital paths and time delays

With various prehospital paths through which patients arrived in the hospital various time delays occurred. Longer time delays occur when more health care providers are involved. When (only) an ambulance is involved, paths and delays are shorter, as shown in other studies [7–9]. If a ST-elevated myocardial infarction is suspected based on the ECG made in the ambulance or if the patient has typical symptoms, a phone call to the hospital with PCI facilities is made, the ECG is digitally send, and the patient is directly transported to the cardiac catheterization laboratory. As a result, the percentage of ACS patients arriving at CCU within 90 min after first medical contact was highest (87 %) when patients were directly transported by ambulance. Within these 90 min lies the optimal time to perform a PCI for patients with ST-elevated myocardial infarction [1].

Similarly, 69 % of all stroke patients who were directly transported by ambulance arrived within 4 h after onset of symptoms at the ED. The overall time window for rt-PA treatment is 4.5 h [2]. Before rt-PA can be delivered, a diagnostic work-up, including neurological examination, imaging and laboratory analysis, is necessary to exclude hemorrhage and diseases mimicking stroke, and to identify other contraindications. Moreover the diagnosis of ischemic stroke needs to be confirmed. Therefore, patients who arrive more than 4 h after the start of the symptoms are too late to be treated with thrombolytic therapy.

The challenge is to identify the patients that will benefit from a fast path by ambulance to the hospital. National protocols for ambulance services exist. However, the correct identification of stroke symptoms is not easy; on the one hand, symptoms can be difficult to recognize and on the other hand, as many as 20 % of presumed stroke symptoms are caused by completely different diseases. The proportion of strokes correctly identified by emergency medical systems dispatchers varies between 45 % and 83 % pointing strongly in the direction of continuous medical educational programs to improve on stroke recognition [10–13]. Another challenge is to educate patients to recognize ACS and stroke, and then call the national emergency number immediately.

Contact with GP

Although patients arrived at the hospital through various prehospital paths, almost half contacted their own GP first. This is far less than in 1998–1999 when 87 % first contacted their GP [8]. In the Netherlands this is usual care, GPs act as gate keepers for hospitals. On the other hand, GPs may receive many patients with complaints which at first sight point in the direction of an ACS or stroke, but which after history taking and physical examination appear to be another disease. This study does not have insight into the number of patients who present themselves to the GP but are not transferred to the hospital. Nevertheless, where the GP was involved or where private transportation was used, time intervals were rather long, as reported before [8, 14]. Reasons for these long time intervals are unclear. It might be that more patients visiting their GP have aspecific symptoms which makes it difficult to ascertain a diagnosis and act quickly. Delays in women may be specifically long as they appear to have aspecific symptoms of myocardial infarction; although findings regarding differences by gender are inconsistent [15, 16]. In contrast to myocardial infarction, classic stroke symptoms do not differ between men and women [17].

This study showed that time intervals of prehospital paths involving a GP cooperative were shorter than when a patients' own GP was involved. Since during office hours patients have to go to their own GP and during the evening, night or in the weekend to a GP cooperative, both organizations are likely to receive similar patients. What may explain differences in time intervals is the way both are organized (e.g. having a direct phone line to ambulance emergency medical services, different triage systems); although other reasons such as patients postponing seeking medical advice until Monday morning when their GP is available, or patients visiting GP cooperative with more serious symptoms, cannot be ruled out.

Almost half of the patients who presented themselves to their GP were subsequently transported by ambulance to the hospital. This indicates that some patients, in terms of time delay, could have benefited from bypassing the GP by calling the national emergency number instead. This confirms that the use of emergency medical systems is crucial to reduce prehospital delay [14]. The difference in contacting the ambulance between GP (~50 %) and GP cooperative (80 % ACS, 64 % stroke) is striking. Further research may give insight into reasons for this difference. Additionally, a study might investigate the effect of educating GPs in choosing the most efficient prehospital path.

There were some strange observations at first sight. A few patients had contact with their own GP and later on with a GP cooperative. Obviously, the provisional diagnosis of ACS or stroke was not made at first visit to the GP. Other reasons were not specifically investigated but this finding adds to the complexity of the prehospital routing of patients. Another finding was that not every patient with a provisional diagnosis of ACS or stroke was transported with an ambulance according to the guidelines. When we looked into this we found many good reasons not to call for an ambulance. For example, 20 out of 27 ACS patients who contacted their own GP first and went to the CCU with private transportation waited more than 6 h (some even days) before seeking medical advice and some patients simply refused to be transported by ambulance (personal communication). These findings add to the complexity of real world prehospital paths.

Patient delay

The prehospital delay strongly depends on the choice of the patient when and where to enter the health care system. It is of interest to know what causes specific care-seeking behavior in patients. Which patients chose to contact their GP, GP cooperative or immediately called the emergency number? This knowledge may lead to more focused interventions in reducing delays. Most of the delay in the overall prehospital paths was due to the patient who waits too long before contacting a health care provider. Although three-quarter of the patients were at home and half of the patients were in the company of a partner when symptoms started, patient delay was long. Almost half of all ACS patients waited more than 4 h before seeking medical advice compared to over 30 % of all stroke patients. Patient delay is a worldwide problem and demographic, social, cognitive and emotional factors, as well as clinical characteristics play a role [18]. Median delays by ACS patients in the US vary between 1.5 and 6 h [18] compared to 3 h in this study. For stroke patients median delays differ from 53 min to 2 h in different studies [19–21]. Median time in the present study was one hour, meaning that 50 % of all patients waited longer than one hour before seeking medical advice. Apparently, patient delay did not change over the last 14 years in the Netherlands [8]. In contrast, overall median time between onset of symptoms and arrival at hospital seems to be reduced, from 5 h and 10 min in 1998–1999 to 4 h in our study. Minimizing patient delay in seeking care in ACS or stroke patients by mass media interventions is disappointing. Public health campaigns aiming to recognize symptoms and to get professional help as early as possible, are marginally successful, last only a few months, or do not influence patient delay at all [7, 22–24].

Door-to-balloon time and door-to-needle time

Although door-to-balloon time for patients with ST-elevated myocardial infarction in need of PCI and door-to-needle time in stroke patients may be improved, in-hospital delays are very small compared to the overall time between onset of symptoms and arrival at hospital. Obviously, door-to-balloon time and door-to-needle time protocols have proven their value. Much more time is to gain in the prehospital phase.

Strengths and limitations

One of the strengths of this study is that data was provided by patients themselves using structured questionnaires together with data extracted from registries. This gives an entire overview of the numerous and complex prehospital paths, which, to our knowledge, has been investigated in only a few studies and in the Dutch situation never to such an extent. The study is limited by a low consecutive recruitment rate. About 21 % of all ACS patients and 37 % stroke patients participated. We did not keep record of the reasons for exclusion. Therefore we do not know the reason for non-participation of each specific patient. During a discussion of the results with healthcare professionals from CCUs and stroke units, it appeared that refusal of the patient was rarely the reason for non-participation. In reality the attending nurse(specialist)s were too busy and forgot to ask patients to participate. We think that it is very unlikely that these reasons are associated with the various pre-hospital paths. The design of the study precluded patients who died before reaching hospital. The characteristics (sex, age) of participants are in line with other Dutch studies [8, 25]. Nevertheless, we cannot exclude with certainty that patient selection was fully absent.

Patients in this study came from three hospitals in a region where prehospital and hospital healthcare providers have regular meetings to optimize care for patients with acute coronary syndrome and stroke. These networks exist throughout the Netherlands where similar guidelines are used. Therefore, our results are probably applicable throughout the country. In other countries organization of emergency medicine may differ [26], resulting into various other paths and time intervals.

Conclusions

Overall, efforts to reduce patient delay may lead to a relatively higher reduction in time between onset of symptoms and arrival in hospital than efforts to reduce delays involving health care providers. However, since reducing patient delay is difficult, and noticeable differences do exist between various prehospital paths where often two or more health care providers are involved, further research into reasons for these differences may yield possibilities to optimize paths and thus reduce overall time delay. Evidence is appearing that in the Dutch situation it is better, as it is in many other countries around the world, to bypass the GP in case of ACS or stroke and directly call the national emergency number.

Abbreviations

ACS: acute coronary syndrome; CCU: coronary care unit; ECG: electrocardiogram; ED: emergency department; GP: general practitioner; IQR: interquartile ranges; MI: myocardial infarction; PCI: percutaneous coronary intervention; rt-PA: recombinant tissue plasminogen activator; SD: standard deviation.

Competing interests

The author(s) declare that they have no competing interests.

Authors' contributions

CD designed the study, performed data analyses and wrote the draft of the article. MZ collected data, performed data analyses and critically read the article. HD collected data and critically read the article. RE, PB, GH contributed to the design of the study and critically read the article. FE critically read the article. All authors read and approved the final manuscript.

Acknowledgments

We thank all patients who participated in the study and all nurses and nurse specialists of the coronary care units, stroke units and emergency departments of all three hospitals (Medisch Spectrum Twente (MST), Enschede; Ziekenhuisgroep Twente (ZGT), locations in Almelo and Hengelo; Streekziekenhuis Koningin Beatrix (SKB), Winterswijk). Employees of ambulance emergency medical services (Ambulance Oost and region Achterhoek NOG Connexxion), GP cooperatives, GPs in the region Twente and Oost-Achterhoek, The Netherlands, are thanked for providing data. Furthermore, J. Smid MSc, collected part of the data. Mrs. M. Raisch is thanked for editing English spelling and grammar. This study is initiated and funded by Regional Network for Emergency Care, Acute Zorg Euregio, Enschede, The Netherlands.

Author details

[1]Department of Health Technology and Services Research (HTSR), MIRA institute for Biomedical Technology and Technical Medicine, University of Twente, RA 5252, PO Box 217, 7500 AE, Enschede, The Netherlands. [2]Department of Neurology, Medisch Spectrum Twente, Enschede, The Netherlands. [3]Department of Cardiology, Thoraxcentrum Twente, Medisch Spectrum Twente, Enschede, The Netherlands. [4]Ambulance Oost, Hengelo, The Netherlands. [5]Regional Network for Emergency Care, Acute Zorg Euregio, Enschede, The Netherlands.

References

1. The Task Force on the management of ST-segemtn elevation acute moycardial infarcton of the European Society of Cardiology (ESC). ESC Guidelines for the management of acute myocardial infarction in patients presenting with ST-segment elevation. Eur Heart J. 2012;33(20):2569–619. doi:10.1093/eurheartj/ehs215.
2. Jauch EC, Saver JL, Adams Jr HP, Bruno A, Connors JJ, Demaerschalk BM, et al. Guidelines for the early management of patients with acute ischemic stroke: a guideline for healthcare professionals from the American Heart Association/American Stroke Association. Stroke. 2013;44(3):870–947. doi:10.1161/STR.0b013e318284056a.
3. Lees KR, Bluhmki E, von Kummer R, Brott TG, Toni D, Grotta JC, et al. Time to treatment with intravenous alteplase and outcome in stroke: an updated pooled analysis of ECASS, ATLANTIS, NINDS, and EPITHET trials. Lancet. 2010;375(9727):1695–703. doi:10.1016/S0140-6736(10)60491-6.
4. Fassbender K, Balucani C, Walter S, Levine SR, Haass A, Grotta J. Streamlining of prehospital stroke management: the golden hour. Lancet Neurol. 2013;12(6):585–96. doi:10.1016/S1474-4422(13)70100-5.
5. Evenson KR, Foraker RE, Morris DL, Rosamond WD. A comprehensive review of prehospital and in-hospital delay times in acute stroke care. Int J Stroke. 2009;4(3):187–99. doi:10.1111/j.1747-4949.2009.00276.x.
6. Herlitz J, Wireklintsundstrom B, Bang A, Berglund A, Svensson L, Blomstrand C. Early identification and delay to treatment in myocardial infarction and stroke: differences and similarities. Scand J Trauma Resusc Emerg Med. 2010;18:48. doi:10.1186/1757-7241-18-48.
7. Bray JE, Straney L, Barger B, Finn J. Effect of public awareness campaigns on calls to ambulance across Australia. Stroke. 2015;46(5):1377–80. doi:10.1161/STROKEAHA.114.008515.
8. Meijer RJ, Hilkemeijer JH, Koudstaal PJ, Dippel DW. Modifiable determinants of delayed hospital admission following a cerebrovascular accident. Ned Tijdschr Geneeskd. 2004;148(5):227–31.
9. Price CI, Rae V, Duckett J, Wood R, Gray J, McMeekin P, et al. An observational study of patient characteristics associated with the mode of admission to acute stroke services in North East England. PLoS One. 2013;8(10):e76997. doi:10.1371/journal.pone.0076997.
10. Buck BH, Starkman S, Eckstein M, Kidwell CS, Haines J, Huang R, et al. Dispatcher recognition of stroke using the National Academy Medical Priority Dispatch System. Stroke. 2009;40(6):2027–30. doi:10.1161/STROKEAHA.108.545574.
11. Jones SP, Carter B, Ford GA, Gibson JM, Leathley MJ, McAdam JJ, et al. The identification of acute stroke: an analysis of emergency calls. Int J Stroke. 2013;8(6):408–12. doi:10.1111/j.1747-4949.2011.00749.x.
12. Caceres JA, Adil MM, Jadhav V, Chaudhry SA, Pawar S, Rodriguez GJ, et al. Diagnosis of stroke by emergency medical dispatchers and its impact on the prehospital care of patients. J Stroke Cerebrovasc. 2013;22(8):e610–4. doi:10.1016/j.jstrokecerebrovasdis.2013.07.039.
13. Watkins CL, Leathley MJ, Jones SP, Ford GA, Quinn T, Sutton CJ, et al. Training emergency services' dispatchers to recognise stroke: an interrupted time-series analysis. BMC Health Serv Res. 2013;13:318. doi:10.1186/1472-6963-13-318.
14. Saver JL, Smith EE, Fonarow GC, Reeves MJ, Zhao X, Olson DM, et al. The "golden hour" and acute brain ischemia: presenting features and lytic therapy in >30,000 patients arriving within 60 minutes of stroke onset. Stroke. 2010;41(7):1431–9. doi:10.1161/STROKEAHA.110.583815.
15. Chen W, Woods SL, Puntillo KA. Gender differences in symptoms associated with acute myocardial infarction: a review of the research. Heart Lung. 2005;34(4):240–7.
16. Alconero-Camarero AR, Munoz-Cacho P, Revuelta JM. Gender similarities and differences in the presentation of symptoms in acute myocardial infarction. Int J Cardiol. 2013;168(3):2968–9. doi:10.1016/j.ijcard.2013.04.119.
17. Stuart-Shor EM, Wellenius GA, Dellolacono DM, Mittleman MA. Gender differences in presenting and prodromal stroke symptoms. Stroke. 2009;40(4):1121–6. doi:10.1161/STROKEAHA.108.543371.
18. Moser DK, Kimble LP, Alberts MJ, Alonzo A, Croft JB, Dracup K, et al. Reducing delay in seeking treatment by patients with acute coronary syndrome and stroke: a scientific statement from the American Heart Association Council on cardiovascular nursing and stroke council. Circulation. 2006;114(2):168–82. doi:10.1161/CIRCULATIONAHA.106.176040.
19. Chang KC, Tseng MC, Tan TY. Prehospital delay after acute stroke in Kaohsiung, Taiwan. Stroke. 2004;35(3):700–4. doi:10.1161/01.STR.0000117236.90827.17.
20. Mandelzweig L, Goldbourt U, Boyko V, Tanne D. Perceptual, social, and behavioral factors associated with delays in seeking medical care in patients with symptoms of acute stroke. Stroke. 2006;37(5):1248–53. doi:10.1161/01.STR.0000217200.61167.39.
21. Mosley I, Nicol M, Donnan G, Patrick I, Dewey H. Stroke symptoms and the decision to call for an ambulance. Stroke. 2007;38(2):361–6. doi:10.1161/01.STR.0000254528.17405.cc.
22. Caldwell MA, Miaskowski C. Mass media interventions to reduce help-seeking delay in people with symptoms of acute myocardial infarction: time for a new approach? Patient Educ Couns. 2002;46(1):1–9.
23. Lecouturier J, Rodgers H, Murtagh MJ, White M, Ford GA, Thomson RG. Systematic review of mass media interventions designed to improve public recognition of stroke symptoms, emergency response and early treatment. BMC Public Health. 2010;10:784. doi:10.1186/1471-2458-10-784.
24. Reeves MJ. Reducing the delay between stroke onset and hospital arrival: is it an achievable goal? JAHA. 2012;1(3):e002477. doi:10.1161/JAHA.112.002477.

25. Lahr MM, Luijckx GJ, Vroomen PC, van der Zee DJ, Buskens E. Proportion of patients treated with thrombolysis in a centralized versus a decentralized acute stroke care setting. Stroke. 2012;43(5):1336–40. doi:10.1161/STROKEAHA.111.641795.

26. Fleischmann T, Fulde G. Emergency medicine in modern Europe. Emerg Med Australas. 2007;19(4):300–2. doi:10.1111/j.1742-6723.2007.00991.x.

17

The association of dairy intake of children and adolescents with different food and nutrient intakes in the Netherlands

Marjo J. E. Campmans-Kuijpers[1], Cecile Singh-Povel[2], Jan Steijns[2] and Joline W. J. Beulens[1*]

Abstract

Background: Dairy products are nutrient-rich foods that may contribute to adequate nutrient intakes. However, dairy intake might also be associated with other food sources that influence nutrient intakes. Therefore, we studied the association of dairy, milk and cheese intake with intake of foods and nutrients from (non)dairy sources.

Methods: Dietary intake was assessed from 2007 to 2010 through two non-consecutive 24-h dietary recalls in 1007 children (7–13 years) and 706 adolescents (14–18 years). Participants were divided into non-consumers of a particular dairy product and tertiles according to their dairy intake (lowest, medium and highest intake). P for trend was calculated by linear regression over the median intakes of non-consumers and the tertiles for dairy, milk and cheese.

Results: In children, higher dairy consumption was associated with higher intakes of fruits (54.8 g ± 22.3; $p < 0.0001$), vegetables (25.0 g ± 14.6; $p = 0.001$) and cereals (18.5 g ± 20.7; $p = 0.01$) and with lower consumption of non-alcoholic beverages (−281 g ± 101; $p = 0.01$): soft drinks (−159 g ± 28.2; $p < 0.0001$) and fruit juices (−40.5 ± 14.8; $p = 0.01$). Results were comparable for milk consumption. In adolescents, similar results were found for milk and dairy consumption, except for the associations with higher fruits and vegetable intake.

In children and adolescents, higher cheese consumption was associated with higher vegetable and non-alcoholic beverages consumption; and lower meat consumption (−7.8 g ± 4.8; $p = 0.05$) in children. Higher cheese consumption was also associated with higher intakes of saturated fat (8.5 g ± 0.9), trans-fatty acids (0.48 g ± 0.06), sodium (614 mg ± 59.3) and several vitamins and minerals .

Conclusions: Higher milk and dairy consumption were associated with lower non-alcoholic beverages consumption, and higher cereal, fruit and vegetable consumption in children, which was also reflected in the nutrient intakes. These findings confirm that the consumption of milk and dairy products might be a marker for healthier eating habits.

Keywords: Dairy, Milk, Food-intake, Children, Adolescents

Background

Dairy products are nutrient-rich foods [1], which remain an important source of micronutrients like calcium, vitamin B2 and B12 [2]. In addition, dairy products provide children with energy, high-quality protein, and essential and nonessential fatty acids.

However, dairy products, and especially cheese and high-fat dairy products, may also contribute to an excess intake of energy, sodium, saturated fatty acids (SFA) and trans-fatty acids (TFA) [2]. Despite its contribution to energy intake, recent meta-analyses showed that high dairy intake was associated with lower adiposity in adolescents, while in younger children no association was found, although heterogeneity of the studies was high [3]. A review on dairy intakes in children and adolescents showed that dairy consumption was not or inversely associated with incidence of dental caries, and hypertension; and positively associated with linear growth and bone health during childhood [2].

Nonetheless, in recent decades, the consumption of milk and dairy products by children and adolescents has waned, with a substantial proportion of youth failing to

* Correspondence: J.Beulens@umcutrecht.nl
[1]Julius Center for Health Sciences and Primary Care, University Medical Center Utrecht, P.O. Box 85500 3508 GA Utrecht, The Netherlands
Full list of author information is available at the end of the article

meet intake recommendations [2]. Whereas most studies found dairy consumption declines further with increasing age, particularly throughout adolescence [2, 4, 5], a British study found no difference in milk-based dairy consumption between middle-childhood (9 to 11 years) and adolescence (15 to 18 years) [6].

In the Netherlands, children aged 4 to 8 years are recommended to consume 400 ml of milk and 10 gram of cheese, whereas for adolescents 600 ml of milk and 20 gram cheese is recommended, both preferably low fat [7]. These recommendations are comparable to other developed countries, where children under the age of 9 years are recommended to use approximately 500 ml dairy products and adolescents > 600 ml dairy per day [2].

In the Dutch National Food Consumption Survey 2007–2010 Dutch children and adolescents consumed insufficient fruit, vegetables, fish and fibre and too much SFAs [8]. Furthermore, the intakes of vitamin A, vitamin C, vitamin E, calcium, magnesium, potassium and zinc were below the recommended amounts for certain children, but without health effects [8]. Increased dairy intake could thus contribute to the adequate intakes of nutrients in Dutch children and adolescents.

However, the contribution of dairy to adequate nutrient intakes also depend on replacement of dairy by other food products in the diet. We are aware of only one study that addressed the relation of dairy consumption with intakes of other food groups in 8 to 10 year old children [9]. This study showed that a low milk intake was associated with higher intake of sugar sweetened beverages. A higher dairy intake was also associated with higher consumption of foods from the bread and cereal group and lower consumption from the meat and alternatives group (including fish, eggs, nuts and seeds). The consumption of milk and dairy products might thus be marker for healthier eating habits. Whether intake of dairy products is associated with intakes of other food sources in diet of adolescents has not been investigated to date. It is similarly unknown how such associations are reflected in nutrient intakes from dairy and non-dairy sources.

The aim of the present research is to study whether milk and dairy products are associated with the intakes of other food products in the diet and whether this is associated with a different nutrient intake from non-dairy products.

Methods
Study population
For this study, data from the Dutch National Food Consumption Survey 2007–2010 were used [8]. The survey was conducted among 3819 children and adults aged 7 to 69 years. The population was divided into six age categories: 7 to 8 years; 9 to 13 years; 14 to 18 years; 19 to 30 years; 31 to 50 years; and 51 to 69 years. For the

current study we included the children 7–13 years ($N = 1007$; response rate 74 %) and adolescents 14–18 years ($N = 706$; response rate 62 %) of this sample. The study population were representative of the general Dutch population according to the levels of education, region, and urbanisation. Recalls were almost equally spread during the week (Saturdays were underrepresented) and during the year (winter was slightly overrepresented). Furthermore, children were overrepresented in the study population. To adjust for these small deviations in sociodemographic characteristics and imbalances in season and the day combination of both consumption days a weighting factor was used. Permission to use the data from the Dutch National Food Consumption Survey 2007–2010 was obtained from National Institute for Public Health and the Environment. Ethical approval and informed consent were deemed unnecessary according to the Dutch legislation [10].

Dietary assessment
The data were collected through two non-consecutive 24-h dietary recalls (using the computer directed interview program EPIC-soft) [11, 12]. Trained dieticians used a multiple pass approach [11–13]. Children aged 7 to 15 years were interviewed face to face by a dietician with at least one of the parents present during home visits. Participants over the age of 15 were interviewed by telephone, at dates and times unannounced to the participants. Each person was interviewed twice with an interval of 2 to 6 weeks. The recalls were spread equally over all days of the week and the four seasons. Interview days were not planned on holidays. The survey consisted of a description of foods by a further specification of the foods using facets and descriptors such as preparation method and fat content. Portion sizes of foods and meals were quantified in several ways: by means of quantities shown by photos, or in household measures, standard units, by weight and/or by volume. Further, the food frequencies of the intakes of dietary supplements, distinguishing between winter time and during the rest of the year, were asked.

Dairy intake
We analyzed overall dairy intake, but also the subcategories of milk and cheese intake, because cheese and milk are used differently in the Dutch diet. Therefore, the intakes of dairy products were divided into three categories: 1. Dairy products (the overall category) 2. Milk and 3. Cheese. Dairy products included milk, milk beverages, yogurt, fromage blanc, petits suisses, cheese products, and milk based desserts. Milk contained only milk and buttermilk. Cheese contained cheese products (including fresh cheeses). The mean intake over the two registered days were calculated. Per age category, participants were

divided into non-consumers of a particular dairy product and three tertiles according to their dairy intake. Non-dairy consumers were those participants who did not consume any dairy products in the two days of the dietary recalls.

Food groups
In this study we used food groups based on EPIC-soft classification [12]. We studied 17 food groups and presented the results of the 13 main food groups, including: 1. Potatoes, 2. Vegetables, 3. Fruits, 4. Dairy products, 5. Cereals, 6. Meats, 7. Fish, 8. Eggs, 9. Fats, 10. Sugar_confectionary, 11. Cakes, 12. Non-alcoholic beverages, and 13. Alcoholic beverages.

The food group 'fruits' included fruits, nuts and olives; the food group term 'fats' was used for fats like margarine and oil. The term 'soft drinks' included carbonated drinks, soft drinks, isotonic drinks and diluted syrups. Further, we used 'fruit juice' as a generic term for fruit and vegetable juices and chocolate spread as a generic term for chocolate spread, flakes and confetti. Since cheese might be replaced with confectionary (sugar, honey or jam) on bread, these intakes were calculated for the cheese category.

Measurement on non-dietary factors
Three age-specific general questionnaires were used to collect characteristics that are relevant on the level of the individual person (e.g. age and sex), the properties on the household (e.g. size and income) and lifestyle characteristics of the participant: the activities, general diet characteristics, consumption frequency of certain specific foods, use of dietary supplements (per season) and so on [8].

Since all participants were under the age of 19, the educational level concerned the head of household and was categorized into three categories; low (primary school, lower vocational, low or intermediate general education); middle (intermediate vocational education and higher general education); high (higher vocational education and university) and a category for incomplete information.

Squash (Short Questionnaire to Assess Health enhancing physical activity) questionnaires were used for adolescents to obtain information on physical activity [14]. For the younger children, questions on activities relevant for this age group (like watching television, computer time, sports at school, walking or cycling to school, sport club activities and playing outdoors) were used. Physical activity up to 5 h/week was inactive; >5 h/week was active.

Tobacco use was gathered through the general questionnaire, but not for children. The information on smoking for adolescents was divided into three categories: current smoking of at least one cigarette, cigar or pipe a day, former smokers and never-smokers.

Body weight and height were reported (not measured) to an accuracy of 0.1 kg and 0.5 cm respectively. Body mass index (BMI) was calculated based on the average body weight and height of both interview days. The basal metabolism rate (BMR) was calculated based on sex, weight, height and age according to the Harris-Bennedict formulas [15]. The energy intake BMR ratio was calculated by dividing the mean energy intake by the BMR.

Statistical analyses
Mean intakes of dairy products were calculated by dividing the intake over the two registered days by two. To study the trends over the intakes of non-consumers and low- and high consumers we divided the participants in non-consumers and tertiles of respectively dairy, milk and cheese intakes. The following items were analyzed for each dairy category: intake of all nutrients, nutrient intake from dairy sources and the nutrient intake from non-dairy sources, the intakes of food groups, specific dairy products and beverages. Estimates (± SE) and P for trend were calculated by linear regression over the median intakes of non-consumers and the tertiles. To generalize the results to the general population, weighting factors to adjust demographic properties, season and the day combination of both consumption days were used as a weighting variable [16]. For this variable the day at which the recall applied to was classified as either weekday (Mon-Tue-Wed-Thu) or as weekend day (Fri-Sat-Sun). In a secondary analysis, these differences were adjusted for energy intake, since a higher dairy intake was associated with a higher energy intake. To assess the robustness of the associations, we adjusted for age, sex and parental educational level and subsequently repeated these analyses without the weighing factors. To correct for potential underreporting we additionally adjusted for BMR. Analyses were performed using SAS 9.2. A p-value of 0.05 was considered significant.

Results
Baseline characteristics
For children aged 7–13 years height, weight and BMI (categories) did not differ over dairy tertiles (Table 1). For adolescents, firstly higher dairy consumption was associated with higher height and weight, although no differences were seen in BMI . Secondly, higher dairy consumption was associated with less frequent achievement of the physical activity norm and less smoking.

Children age 7–13 years
Among children aged 7–13 years, a higher dairy consumption (693 g ±34.4 in third tertile; p-for-trend < 0.0001) was significantly associated with higher consumption of vegetables (25.0 g ±14.6; $p = 0.001$), fruits

Table 1 Baseline characteristics of the study population (DNFCS 2007–2010)

Age	7–13 years				14–18 years			
	Non-dairy consumers	Tertile 3	mean	P for trend	Non-dairy consumers	Tertile 3	mean	P for trend
N	17	330	1007		21	228	706	
Males (N/%)	9 (52.9 %)	184 (55.7 %)	504 (50.1 %)		13 (61.9 %)	141 (61.8 %)	352 (49.9 %)	
Height (cm) M/F	139.9(8.7)/ 141.5(16.5)	147.8(14.4)/ 147.0(14.0)	146.1(14.1)/ 146.3(13.8)	0.09	173.9(8.1)/ 168.8(5.0)	180.1(8.5)/ 170.6(6.6)	178.9(9.1)/ 169.1(6.5)	<0.0001
Weight (kg) M/F	31.3(8.0)/ 36.1(10.6)	38.7(12.0)/ 39.6(11.7)	38.0(11.9)/ 39.2(12.3)	0.47	64.9(10.9)/ 74.3(20.7)	67.7(10.9)/ 61.0(9.1)	67.4(12.5)/ 60.9(10.8)	0.02
BMI (kg/m^2) M/F	15.9(2.8)/ 17.8(3.6)	17.3(2.8)/ 18.0(2.8)	17.4(2.8)/ 17.9(3.1)	0.57	21.5(3.7)/ 26.0(6.6)	20.9(3.0)/ 20.9(2.8)	21.0(3.1)/ 21.3(3.4)	0.37
EI/BMR	1.58(0.20)	1.79(0.24)	1.69 (0.23)	<0.0001	1.13 (0.26)	1.57(0.27)	1.46(0.27)	<0.0001
BMI category				0.75				0.45
Seriously underweight	3 (17.6 %)	5 (1.5 %)	28 (2.8)		0 (0.0 %)	3 (1.3 %)	10(1.4 %)	
Underweight	3 (17.6 %)	19 (5.8 %)	70(7.0 %)		1 (4.8 %)	12 (5.3 %)	48(6.8 %)	
Normal weight	8 (47.1 %)	246 (74.5 %)	715(71.2 %)		12 (57.1 %)	183 (80.3 %)	533(75.5 %)	
Overweight	3 (17.6 %)	52 (15.8 %)	160(15.9 %)		6 (28.6 %)	25 (11.0 %)	95(13.5 %)	
Obese	0 (0.0 %)	8 (2.4 %)	33(3.3 %)		2 (9.5 %)	5 (2.2 %)	20(2.8 %)	
Size of household				0.17				0.68
1	0 (0.0 %)	0 (0.0 %)	0(0.0 %)		1 (4.8 %)	4 (1.8 %)	11(1.6 %)	
2 and 3	1 (5.9 %)	76 (23.0 %)	244(24.8 %)		5 (23.8 %)	50 (21.9 %)	169(24.3 %)	
4	12 (70.6 %)	146 (44.2 %)	446(45.4 %)		11 (52.4 %)	102 (44.7 %)	325(46.8 %)	
5+	4 (23.5 %)	108 (32.7 %)	292(29.7 %)		4 (19.0 %)	72 (31.6 %)	190(27.3 %)	
Education level[a]				0.22				0.29
Low	3 (17.6 %)	48 (17.4 %)	127(12.6 %)		3 (14.3 %)	102 (44.7 %)	297(42.1 %)	
Moderate	0 (0.0 %)	13 (4.7 %)	52(5.2 %)		1 (7.1 %)	18 (7.9 %)	54(7.7 %)	
High	1 (5.9 %)	29 (10.5 %)	97(9.6 %)		1 (7.1 %)	8 (3.5 %)	18(2.5 %)	
Student/schoolgoing	4 (23.5 %)	88(31.8 %)	271(26.9 %)		19 (90.5 %)	213 (93.4 %)	644(91.2 %)	
Native country[b]	17(100 %)	324(98.2 %)	989(98.2 %)	0.023	21 (100 %)	223 (97.8 %)	688(97.5 %)	0.94
Physical activitity false (N/%)[c]	3 (17.6 %)	69 (24.9 %)	205(20.4 %)	0.43	15 (71.4 %)	144 (63.2 %)	497(70.4 %)	0.01
Smoking habits (yes/former/never)	0//0/4	0/1/89	0/2/275	0.37	3/0/18	16/8/204	66/28/612	0.04
Alcohol consumption yes(N/%)	0 (0.0 %)	1 (0.4 %)	9 (3.3 %)	0.24	6 (0.8 %)	112 (49.1 %)	335(47.5 %)	0.20

[a]Education level of parents was divided into low (intermediate general education); moderate (higher vocational education) and high (university)
[b]Native country: percentage of people from Dutch origin
[c]Physical Activity: indication whether the participant meets the physical activity guideline (false/true)
Education level, Physical Activity, Smoking habits and alcohol consumption: 730 missings

(54.8 g ±22.3; $p < 0.0001$), cereals (18.5 g ±20.7; $p = 0.01$) and fats (3.0 g ±3.7;$p = 0.01$) and lower consumption of non-alcoholic beverages (−281 g ±101; $p < 0.0001$) (Table 2): in particular soft drinks (−159 g ±28.2; $p < 0.0001$), fruit juices (−40.5 g ±14.8; $p = 0.01$) and coffee or tea (−15.5 g ±11.0; $p = 0.01$) than non-dairy consumers (data not presented). This higher dairy consumption was associated with significantly higher intakes of energy (392 kcal ±122; $p < 0.0001$), protein, fat, fibre, calcium, folate, iodine, potassium, magnesium, phosphorus, selenium, zinc, retinol activity equivalents and vitamins B1, B2, B6 and B12 compared to non-dairy consumers (Table 3).

Higher dairy consumption was associated with significantly lower nutrient intake from non-dairy sources such as energy (−229 kcal ±126), (vegetable) protein (−0.81 g ±2.0), and higher intakes of fibre (1.18 g ±1.2), iron (0.28 mg ±0.64), folate (31.6 µg ±19.6), iodine (23.0 µg ±12.7), retinol equivalents (109 µg ±132), and vitamin D (0.73 µg ±0.38)(Data not shown). Only 17 children (1.7 %) did not consume any dairy on both recall days.

Table 2 Per tertile dairy, milk and cheese consumption the intakes of food groups in gram for children aged 7 to 13 years

Per tertile dairy	Non consumers		Tertile1		Tertile2		Tertile3			Overall		
	Estimate	St error	Estimate	St error	Estimate	St error	Estimate	St error	p-value	Estimate	St error	p-value
N	17			330		330		330			1007		
Potatoes	87.9	18.1	−10.4	18.5	−5.7	18.5	−5.2	18.5	0.78	0.007	0.008	0.40
Vegetables	50.5	14.3	12.1	14.6	21.3	14.6	25.0	14.6	0.09	0.02	0.006	0.001
Fruits	46.5	21.8	31.0	22.3	46.3	22.3	54.8	22.3	0.01	0.04	0.01	<.0001
Dairy products	0.0	33.6	154.2	34.3	385.5	34.3	693.2	34.4	<.0001	0.81	0.02	<.0001
Cereals	170	20.2	2.8	20.7	4.1	20.6	18.5	20.7	0.37	0.02	0.009	0.01
Meats	78.9	14.2	6.7	14.5	9.6	14.5	2.3	14.5	0.87	−0.005	0.006	0.38
Fish	2.4	5.9	1.6	6.0	7.9	6.0	4.2	6.0	0.48	0.004	0.003	0.09
Eggs	1.2	4.0	6.2	4.1	6.6	4.1	7.9	4.1	0.06	0.003	0.002	0.09
Fats	18.8	3.7	0.3	3.7	3.4	3.7	3.0	3.7	0.42	0.004	0.002	0.01
Sugar_confectionary	85.9	14.7	−5.5	15.0	−9.2	15.0	−4.0	15.0	0.79	0.001	0.007	0.82
Cakes	51.4	13.0	4.4	13.3	7.4	13.3	5.6	13.3	0.67	0.002	0.006	0.68
Non_alcoholic_beverage	1111	99.1	−1.6	101	−143	101	−281	101	0.01	−0.42	0.04	<.0001
Alcoholic_beverage	0.0	3.7	1.3	3.8	0.4	3.8	1.8	3.8	0.63	0.001	0.002	0.63
Per tertile milk	Non consumers		Tertile1		Tertile2		Tertile3			Overall		
N	335			221		227		224			1007		
Potatoes	80.3	3.9	3.7	6.1	−1.7	6.0	0.4	6.1	0.94	−0.002	0.01	0.83
Vegetables	62.1	3.0	8.8	4.8	11.7	4.8	13.3	4.8	0.01	0.02	0.008	0.01
Fruits	85.6	4.7	−9.2	7.3	6.0	7.3	21.8	7.3	0.003	0.04	0.01	0.001
Dairy products	267	11.5	43.3	18.0	163	18.0	396	18.1	<.0001	0.68	0.03	<.0001
Cereals	172	4.3	−0.8	6.7	7.4	6.7	17.5	6.8	0.01	0.03	0.01	0.005
Meats	89.6	3.0	−6.0	4.7	−7.4	4.7	−6.7	4.7	0.16	−0.01	0.008	0.15
Fish	5.8	1.3	1.8	2.0	1.4	2.0	1.8	2.0	0.37	0.003	0.003	0.44
Eggs	7.7	0.9	0.2	1.3	−0.9	1.3	2.1	1.3	0.13	0.003	0.002	0.25
Fats	20.0	0.8	1.1	1.2	1.5	1.2	2.0	1.2	0.11	0.003	0.002	0.11
Sugar_confectionary	85.0	3.1	−11.1	4.9	−4.4	4.9	−7.9	4.9	0.11	−0.009	0.008	0.28
Cakes	57.3	2.8	−1.2	4.3	5.2	4.3	−4.8	4.3	0.27	−0.004	0.007	0.57
Non_alcoholic_beverage	1046	21.6	−18.3	33.8	−105	33.6	−206	33.9	<.0001	−0.37	0.06	<.0001
Alcoholic_beverage	0.4	0.8	1.4	1.2	2.2	1.2	−0.3	1.2	0.82	0.0000	0.002	1.00
Per tertile cheese	Non consumers		Tertile1		Tertile2		Tertile3			Overall		
N	308			233		233		233			1007		
Potatoes	92.0	3.9	−7.1	6.0	−15.6	6.0	−26.0	6.0	<.0001	−0.04	0.01	<.0001
Vegetables	63.2	3.1	5.5	4.8	9.4	4.8	13.0	4.8	0.01	0.02	0.008	0.005
Fruits	80.6	4.8	13.0	7.4	15.3	7.3	11.5	7.4	0.12	0.02	0.01	0.13
Dairy products	395	14.5	−22.6	22.1	−24.6	22.1	75.6	22.2	0.001	0.12	0.04	0.001
Cereals	154	4.2	12.5	6.4	25.5	6.4	66.7	6.5	0.0001	0.11	0.01	<.0001
Meats	89.1	3.1	−1.6	4.7	−8.0	4.7	−7.8	4.8	0.10	−0.02	0.008	0.049
Fish	8.9	1.3	−3.1	2.0	−3.1	2.0	−2.6	2.0	0.19	−0.004	0.003	0.24
Eggs	9.0	0.9	−2.2	1.3	−2.1	1.3	−0.7	1.4	0.80	0.000	0.002	0.88
Fats	21.3	0.8	−1.0	1.2	−0.7	1.2	0.6	1.2	0.63	0.001	0.002	0.58
Sugar_confectionary	87.9	3.2	−14.0	4.9	−11.0	4.9	−10.2	4.9	0.04	−0.01	0.008	0.09
Cakes	61.4	2.8	−6.0	4.3	−2.0	4.3	−10.4	4.4	0.02	−0.01	0.007	0.053

Table 2 Per tertile dairy, milk and cheese consumption the intakes of food groups in gram for children aged 7 to 13 years *(Continued)*

Non_alcoholic_beverage	933	22.5	30.1	34.5	44.0	34.4	99.3	34.6	0.004	0.16	0.06	0.005
Alcoholic_beverage	1.2	0.8	−0.9	1.2	−1.1	1.2	1.4	1.2	0.25	0.002	0.002	0.35

A *p*-value of 0.05 was considered significant

Tertile 1,2 and 3 represent respectively the lowest, medium and highest consumers of dairy, milk and cheese. P for trend is the p for trend over non-consumers and all three tertiles

For milk consumption, we observed similar associations with higher consumption of vegetables and fruits (Table 2) and with lower consumption of soft drinks (−159 g ±28.2), fruit juice (−40.5 g ±14.8) and less tea or coffee (−15.5 g ±11.0) as found for total dairy consumption. As milk contained only milk and buttermilk, higher milk consumption was also associated with lower intakes of other milk beverages (−13.7 g ±7.7) and especially less yoghurt (−68.5 g ±14.6). Comparable to higher dairy intake, higher milk intake was significantly associated with the same nutrients as for dairy consumption (Additional file 1). 335 children (33.3 %) did not drink any milk on both recall days.

For cheese consumption we observed associations similar to dairy with a higher consumption of vegetables, cereals and non-alcoholic beverages, but lower consumption of potatoes (−26.0 g ±6.0) and meat (−7.8 g ±4.8) than non-cheese consumers (Table 2). A higher cheese consumption was associated with lower consumption of chocolate spread (data not shown). Higher cheese consumption was significantly associated with higher intakes of energy, protein, SFAs, TFAs, calcium, sodium and several vitamins and minerals such as potassium, zinc and vitamin A (Additional file 2). 308 children (30.6 %) did not consume any cheese on both recall days.

Adolescents age 14–18 years

In adolescents, similar results were found as for children except for the significant associations of dairy and milk consumption with higher fruit and vegetables intakes. Higher dairy consumption was associated with higher consumption of cereals (50.3 g ±22.8; p-for-trend = 0.01), and lower intakes of non-alcoholic beverages (−299 g ±116; $p < 0.0001$) (Table 4): in particular soft drinks (−96.5 g ±94.2; $p = 0.0001$) and coffee or tea (−15.3 g ±54.4; $p < 0.0001$) than non-dairy consumers (Data not presented). High dairy consumption was associated with significantly higher intakes of energy, animal protein, fat, fibre, calcium and other dairy predominant nutrients. Higher dairy consumption was associated with significantly higher intakes of nutrients from non-dairy products such as vegetable protein (5.3 g ±2.3), fibre (3.8 g ±1.42), iron (1.01 mg ±0.67), folate (58.1 μg ±20.0), potassium (269 mg ±177), magnesium (22.5 mg ±19.9) and vitamin D (0.94 μg ±0.37) and lower energy intakes

(−309 kcal ±166) from non-dairy products. (data not shown) 3 % ($N = 21$) adolescents did not consume any dairy on both recall days.

Higher milk consumption was associated with lower consumption of non-alcoholic beverages (Table 4), soft drinks (−159 g ±44.8) and coffee or tea (−93.2 g ±25.7) (Data not presented) and higher intakes of fish (4.8 g ±2.3) than non-milk consumers. Comparable to children, higher milk consumption in adolescents was significantly associated with higher intakes of energy and other milk nutrients (Additional file 3). 32.7 % ($N = 231$) of the adolescents did not drink any milk on both recall days.

Comparable to children, higher cheese consumption by adolescents was associated with higher consumption of vegetables, cereals, and non-alcoholic beverages and lower intakes of potatoes (Table 4) and chocolate spread (5 g) (Data not presented). In contrast to children, higher cheese consumption was associated with higher fruit and fat consumption, but not with lower meat consumption. Higher cheese consumption was again associated with higher intakes of energy, protein, SFA, TFA, calcium, sodium and other dairy nutrients (Additional file 4). 27.2 % ($N = 192$) of the adolescents did not consume any cheese on both recall days.

Adjustments

Adjustment for energy intake did not alter our results, although higher dairy consumption was associated lower intakes of vitamin C and vitamin E than non-dairy consumers and the associations with SFA and sodium lost significance in children (Table 3) and the association between higher dairy consumption with TFA and sodium lost significance in adolescents (Table 5). Additional correction for age, sex and education of parents did not alter the results in children with the exception of milk intake, which was no longer associated with fruit and cereals; and cheese intake was no longer associated with potatoes and meats.

In adolescents, only in the dairy category cereals lost significance, and the association with meat became significant for dairy, milk and cheese (data not shown).

Additional correction for BMR did not alter any of the results. Analyses without the weighting factors to adjust demographic properties, season and the day combination of both consumption days did not change the results.

Table 3 Total nutrient intake over tertiles dairy consumption in children aged 7–13 years

Per tertile dairy	Non-dairy consumers		Tertile 1		Tertile 2		Tertile 3			Overall		p for trend	p for trend energy corrected
	Estimate	St. error	Estimate	St. error	Estimate	St. error	Estimate	St. error	p-value	Estimate	St. error	p for trend	p for trend energy corrected
N	17		330		330		330			1007		1007	1007
Consumed quantity(g)	1836	125	150	128	270	128	465	128	0.0003	0.48	0.06	<.0001	<.0001
Energy (kcal)	1852	120	128	122	210	122	392	122	0.001	0.40	0.05	<.0001	<.0001
Total protein(g)	48.9	4.6	8.2	4.7	17.7	4.7	27.8	4.7	<.0001	0.03	0.002	<.0001	<.0001
Vegetable protein(g)	27.6	1.96	−2.5	2.0	−1.8	2.0	−0.54	2.0	0.79	0.003	0.001	0.003	0.03
Animal protein(g)	21.4	3.9	10.6	4.0	19.3	4.0	28.2	4.0	<.0001	0.03	0.002	<.0001	0.29
Total fat(g)	66.7	6.5	9.9	6.7	11.0	6.7	15.3	6.7	0.02	0.009	0.003	0.002	<.0001
Saturated fatty acids(g)	19.7	2.6	8.2	2.6	9.4	2.6	12.7	2.6	<.0001	0.007	0.001	<.0001	0.37
Mono-unsaturated fatty acids cis(g)	26.5	2.6	1.54	2.6	1.05	2.6	1.72	2.6	0.51	0.0004	0.001	0.75	<.0001
Poly-unsaturated fatty acids(g)	15.9	1.59	−1.27	1.62	−1.21	1.62	−1.31	1.63	0.42	0.0002	0.001	0.80	<.0001
Trans fatty acids(g)	0.56	0.19	0.00	0.19	0.67	0.19	0.85	0.19	<.0001	0.0004	0.000	<.0001	0.048
N-3 fish fatty acids (EPA + DHA.mg)	28.7	53.7	21.4	54.9	72.6	54.9	41.5	54.9	0.45	0.03	0.02	0.15	0.31
Total carbohydrates(g)	256	16.4	1.23	16.7	9.3	16.7	33.7	16.7	0.04	0.05	0.007	<.0001	0.80
Mono- and disaccharides(g)	135	11.7	−1.25	12.0	7.0	12.0	26.2	12.0	0.03	0.04	0.005	<.0001	0.00
Polysaccharides(g)	120	8.5	2.6	8.70	2.4	8.7	7.6	8.7	0.38	0.008	0.004	0.047	<.0001
Fibre(g)	15.3	1.23	−0.23	1.25	1.06	1.25	2.4	1.26	0.053	0.004	0.001	<.0001	0.00
Alcohol(g)	0.00	0.08	0.04	0.08	0.02	0.08	0.05	0.08	0.56	0.000	0.000	0.74	0.77
Calcium(mg)	387	67.7	231	69.2	485	69.2	887	69.2	<.0001	0.99	0.03	<.0001	<.0001
Copper(mg)	0.87	0.07	0.02	0.07	0.08	0.07	0.14	0.07	0.04	0.000	0.0003	<.0001	0.47
Iron(mg)	8.2	0.64	−0.31	0.66	0.21	0.66	0.90	0.66	0.17	0.002	0.0003	<.0001	0.11
Folate equivalents(µg)	135	19.8	27.8	20.3	47.9	20.3	77.7	20.3	0.0001	0.08	0.009	<.0001	<.0001
Iodine(µg)	107	12.9	21.2	13.2	43.5	13.2	64.1	13.2	<.0001	0.07	0.006	<.0001	<.0001
Potassium(mg)	2075	168	74.5	171	460	171	942	171	<.0001	1.29	0.07	<.0001	<.0001
Magnesium(mg)	225	16.9	−9.3	17.2	21.1	17.2	68.5	17.3	<.0001	0.11	0.008	<.0001	0.0004
Sodium(mg)	1802	184	405	188	494	188	636	189	0.0008	0.38	0.08	<.0001	0.61
Phosphorus(mg)	788	73.2	204	74.8	443	74.8	751	74.8	<.0001	0.83	0.03	<.0001	<.0001
Selenium(µg)	25.2	3.3	6.5	3.4	9.9	3.4	11.8	3.4	0.0004	0.009	0.001	<.0001	0.02
Zinc(mg)	5.8	0.71	1.53	0.72	2.5	0.72	3.9	0.72	<.0001	0.004	0.0003	<.0001	<.0001
Retinol activity equivalents(µg)	445	131	89.1	134	216	134	283	134	0.04	0.30	0.06	<.0001	0.004
Vitamin B1(mg)	0.89	0.12	−0.02	0.13	0.09	0.13	0.17	0.13	0.17	0.000	0.0001	<.0001	0.02
Vitamin B2(mg)	0.71	0.12	0.26	0.12	0.66	0.12	1.22	0.12	<.0001	0.001	0.0001	<.0001	<.0001
Vitamin B6(mg)	1.29	0.21	0.16	0.22	0.33	0.22	0.50	0.22	0.02	0.001	0.0001	<.0001	0.002
Vitamin B12(µg)	1.27	0.44	1.15	0.45	2.3	0.45	3.3	0.45	<.0001	0.003	0.0002	<.0001	<.0001
Vitamin C(mg)	98	12.5	−14.6	12.7	−14.4	12.7	−18.2	12.8	0.16	−0.006	0.006	0.24	0.001
Vitamin D(µg)	1.83	0.38	0.37	0.39	0.80	0.38	0.88	0.39	0.02	0.001	0.0002	<.0001	0.08
Vitamin E(mg)	11.9	1.26	−0.94	1.29	−0.54	1.29	−0.35	1.29	0.79	0.001	0.001	0.15	0.01

A p-value of 0.05 was considered significant
Tertile 1,2 and 3 represent respectively the lowest, medium and highest dairy consumers
P for trend is the p for trend over non-consumers and all three tertiles

Table 4 Per tertile dairy. milk and cheese consumption the intakes of food groups in gram for children aged 14 to 18 years

Per tertile dairy	Non consumers		Tertile1		Tertile2		Tertile3		Overall		
	Estimate	St error	Estimate	St error	Estimate	St error	Estimate	St error	Estimate	St error	p-value
N	21		228		229		228			706	
Potatoes	96.2	17.3	−7.1	18.2	6.8	18.3	−0.63	18.2	0.01	0.02	0.46
Vegetables	83.5	13.3	8.2	13.9	3.6	14.0	12.7	13.9	0.01	0.01	0.36
Fruits	35.9	19.9	50.9	20.9	45.0	20.9	55.6	20.9	0.02	0.02	0.19
Dairy products	0.00	29.7	127.1	31.2	354	31.3	707	31.1	1.26	0.03	<.0001
Cereals	192	21.7	27.4	22.8	21.1	22.8	50.3	22.8	0.06	0.02	0.007
Meats	116	13.1	−13.7	13.8	−10.2	13.8	−16.1	13.7	−0.009	0.01	0.47
Fish	2.9	4.6	4.0	4.8	2.4	4.8	6.0	4.8	0.005	0.004	0.23
Eggs	5.4	3.2	3.6	3.4	1.30	3.4	2.8	3.4	−0.001	0.003	0.81
Fats	16.7	3.6	7.6	3.8	5.9	3.8	8.1	3.8	0.003	0.003	0.35
Sugar_confectionary	48.7	10.8	11.5	11.3	7.4	11.3	15.8	11.3	0.01	0.01	0.23
Cakes	31.5	10.7	19.6	11.3	23.4	11.3	25.8	11.3	0.02	0.01	0.06
Non_alcoholic_beverage	1504	111	−30.4	116	−155	117	−299	116	−0.58	0.10	<.0001
Alcoholic_beverage	221	83.8	−166.5	88.0	−124	88.2	−120	87.9	0.05	0.08	0.53
Per tertile milk	Non consumers		Tertile1		Tertile2		Tertile3		Overall		
N	231		160		157		158			706	
Potatoes	89.2	5.5	4.9	8.7	23.1	8.8	2.3	8.6	0.02	0.02	0.40
Vegetables	83.0	4.2	16.7	6.7	13.8	6.7	7.9	6.6	0.02	0.02	0.33
Fruits	80.8	6.4	11.6	10.1	−1.82	10.2	8.1	9.9	0.009	0.02	0.71
Dairy products	205	14.0	91.4	22.2	213	22.3	500	21.8	1.20	0.05	<.0001
Cereals	226	7.0	−14.1	11.0	−10.6	11.1	14.9	10.8	0.04	0.03	0.16
Meats	105	4.2	−2.5	6.6	0.98	6.7	−7.6	6.5	−0.01	0.02	0.34
Fish	5.0	1.47	0.89	2.3	3.1	2.3	4.8	2.3	0.01	0.01	0.02
Eggs	8.4	1.03	0.54	1.63	−0.91	1.64	−1.89	1.60	−0.005	0.004	0.17
Fats	23.8	1.16	−1.49	1.83	0.58	1.85	0.16	1.81	0.002	0.004	0.67
Sugar_confectionary	57.6	3.5	4.4	5.4	2.2	5.5	4.1	5.4	0.008	0.01	0.55
Cakes	49.9	3.4	6.6	5.4	2.2	5.5	8.1	5.4	0.02	0.01	0.23
Non_alcoholic_beverage	1452	35.5	−52.2	56.1	−153	56.5	−267	55.3	−0.67	0.13	<.0001
Alcoholic_beverage	91.6	26.9	−23.1	42.4	2.1	42.7	7.7	41.8	0.04	0.10	0.72
Per tertile cheese	Non consumers		Tertile1		Tertile2		Tertile3		Overall		
N	192		165		179		170			706	
Potatoes	101	6.1	−3.9	9.0	5.8	8.8	−22.2	8.9	−0.04	0.02	0.03
Vegetables	84.2	4.7	0.99	6.9	10.0	6.7	18.3	6.8	0.04	0.01	0.003
Fruits	65.8	7.0	28.5	10.3	15.2	10.0	35.0	10.2	0.06	0.02	0.01
Dairy products	355	20.8	22.0	30.6	34.6	29.8	74.3	30.1	0.16	0.07	0.01
Cereals	205	7.5	−3.2	11.0	10.9	10.7	69.7	10.8	0.16	0.02	<.0001
Meats	109	4.6	−6.4	6.8	−3.9	6.6	−13.4	6.7	−0.03	0.01	0.08
Fish	9.1	1.63	−2.6	2.4	−1.87	2.3	−4.4	2.4	−0.01	0.005	0.11
Eggs	6.9	1.14	2.3	1.68	1.28	1.64	0.31	1.66	−0.001	0.004	0.86
Fats	21.9	1.28	−1.44	1.88	4.4	1.83	3.6	1.85	0.01	0.004	0.004
Sugar_confectionary	57.3	3.8	7.7	5.6	4.2	5.5	−1.00	5.5	−0.01	0.01	0.59
Cakes	57.3	3.8	−2.9	5.6	−7.9	5.5	−3.8	5.5	−0.01	0.01	0.39

Table 4 Per tertile dairy. milk and cheese consumption the intakes of food groups in gram for children aged 14 to 18 years *(Continued)*

Non_alcoholic_beverage	1291	39.8	−37.7	58.5	113	56.9	140	57.6	0.40	0.12	0.001
Alcoholic_beverage	63.9	29.7	23.9	43.6	−9.1	42.5	88.7	43.0	0.16	0.09	0.08

A *p*-value of 0.05 was considered significant

Tertile 1,2 and 3 represent respectively the lowest, medium and highest consumers of dairy, milk and cheese. P for trend is the p for trend over non-consumers and all three tertiles

Discussion

In this Dutch sample of children and adolescents, higher dairy consumption was associated with higher intakes of cereals and lower consumption of non-alcoholic beverages, especially soft drinks. Among children higher dairy consumption was associated with higher intakes of vegetables and fruits, but less fruit juices. Higher cheese intakes were associated with higher consumption of vegetables and non-alcoholic beverages and lower consumption of potatoes in both age categories and with lower meat consumption in children. These associations were also reflected in the nutrient intakes such as protein, fat, MUFA, calcium, vitamin B2, and vitamin B12.

These findings confirm that competing foods such as soda may replace dairy products as mentioned by Nicklas [17] and that higher consumption of dairy foods might be a marker for healthier eating habits [9]. This knowledge might be helpful for recommendations to ensure adequate nutrient intakes in children and adolescents.

In the Netherlands, children aged 4 to 8 years are recommended to consume 400 ml of milk and 10 gram cheese, while for adolescents 600 ml of milk and 20 gram cheese is recommended, both preferably low fat [7]. Our results show that 30 % of the children and adolescents did not consume milk and over 27 % did not consume cheese on the two days. Therefore, a substantial proportion of children and especially adolescents may fail to meet these recommendations. The consumption of dairy products was highest in children and decreased with age [8]. In other developed countries the proportion of children and adolescents meeting dairy product intake recommendation also tends to decrease with age [2, 4, 5], although Green et al. found no difference in milk-based dairy consumption between middle-childhood and adolescence [6].

The Dutch National Food Consumption Survey 2007–2010 [8] showed that the consumption of fruits, vegetables, fish and fibre is insufficient in children and adolescents. We found that higher dairy consumption in children and higher cheese consumption in adolescents was associated with higher intakes of fruits and vegetables. This is in line with a previous study in Australian children (aged 8 to 10 years) which also found that dairy intake was associated with higher intakes of bread and cereals and lower intakes of meat [9]. Although this study also observed slightly higher intakes of fruit and vegetables with higher dairy intake,

these associations did not reach significance, like the adolescents in our study. Overall, our results and the study by Rangan et al. suggests that dairy may contribute to nutrient intakes by contributing nutrients from dairy itself, but also through associations with nutrient intakes from non-dairy food groups. Indeed, in our study higher dairy consumption was associated with increased nutrient intake from non-dairy sources such as fibre, protein, iodine and vitamin D. Moreover, higher dairy and milk consumption was associated with lower consumption of soft drinks and coffee or tea, suggesting that dairy products were mainly replaced by these foods. This is in line with other studies reporting that lower intakes of milk were indeed associated with higher intakes of softdrinks in adolescents [9, 18].

The Dutch National Food Consumption Survey 2007–2010 [8] showed potential inadequacies for vitamin A, C and E, potassium, magnesium and zinc for both children and adolescents. Especially adolescents do not seem to meet the age-specific higher calcium requirements. In contrast, the proportion of SFAs in the diet and sodium intake are too high in both children and adolescents. As a higher dairy intake was associated with higher intakes of vitamin A, calcium, potassium, magnesium and zinc, dairy could thus contribute to the adequate intakes of these nutrients. In addition, dairy intakes were associated with higher intakes of fruits, vegetables, and cereals and could indirectly contribute to higher intakes of vitamin B1 and fibre in children. For vitamin C, we observed opposite results for adolescents and children, with higher dairy intakes, intake of vitamin C was higher among adolescents and lower among children. Consistent with our results, Rangan et al. also showed higher intakes nutrients from dairy, like calcium, potassium, magnesium, zinc, vitamin A and vitamin B2 [9]. However, they did not detect significant associations for vitamin B1, C and fibre. This could be due to the fact that they found no significant associations of dairy consumption with fruit and vegetable intake, while we did in children. Another difference is the adjustment for age, sex and education that was performed by Ragnan, while we only adjusted for energy intake. However, we adjusted for age, sex and parental education in sensitivity analyses and this did not fully explain our results.

On the other hand, higher dairy consumption was also associated with higher energy intake and higher SFAs and TFAs in the diet and with higher sodium intake for

Table 5 Total nutrient intake over tertiles dairy consumption in children aged 14–18 years

Per tertile dairy	Non-dairy consumers		Tertile 1		Tertile 2		Tertile 3			Overall			
	Estimate	St. error	Estimate	St. error	Estimate	St. error	Estimate	St. Error	p-value	Estimate	St. error	p for trend	p for trend energy corrected
N	21		228		229		228			706			
Consumed quantity (g)	2491	161	3.3	169	139	170	398	169	0.02	0.83	0.15	<.0001	0.04
Energy (kcal)	1879	150	335	157	441	158	726	157	<.0001	0.92	0.14	<.0001	xx
Total protein(g)	60.6	4.7	8.8	5.0	16.0	5.0	30.9	5.0	<.0001	0.05	0.004	<.0001	<.0001
Vegetable protein(g)	28.2	2.2	2.0	2.3	2.3	2.3	5.5	2.3	0.02	0.008	0.002	0.0002	0.08
Animal protein(g)	30.9	3.7	8.1	3.9	15.1	3.9	26.7	3.9	<.0001	0.04	0.003	<.0001	<.0001
Total fat(g)	71.0	7.3	13.9	7.7	17.2	7.7	25.0	7.6	0.001	0.03	0.007	<.0001	0.00
Saturated fatty acids(g)	22.0	2.7	8.7	2.8	10.0	2.8	15.4	2.8	<.0001	0.02	0.003	<.0001	0.03
Mono-unsaturated fatty acids cis(g)	27.3	2.9	3.2	3.0	4.2	3.0	6.0	3.0	0.047	0.007	0.003	0.01	<.0001
Poly-unsaturated fatty acids(g)	15.5	1.78	1.27	1.87	1.86	1.88	1.89	1.87	0.31	0.002	0.002	0.31	<.0001
Trans fatty acids(g)	1.11	0.16	0.17	0.17	0.25	0.17	0.41	0.17	0.02	0.0005	0.15	0.0004	0.69
N-3 fish fatty acids (EPA + DHA.mg)	41.6	49.9	55.0	52.4	21.9	52.5	60.1	52.3	0.25	0.02	0.05	0.60	0.64
Total carbohydrates(g)	223	18.2	53.4	19.1	62.6	19.2	99.2	19.1	<.0001	0.11	0.02	<.0001	0.13
Mono- and disaccharides(g)	94.5	11.6	41.9	12.2	45.2	12.2	71.9	12.2	<.0001	0.08	0.01	<.0001	0.001
Polysaccharides(g)	129	10.1	11.5	10.6	17.5	10.6	27.4	10.6	0.01	0.04	0.009	0.0001	0.002
Fibre(g)	16.4	1.38	1.83	1.45	2.6	1.45	5.1	1.45	0.0004	0.007	0.001	<.0001	0.08
Alcohol(g)	9.7	3.9	−6.2	4.12	−5.1	4.1	−4.7	4.1	0.26	0.001	0.004	0.71	0.02
Calcium(mg)	374	67.1	296	70.6	553	70.7	1026	70.4	<.0001	1.63	0.06	<.0001	<.0001
Copper(mg)	0.99	0.08	0.07	0.08	0.12	0.08	0.24	0.08	0.00	0.000	0.07	<.0001	0.79
Iron(mg)	8.9	0.65	0.23	0.68	0.62	0.69	1.58	0.68	0.02	0.003	0.61	<.0001	0.64
Folate equivalents(µg)	160	19.5	43.9	20.5	55.9	20.5	108	20.5	<.0001	0.15	0.02	<.0001	<.0001
Iodine(µg)	149	12.6	2.4	13.3	16.9	13.3	51.6	13.3	0.0001	0.10	0.01	<.0001	<.0001
Potassium(mg)	2217	179	296	188	697	189	1336	188	<.0001	2.3	0.17	<.0001	<.0001
Magnesium(mg)	241	19.9	18.5	21.0	55.4	21.0	113	20.9	<.0001	0.21	0.02	<.0001	<.0001
Sodium(mg)	2312	187	264	196	348	197	607	196	0.002	0.80	0.18	<.0001	0.63
Phosphorus(mg)	981	86.9	212	91.4	438	91.5	836	91.2	<.0001	1.38	0.08	<.0001	<.0001
Selenium(µg)	36.9	3.1	2.3	3.3	3.4	3.3	7.9	3.3	0.02	0.01	0.003	<.0001	0.45
Zinc(mg)	8.5	0.67	0.25	0.70	1.03	0.71	3.0	0.70	<.0001	0.006	0.63	<.0001	<.0001
Retinol activity equivalents(µg)	471	161	189	169	209	170	289	169	0.09	0.27	0.15	0.08	0.64
Vitamin B1(mg)	0.94	0.11	0.10	0.12	0.14	0.12	0.29	0.12	0.02	0.0004	0.11	<.0001	0.05
Vitamin B2(mg)	0.83	0.13	0.26	0.14	0.61	0.14	1.33	0.14	<.0001	0.002	0.13	<.0001	<.0001
Vitamin B6(mg)	1.77	0.22	0.07	0.24	0.19	0.24	0.47	0.24	0.05	0.001	0.21	<.0001	0.12
Vitamin B12(µg)	2.1	0.45	0.96	0.47	1.56	0.47	3.0	0.47	<.0001	0.005	0.43	<.0001	<.0001
Vitamin C(mg)	75.2	12.5	19.5	13.1	17.8	13.2	28.2	13.1	0.03	0.02	0.01	0.04	0.28
Vitamin D(µg)	1.97	0.36	0.72	0.38	0.79	0.38	1.11	0.38	0.003	0.001	0.34	0.002	0.59
Vitamin E(mg)	11.5	1.52	1.26	1.60	1.83	1.60	2.2	1.59	0.17	0.002	0.001	0.10	0.01

A p-value of 0.05 was considered significant
Tertile 1,2 and 3 represent respectively the lowest, medium and highest dairy consumers
P for trend is the p for trend over non-consumers and all three tertiles

cheese consumption. Approximately 65 % of milk fatty acids are saturated [19]. Therefore, dairy products may contribute to the excess intake of SFA in the Dutch population. A high intake of saturated fat is associated with increased risks of cardiovascular diseases and other chronic diseases [20]. In addition, a high sodium intake is associated with an increased risk of hypertension and cardiovascular disease [21]. Despite the contribution of dairy to high intakes of SFAs, TFAs and sodium, prospective cohort studies generally reported neutral or inverse associations between dairy intake and cardiovascular disease [22–24]. This could be due to counteracting effect of other nutrients in dairy such as potassium [25] and magnesium [26] that are associated with a decreased risk of hypertension. The association of calcium with risk of cardiovascular disease is still debated [27], but the effects in the range of habitual dietary intake is likely minimal [28]. Finally, the contribution of high dairy intake to excess energy intake may contribute to adiposity. Despite this, high dairy intake was associated with lower adiposity in adolescents and no association was found in children [3]. Furthermore, dairy products showed associations with linear growth and bone health during childhood [2, 29]. In line with these results, BMI of children and adolescents did not differ according to dairy intake in our study. Since physical activity was higher with higher dairy intake, this could to some extent explain why BMI was not higher with higher dairy and energy intake. Another explanation could be underreporting of dietary intake, and thus also dairy intake, in the non-dairy consumers. We have compared potential underreporting over the dairy categories based on the ratio of energy intake to basal metabolic rate. We indeed observed that this ratio was lower among non-dairy consumers, which could indicate a higher level of underreporting in that category. However, as their physical activity level for adolescents was also lower, this may also explain the differences in ratio of energy intake to basal metabolic rate, but not for children.

Strengths of this study include the dietary assessment using a validated non-consecutive 24-h recall method [11, 12] and the adequate representation of Dutch children and adolescents. However, although two recalls are sufficient to estimate mean intake, one would ideally use more recall days to rank participants correctly from high to low intake. The use of two recall days may lead to misclassification over the dairy categories and probably underestimates the true dairy intake for the non-consumers and overestimates the true dairy intake for the highest tertile. Furthermore the percentage of absolute non-consumers is probably somewhat lower as some people who did not report dairy on one of the recall days may occasionally still consume dairy. Therefore, the percentage of children or adolescents not meeting the dairy recommendations should be interpreted with caution. A further limitation of this study is the use of self-reported height and weight [30].

Conclusions

Higher milk and dairy consumption were associated with lower non-alcoholic beverages consumption, and higher cereal, fruit and vegetable consumption in children, which was also reflected in the nutrient intakes. These findings confirm that the consumption of milk and dairy products might be marker for healthier eating habits. This knowledge might be helpful for recommendations to ensure adequate nutrient intakes in children and adolescents.

Additional files

Additional file 1: Total nutrient intake over tertiles milk consumption in children aged 7–13 years. A p-value of 0.05 was considered significant. Tertile 1,2 and 3 represent respectively the lowest, medium and highest milk consumers. P for trend is the p for trend over non-consumers and all three tertiles. (DOCX 19 kb)

Additional file 2: Total nutrient intake over tertiles cheese consumption in children aged 7–13 years. A p-value of 0.05 was considered significant. Tertile 1,2 and 3 represent respectively the lowest, medium and highest cheese consumers. P for trend is the p for trend over non-consumers and all three tertiles. (DOCX 18 kb)

Additional file 3: Total nutrient intake over tertiles milk consumption in children aged 14–18 years. A p-value of 0.05 was considered significant. Tertile 1,2 and 3 represent respectively the lowest, medium and highest milk consumers. P for trend is the p for trend over non-consumers and all three tertiles. (DOCX 22 kb)

Additional file 4: Total nutrient intake over tertiles cheese consumption in children aged 14–18 years. A p-value of 0.05 was considered significant. Tertile 1,2 and 3 represent respectively the lowest, medium and highest cheese consumers. P for trend is the p for trend over non-consumers and all three tertiles. (DOCX 19 kb)

Abbreviations
BMI: body mass index; BMR: basal metabolism rate; MUFA: mono-unsaturated fatty acids; SFA: saturated fatty acids; TFA: trans-fatty acids.

Competing interests
This study was funded by FrieslandCampina, Amersfoort, The Netherlands. Cecile Singh-Povel and Jan Steijns are employed by FrieslandCampina. There are no conflicts of interest to disclose for any of the authors.

Authors' contributions
The authors' responsibilities were as follows- JS, CSP and JWB proposed the research question, MJCK and JWB conducted the research, MJCK analyzed the data and drafted the manuscript. JWB had primary responsibility for final content. All authors interpreted the data and critically revised the manuscript. All authors read and approved the final manuscript.

Acknowledgements
This study was funded by FrieslandCampina. JS and CSP are employees of this company.

Author details
[1]Julius Center for Health Sciences and Primary Care, University Medical Center Utrecht, P.O. Box 85500 3508 GA Utrecht, The Netherlands. [2]FrieslandCampina, Amersfoort, The Netherlands.

References

1. Vissers PA, Streppel MT, Feskens EJ, et al. The contribution of dairy products to micronutrient intake in the Netherlands. J Am Coll Nutr. 2011; 30(5 Suppl 1):415S–21.

2. Dror DK, Allen LH. Dairy product intake in children and adolescents in developed countries: trends, nutritional contribution, and a review of association with health outcomes. Nutr Rev. 2014;72(2):68–81.

3. Dror DK. Dairy consumption and pre-school, school-age and adolescent obesity in developed countries: a systematic review and meta-analysis. Obes Rev. 2014;15(6):516–27.

4. Baird DL, Syrette J, Hendrie GA, et al. Dairy food intake of Australian children and adolescents 2–16 years of age: 2007 Australian National Children's Nutrition and Physical Activity Survey. Public Health Nutr. 2012;15(11):2060–73.

5. Parker CE, Vivian WJ, Oddy WH, et al. Changes in dairy food and nutrient intakes in Australian adolescents. Nutrients. 2012;4(12):1794–811.

6. Green BP, Turner L, Stevenson E, et al. Short communication: patterns of dairy consumption in free-living children and adolescents. J Dairy Sci. 2015; 98(6):3701–5.

7. Dutch Food Institution (Stichting Voedingscentrum). Accessed: 1-7-2014.

8. van Rossum CTM, Fransen HP, Verkaik-Kloosterman J, et al. Dutch national food consumption survey 2007–2010: diet of children and adults aged 7 to 69 years. Bilthoven: National Institute for Public Health and the Environment; 2011. RIVM report 350050006/2011, 1–143.

9. Rangan AM, Flood VM, Denyer G, et al. Dairy consumption and diet quality in a sample of Australian children. J Am Coll Nutr. 2012;31(3):185–93.

10. Dutch legislation medical scientific research on human beings. Accessed: http://www.st-ab.nl/wetten/0609_Wet_medisch-wetenschappelijk_ onderzoek_met_mensen.htm.

11. Slimani N, Deharveng G, Charrondiere RU, et al. Structure of the standardized computerized 24-h diet recall interview used as reference method in the 22 centers participating in the EPIC project. European Prospective Investigation into Cancer and Nutrition. Comput Methods Programs Biomed. 1999;58(3):251–66.

12. Slimani N, Ferrari P, Ocke M, et al. Standardization of the 24-h diet recall calibration method used in the european prospective investigation into cancer and nutrition (EPIC): general concepts and preliminary results. Eur J Clin Nutr. 2000;54(12):900–17.

13. Slimani N, Casagrande C, Nicolas G, et al. The standardized computerized 24-h dietary recall method EPIC-Soft adapted for pan-European dietary monitoring. Eur J Clin Nutr. 2011;65 Suppl 1:S5–15.

14. Wendel-Vos GC, Schuit AJ, Saris WH, et al. Reproducibility and relative validity of the short questionnaire to assess health-enhancing physical activity. J Clin Epidemiol. 2003;56(12):1163–9.

15. Harris JA, Benedict FG. A biometric study of human basal metabolism. Proc Natl Acad Sci. 1918;4(12):370–3.

16. Souverein OW, Dekkers AL, Geelen A, et al. Comparing four methods to estimate usual intake distributions. Eur J Clin Nutr. 2011;65 Suppl 1:S92–101.

17. Nicklas TA, Jahns L, Bogle ML, et al. Barriers and facilitators for consumer adherence to the dietary guidelines for Americans: the HEALTH study. J Acad Nutr Diet. 2013;113(10):1317–31.

18. Mathias KC, Slining MM, Popkin BM. Foods and beverages associated with higher intake of sugar-sweetened beverages. Am J Prev Med. 2013;44(4):351–7.

19. Jensen RG. The composition of bovine milk lipids: January 1995 to December 2000. J Dairy Sci. 2002;85(2):295–350.

20. Yu S, Derr J, Etherton TD, et al. Plasma cholesterol-predictive equations demonstrate that stearic acid is neutral and monounsaturated fatty acids are hypocholesterolemic. Am J Clin Nutr. 1995;61(5):1129–39.

21. Aaron KJ, Sanders PW. Role of dietary salt and potassium intake in cardiovascular health and disease: a review of the evidence. Mayo Clin Proc. 2013;88(9):987–95.

22. Soedamah-Muthu SS, Ding EL, Al-Delaimy WK, et al. Milk and dairy consumption and incidence of cardiovascular diseases and all-cause mortality: dose–response meta-analysis of prospective cohort studies. Am J Clin Nutr. 2011;93(1):158–71.

23. de Oliveira Otto MC, Mozaffarian D, Kromhout D, et al. Dietary intake of saturated fat by food source and incident cardiovascular disease: the Multi-Ethnic Study of Atherosclerosis. Am J Clin Nutr. 2012;96(2):397–404.

24. Kratz M, Baars T, Guyenet S. The relationship between high-fat dairy consumption and obesity, cardiovascular, and metabolic disease. Eur J Nutr. 2013;52(1):1–24.

25. Adrogue HJ, Madias NE. The impact of sodium and potassium on hypertension risk. Semin Nephrol. 2014;34(3):257–72.

26. Qu X, Jin F, Hao Y, et al. Magnesium and the risk of cardiovascular events: a meta-analysis of prospective cohort studies. PLoS One. 2013;8(3), e57720.

27. Rautiainen S, Wang L, Manson JE, et al. The role of calcium in the prevention of cardiovascular disease--a review of observational studies and randomized clinical trials. Curr Atheroscler Rep. 2013;15(11):362.

28. Wang L, Manson JE, Song Y, et al. Systematic review: vitamin D and calcium supplementation in prevention of cardiovascular events. Ann Intern Med. 2010;152(5):315–23.

29. de Beer H. Dairy products and physical stature: a systematic review and meta-analysis of controlled trials. Econ Hum Biol. 2012;10(3):299–309.

30. Jansen W, van de Looij-Jansen PM, Ferreira I, et al. Differences in measured and self-reported height and weight in Dutch adolescents. Ann Nutr Metab. 2006;50(4):339–46.

18

Determinants of anemia among 6–59 months aged children in Bangladesh: evidence from nationally representative data

Jahidur Rahman Khan[1*], Nabil Awan[2] and Farjana Misu[3]

Abstract

Background: Anemia is a global public health problem but the burden of anemia is disproportionately borne among children in developing countries. Anemia in early stages of life has serious consequences on the growth and development of the children. We examine the prevalence of anemia, possible association between anemia and different socio-economic, demographic, health and other factors among children with ages from 6 to 59 months from the nationally representative 2011 Bangladesh Demographic and Health Survey (BDHS).

Methods: Data on hemoglobin (Hb) concentration among the children aged 6–59 months from the most recent BDHS (2011) were used. This nationally representative survey allowed a multistage stratified cluster sampling design and provided data on a wide range of indicators such as fertility, mortality, women and child health, nutrition and other background characteristics. Anemia status was determined using hemoglobin level (<11.0 g/dl), and weighted prevalence of childhood anemia along with 95 % confidence intervals were provided. We also examined the distribution of weighted anemia prevalence across different groups and performed logistic regression to assess the association of anemia with different factors.

Results: A total of 2171 children aged 6–59 months were identified for this analysis, with weighted prevalence of anemia being 51.9 % overall- 47.4 % in urban and 53.1 % in rural regions. Results of a multivariable logistic regression analysis showed that, children below 24 months of age (odds ratio, [OR] 3.01; 95 % confidence interval [CI] 2.38-3.81), and those from an anemic mother (OR 1.80; 95 % CI 1.49-2.18) were at higher risk of anemia. Childhood anemia was significantly associated with chronic malnutrition of child, source of drinking water, household wealth and geographical location (defined by division).

Conclusions: A high prevalence of anemia among 6–59 months aged children was observed in Bangladesh. Given the negative impact of anemia on the development of children in future, there is an urgent need for effective and efficient remedial public health interventions.

Keywords: Anemia, 6–59 months, Children, Determinants, Bangladesh

* Correspondence: jkhan@isrt.ac.bd
[1]Centre for Nutrition and Food Security, International Centre for Diarrhoeal Disease Research, Bangladesh (icddr, b), Dhaka, Bangladesh
Full list of author information is available at the end of the article

Background

Anemia is a prevalent public health problem which affects about a quarter of the world population [1], notably pre-school aged (PreSAC) children with global prevalence in the 0–5 year-old age group rising to 47.4 % [2]. According to World Health Organization (WHO) criteria, anemia ranks as a severe public health problem (defined as a prevalence of ≥ 40 %). Anemia can adversely affect cognitive advancement, performance in school, physical and behavioral growth, and immunization ability of children against disease [3–6]. It remains a major cause of mortality and morbidity in developing countries where resources to determine the underlying etiology remain poor [3]. According to WHO, Africa has the highest anemia prevalence overall for PreSAC, non-pregnant and pregnant women, where the Asian region shows the highest number of people being affected with 58 % of the anemia burden exists for PreSAC [2]. According to recent information from the South Asian region, the prevalence of anemia among children 6–35 months aged was about 79 % in India. In Nepal, the prevalence among children <5 years was 46 %. The national overall prevalence of Anemia in Bangladesh was approximately 51 % in 2011 [7].

Anemia in children is of particular interest since it can negatively and irreversibly impact their future development. Although the etiology of anemia among children is multi-factorial, the most significant correlates to the onset of childhood anemia is iron deficiency with a smaller proportion due to deficiencies of such micronutrients as folate, Vitamin A and B12 [8–10]. Prevalence of iron deficiency anemia in developing countries varies; Villalpando notes it is frequently four times higher than in developed countries [8].

Several surveys in the past have shown that anemia is a severe problem in Bangladesh among children. In Bangladesh, prevalence of anemia varied across the different surveys which were focused on slightly different populations. According to the Nutritional Surveillance Project (NSP), prevalence of anemia was 47 % in 2001 and 68 % in 2004 among 6–59 months aged children [11]. Anemia tends to reduce with age, and another study notes 64 % prevalence in children aged 6–23 months, and 42 % in children aged 24–59 months in Bangladesh [12]. On the other hand, National Micronutrient Survey in 2011–12 showed an anemia prevalence of only 33 % among 6–59 months aged children, although methodology was different than in other studies [13]. The prevalence of anemia is higher among younger children because their nutritional requirements for growth are high. The underlying causes of anemia among children are multi-factorial and there is no study which works with national level data on anemia and associated factors.

In this study, we performed a comprehensive investigation of childhood anemia and its determinants among the PreSAC children in Bangladesh. Our aim is to estimate the national prevalence of anemia and explore the factors associated with anemia as a basis for prevention and control programs. Moreover, the study can help public health policymakers determine priorities for intervention.

Methods

Data on 7481 children with ages from 6 to 59 months born in the last 5 years were extracted from 2011 Bangladesh Demographic and Health Survey (BDHS). This national level survey was designed to provide data on basic indicators of fertility regulation, maternal health, child health, nutritional status of mothers and children, awareness and attitude towards HIV/AIDS, and the prevalence of non-communicable diseases. Enumeration areas (EAs) from the population census 2011 were primary sampling units (PSUs) for this survey, with PSUs designed to produce separate estimates of key indicators for each of the seven divisions such as Dhaka, Chittagong, Rajshahi, Rangpur, Khulna, Barisal and Sylhet. Data collection took place over a five month period from July 8 to December 27, 2011. By using the stratified, two-stage cluster design, where, a total of 600 clusters (including 207 clusters in urban areas and 393 clusters in rural areas) were chosen in first stage [14]. In the second stage of sampling, a systematic sample of 30 households (HHs) was selected on average per cluster. Detailed information about the survey can be found in the 2011 BDHS report [14]. Hemoglobin testing was carried out among children aged 6–59 months in every third household in the BDHS sample using HemoCue rapid testing methodology. For the test, a drop of capillary blood was taken from a child's fingertip or heel and was drawn into the microcuvette which was then analyzed using the photometer that displays the hemoglobin concentration [14]. After selecting only children from *de jure* households and excluding children with missing information on hemoglobin or any of the other key predictors considered in this study, 2171 children of 6–59 months aged from the 2011 survey were retained for the final analysis. Data selection procedure is given in Fig. 1 in the form of a flow chart.

Ethics approval

Our study was wholly based on an analysis of existing public domain health survey datasets obtained from BDHS 2011, which is freely available online with all identifier information removed. The main author communicated with MEASURE DHS and ICF International and permission was granted to download and use the data. The BDHS 2011 was reviewed and approved by the

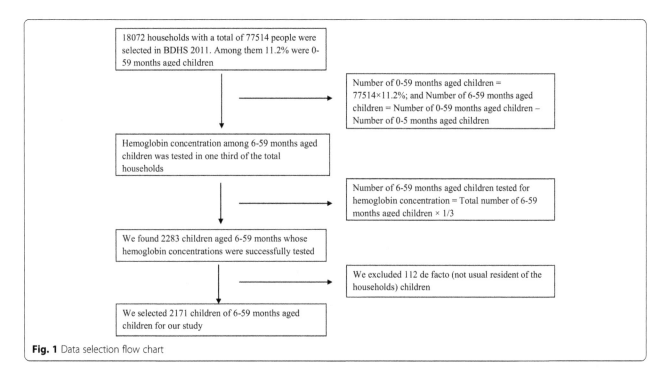

Fig. 1 Data selection flow chart

ICF Macro Institutional Review Board and the National Research Ethics Committee of the Bangladesh Medical Research Council. This survey was conducted by the National Institute of Population Research and Training (NIPORT) of the Ministry of Health and Family Welfare and implemented by Mitra and Associates, Bangladesh. The technical assistance for the survey was provided by ICF International of Calverton, Maryland, USA, as a part of its international Demographic and Health Survey program (MEASURE DHS). The U.S. Agency for International Development (USAID) provided financial support to complete the survey.

Measurement of variables
Outcome variables
Anemia was considered as the outcome variable. Hemoglobin concentration is the most reliable indicator of anemia at the population level [1]. According to WHO's criteria, 6–59 months aged children with hemoglobin level less than 11.0 g/dl are considered as anemic [1].

Explanatory variables
A number of health, demographic and socio economic factors are associated with children's nutritional status. Maternal age (<20, 20–29, 30–39,≥40), parental educational (no education, primary, secondary, higher), sex of the children, age of the children (6–23 months, 24–59 months), number of living children (1, 2, 3, >3), number of household members (≤4, 5–8, ≥9), number of eligible children (1, >1), currently breastfeeding (yes, no),

mother's anemia (yes, no), mother's Body Mass Index, BMI (<18.5 kg/m^2, ≥18.5 kg/m^2), size of the children at birth (small, average, large), household toilet facilities and source of drinking water (both binary variables broken down into improved and non-improved), presence of fever (yes, no) or diarrhea (yes, no) within last 2 weeks from date of interview are all considered potentially important factors in analyzing nutritional status of under five aged children and were included in the analysis. According to BDHS, a household water connection (piped), public standpipe, borehole, protected dug well or spring or rainwater collection is considered to be an 'improved' source of drinking water. Similarly, the 'improved' toilet facilities are considered to be flush toilets, ventilated improved pit latrines, traditional pit latrines with a slab, or composting toilets [14]. A Z-score cut-off point of less than −2 standard deviation (SD) is used to classify child malnutrition status such as low weight-for-age (underweight), low height-for-age (stunting) and low weight-for-height (wasting) according to WHO criteria. A wealth index was calculated using principle component analysis of asset variables and then categorized into terciles (poor, middle, rich). Place of residence (rural, urban) and geographic region based on seven divisions in Bangladesh (Barisal, Chittagong, Dhaka, Khulna, Rajshahi, Rangpur and Sylhet) were also included as covariates.

Statistical analysis
Descriptive statistics of each of the selected variables and distribution of anemia by different factors were

shown with 95 % CI by adjusting sampling weight. The BDHS 2011 sample was a two-stage stratified cluster sample; sampling weights were calculated based on sampling probabilities separately for each sampling stage and cluster. Due to the non-proportional allocation of sample to divisions and urban and rural areas, and the differences in response rates in sample, sampling weights were adjusted to ensure the representativeness of the survey results at national level. Adjustment for clustering in the sample removes underestimation of variability in the estimates by adjusting standard errors, and weighting the data adjusts for under sampling and oversampling within strata. A detailed description of the weighting procedure can be found in the BDHS report [14]. Logistic regression was applied and ORs with 95 % CI were used to evaluate the factors associated with anemia among 6–59 months aged children. Factors exhibiting a significant association with anemia (p-value <0.05) in univariate models were selected for developing multivariable logistic regression model. Statistical analyses were performed using the R statistical software (version 3.0.1; The R Foundation for Statistical Computing).

Results

A total of 2171 children between the ages of 6–59 months were identified. Among the eligible children male and female ratio were 51:49. Over two thirds of the samples were aged 24–59 months (67.2 %). The prevalence of anemia among children of aged 6–59 months was 51.9 % (95 % CI 49.4-54.5). Prevalence of stunting and underweight status in the children was over a third while the prevalence of wasting was approximately 16 %. The majority of the mothers of the children were at 20–29 years of age and 12.4 % was less than 20 years. Among the selected households, more than half had 5–8 members, with 1-2 children and one 6–59 months aged child. About 98.4 % households had access to improved water sources, while only 51.0 % households had access to improved toilet facilities. The proportion of no formal education among the children's fathers was higher than the mothers. About 44.1 % of children's mothers were anemic and 30.2 % were malnourished (BMI <18.5 kg/m^2) at the time of the survey. More than three-quarters (78.8 %) respondents lived in rural residences reflecting the changing demographics of Bangladesh, and 37.1 % of children lived in households of 'poor' economic class. Most of the selected respondents (30.7 %) lived in Dhaka division in contrast to Barisal division (5.7 %) (Table 1).

Table 2 shows prevalence of anemia by different factors. The prevalence of anemia varied significantly (p < 0.001) by age. For the children aged between 6 to 23 months the prevalence was 28 % greater than the children of age 24–59 months. The percentage of anemic children varied with educational status of parents. The prevalence of anemia was significantly higher for parents with no formal education compared to the higher educated parents. For stunted children the prevalence of anemia was significantly (p = 0.031) higher than in non-stunted children. But we did not find any significant difference in anemia prevalence among the wasted and underweight children. Children who continued breastfeeding were more anemic than the non breast fed children (58.6 % vs. 40.2 %, p < 0.001). The prevalence of anemia among children was significantly (p < 0.001) higher for anemic mothers (61.6 %) and malnourished mothers (58.0 %). There was a significant (p < 0.01) difference of anemia prevalence between children from households with access to an improved water source (51.1 %) and those without such access (74.3 %). But there was no significant difference in anemia prevalence by toilet facilities of households. The prevalence of anemia among children who suffered from fever in last 2 weeks was about nine percent higher than others. Not surprisingly, children from poor and middle economic class families were more anemic than children from rich families. Moreover, the prevalence of anemia was significantly higher among children in rural areas (53.1 %), compared to the urban areas (47.4 %).

Figure 2 shows that the administrative division-wise prevalence of anemia. Barisal, a division from the southern region of the country had the highest prevalence of anemia among children under the age of 5. A northern region Rangpur, also showed similar pattern. The results indicated that about 6 out of 10 children in the Barisal and Rangpur division were anemic; with prevalence estimates for these two regions being 60.4 % and 58.9 % respectively. The lowest prevalence was recorded in Dhaka division, 47.8 %, while for Chittagong, Rajshshi, Khulna and Sylhet rates of anemia were above 50 %. Relative to the WHO cut-off 40 %, all divisions showed concerning levels of anemia.

Table 3 shows the odds ratios from simple and multivariable logistic regression analysis for assessing associations between different factors and anemia among children aged 6–59 months in Bangladesh. Age of the children is recognized as an important factor for childhood anemia, and results showed that children with age between 6–23 months were more at risk of suffering from anemia than 23–59 months aged children, OR 3.01 (95 % CI: 2.38-3.81, p < 0.001). Adjusting for other factors, anemic mother's children were 80 % more likely to be anemic compared to children of non-anemic mothers. Similarly, children from undernourished mothers' were 43 % more likely to be anemic than others. Moreover, parental education was associated with lower rates of PreSAC anemia: children of parents with no formal education were at high risk of anemia compared to the

Table 1 Descriptive statistics of selected variables

Variables	Weighted Estimate (Mean/Proportion)	95 % CI
Anemia (Hb < 11.0 g/dl)		
No	48.1	45.5-50.6
Yes	51.9	49.4-54.5
Household characteristics		
Number of HH members		
≤4	31.5	28.7-34.2
5-8	54.2	51.4-57.1
≥9	14.3	12.0-16.7
Number of under-5 children		
One	60.9	57.8-64.0
More than one	39.1	36.0-42.2
Number of living children	2.4	2.3-2.5
1	28.5	26.1-31.0
2	32.9	30.3-35.4
3	19.5	17.3-21.8
>3	19.1	16.7-21.4
Toilet facilities		
Improved	51.0	47.7-54.4
Non-improved	49.0	45.6-52.3
Water source		
Improved	98.4	97.7-99.2
Non-improved	1.6	0.9-2.3
Wealth index		
Poor	37.1	33.9-40.4
Middle	31.8	29.0-34.5
Rich	31.1	28.0-34.2
Parental characteristics		
Maternal age (*years*)		
<20	12.4	10.8-14.1
20-29	62.2	59.7-64.7
30-39	22.4	20.1-24.7
≥40	3.0	2.1-3.9
Maternal education		
No education	20.3	17.9-22.7
Primary	33.2	30.3-36.1
Secondary	39.9	36.6-43.1
Higher	6.6	5.3-7.9
Father's education		
No education	29.9	27.1-32.8
Primary	30.4	27.8-32.9
Secondary	27.8	25.3-30.3
Higher	11.9	10.2-13.7
Maternal anemia		

Table 1 Descriptive statistics of selected variables (*Continued*)

Anemic	44.1	41.3-47.0
Not anemic	55.9	53.0-58.7
Mother's BMI		
<18.5 kg/m^2	30.2	27.4-33.0
≥18.5 kg/m^2	69.8	67.0-72.6
Child's characteristics		
Sex of children		
Male	51.0	48.4-53.5
Female	49.0	46.5-51.5
Age of the children (*months*)		
6-23 months	32.8	30.8-34.9
24-59 months	67.2	65.1-69.2
Size of children at birth		
Large	13.3	11.5-15.1
Average	68.5	66.2-70.9
Small	18.2	16.3-20.1
Continuous breastfeeding		
No	36.1	33.5-38.7
Yes	63.9	61.3-66.6
Diarrhea in last 2 weeks		
No	94.9	93.8-96.0
Yes	5.1	4.0-6.2
Fever in last 2 weeks		
No	61.3	58.9-63.8
Yes	38.7	36.2-41.1
Stunting		
No (HAZ ≥ −2 SD)	57.8	55.0-60.7
Yes (HAZ < −2 SD)	42.2	39.4-45.0
Under-weight		
No (WAZ ≥ −2 SD)	61.8	59.0-64.6
Yes (WAZ < −2 SD)	38.3	35.4-41.1
Wasting		
No (WHZ ≥ −2 SD)	83.6	81.8-85.5
Yes (WHZ < −2 SD)	16.4	14.5-18.2
Community characteristics		
Place of residence		
Urban	21.2	18.6-23.7
Rural	78.8	76.3-81.4
Division		
Barisal	5.4	3.9-7.0
Chittagong	22.2	17.4-26.9
Dhaka	30.7	25.2-36.2
Khulna	9.4	6.9-11.8

Table 1 Descriptive statistics of selected variables *(Continued)*

Rajshahi	12.7	9.5-16.0
Rangpur	11.5	8.6-14.4
Sylhet	8.1	5.8-10.4

WAZ (Weight for Age Z-score), HAZ (Height for Age Z-score), and WHZ (Weight for Height Z-score) was calculated with WHO Anthro and WHO Child Growth Standards

children of educated parents. Stunting or chronic malnutrition also displayed significant associations with anemia among the PreSAC population. Children who suffered from chronic malnutrition were more likely to be anemic, OR 1.38 (95 % CI: 1.13-1.69, *p* < 0.01). Children who suffered from fever in the 2 weeks prior to measurement were 28 % more likely to manifest anemia. Source of drinking water and toilet facilities of the household are thought to be strong household level predictors of childhood anemia. Children from households without access to 'improved' water sources and toilet facilities were 1.34 and 2.48 times more likely than others to be anemic. Compared to children of poor households according to the composite wealth index, middle and rich household's children were 26 % and 34 % less likely to be anemic. The likelihood of being anemic was 1.21 times higher for rural children than the urban children. Children from Dhaka and Sylhet divisions were less likely to be anemic than the children from Barisal division, which had the highest anemia prevalence among all the divisions.

Discussion

Childhood anemia is a major public health challenge in Bangladesh. Our results reveal that about 52 % of the children aged 6–59 months nationally are anemic, which is consistent with previously reported national prevalence of anemia (51 %) [14]. The findings confirm previous Bangladeshi studies showing high prevalence of anemia among the under-5 children [15], although the current study shows higher levels than, for example, the National Micronutrient Survey [13]. The study confirmed prevalence estimates differed by a number of key variables associated with anemia, as well as regional variation. Our analysis demonstrates that the age of child, chronic malnutrition status of child, mother's anemia status, source of water of household, wealth index have statistically significant associations with childhood anemia.

This study reveals that, the prevalence of anemia amongst every young (those under 2 in the PreSAC sample) was higher than in the overall population. This would likely be due to the high prevalence of maternal micronutrient deficits [16] as well as low concentrations of iron in breast milk, insufficient to meet daily requirements of iron for the children [8]. The likelihood of

anemia is significantly higher among children less than 2 years old compared to those aged 2–5 years. These findings are consistent with previously reported results [9, 17–20].

Household's source of drinking water showed an association with anemia in the PreSAC sample although the percentage of households which had no access to improved water source was only 1.58 %. But among those households, about 74 % of children presented with anemia. These elevated levels could be associated with higher rates of infectious diseases, although presence of fever was controlled in this study. The study's findings in relation to quality of water supply were consistent with previous research [21, 22]. Younger children and those with fever in the previous 2 weeks were also more likely to be anemic. According to [23], fever is common symptom of acute and chronic diseases which have been associated with lower hemoglobin levels as well as anemia.

The prevalence of anemia among children of low height for age (stunted) was high. Stunting, as an indicator of chronic malnutrition, is positively associated with childhood anemia [21, 22, 24, 25], and this association was found in the current study. Nutritional inadequacies may also impair immunity which in turn can have associations with low concentrations of hemoglobin (anemia).

Maternal anemia was highly associated with the occurrence of childhood anemia and the prevalence of anemia among the children of anemic mothers was almost 62 %, again corroborating several previous findings [26–28]. The underlying reasons may be mothers and children share common home environment, socioeconomic, and dietary conditions, and maternal/child anemia may reflect the common nutritional status of the household. Moreover, maternal iron deficiency is associated with low birth weight; even children born with adequate weight have reduced iron reserves when their mothers are anemic [29, 30].

Children of the rich and middle class households had lower prevalence of anemia compared to the poor households, plausibly reflecting improved household nutritional status [31]. This finding is also consistent with previous studies [32, 33].

The study also revealed that children of non-educated, primary and secondary educated parents were more likely to be anemic than children of parents with higher education. Level of education is confounded with socioeconomic status in general, but may also reflect in relatively poorer understanding of optimum child care and nutritional practices. Again, the study results in this regard are consistent with literature [1]. This study also shows an association between maternal age and PreSAC anemia, with older mothers less likely to have anemic children. This is plausibly due to a number of factors,

Table 2 Prevalence of anemia by different factors

Variables	Weighted Prevalence	95 % CI	p-value*
Household characteristics			
Number of HH members			
≤4	49.5	45.0-54.1	0.408
5-8	53.3	50.2-56.4	
≥9	52.1	45.2-59.0	
Number of under-5 children			
One	51.5	48.4-54.5	0.642
More than one	52.7	48.3-57.1	
Number of living children			
1	54.8	50.1-59.5	0.078
2	47.1	42.6-51.7	
3	54.0	48.4-59.7	
>3	53.8	48.0-59.6	
Toilet facilities			
Improved	49.5	45.7-53.2	0.140
Non-improved	53.6	49.8-57.4	
Water source			
Improved	51.1	48.5-53.8	<0.01
Non-improved	74.3	60.8-87.8	
Wealth index			
Poor	57.9	53.8-62.0	<0.001
Middle	52.4	47.9-56.9	
Rich	44.3	40.0-48.7	
Parental characteristics			
Maternal age *(years)*			
<20	65.6	59.0-72.3	<0.001
20-29	50.2	46.9-53.6	
30-39	48.8	43.6-53.9	
≥40	54.2	40.3-68.1	
Maternal education			
No education	51.4	45.8-56.9	0.012
Primary	53.8	49.5-58.0	
Secondary	53.2	49.2-57.2	
Higher	37.0	28.1-45.9	
Father's education			
No education	51.3	46.5-56.1	<0.01
Primary	56.2	51.6- 60.8	
Secondary	52.3	47.8-56.8	
Higher	41.6	34.8-48.4	
Maternal anemia			
Anemic	61.6	58.2-65.0	<0.001
Not anemic	44.3	40.9-47.6	

Table 2 Prevalence of anemia by different factors *(Continued)*

Mother's BMI			
<18.5 kg/m²	58.0	53.2-62.8	<0.01
≥18.5 kg/m²	49.2	46.3-52.1	
Child's characteristics			
Sex of children			
Male	53.0	49.6-56.5	0.363
Female	50.8	47.2-54.4	
Age of the children *(months)*			
6-23 months	70.8	66.8-74.8	<0.001
24-59 months	42.7	39.6-45.8	
Size of children at birth			
Large	55.5	49.1-62.0	0.447
Average	51.0	47.84-54.2	
Small	52.8	47.1-58.5	
Continuous breastfeeding			
No	40.2	36.2-44.1	<0.001
Yes	58.6	55.4-61.8	
Diarrhea in last 2 weeks			
No	51.9	49.3-54.5	0.815
Yes	53.3	41.7-64.8	
Fever in last 2 weeks			
No	48.8	45.6-52.1	<0.01
Yes	56.9	53.0-60.7	
Stunting			
No (HAZ ≥ −2 SD)	49.2	46.1-52.3	0.031
Yes (HAZ < −2 SD)	55.0	50.7-59.3	
Under-weight			
No (WAZ ≥ −2 SD)	51.5	48.4-54.7	0.905
Yes (WAZ < −2 SD)	51.8	47.7-55.9	
Wasting			
No (WHZ ≥ −2 SD)	51.8	49.0-54.6	0.822
Yes (WHZ < −2 SD)	51.1	45.2-56.9	
Community characteristics			
Place of residence			
Urban	47.4	42.7-52.2	0.046
Rural	53.1	50.1-56.2	

*p-value obtained from chi-square test of contingency table

with timing of childbearing being associated with socioeconomic status and household wealth [34].

Higher prevalence of anemia was found in rural regions of Bangladesh. This can also be linked to malnutrition due to limited availability of nutritious foods due to lower socioeconomic status, and lack of access to hygienic sanitation facilities [35], associated with elevated

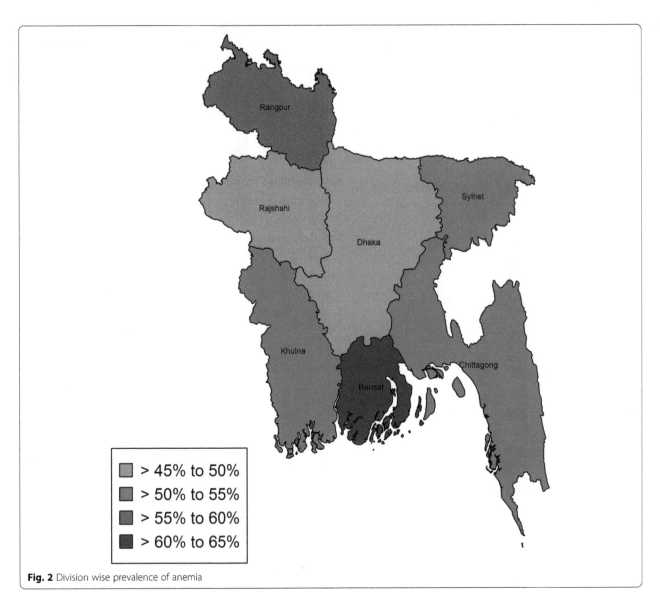

> 45% to 50%
> 50% to 55%
> 55% to 60%
> 60% to 65%

Fig. 2 Division wise prevalence of anemia

rates of disease which in turn is associated with increased risk of anemia. The high prevalence of anemia in rural sectors especially in the southern division Barisal and northern division Rangpur can be linked to the fact that most of the areas in these regions are rural. Demographic changes in Bangladesh are seeing the increased concentration of industries associated with economic growth and thus higher socioeconomic status into the major population centres, Dhaka and Chittagong. Although all of the divisions sampled were at high risk of anemia, the low prevalence observed in Dhaka division, could be due to the high proportion of urban residents in the Dhaka region.

Limitations
Detail on infant and PreSAC feeding was not available for our sample, which limits the insight that can be drawn from the data. Moreover, the BDHS survey does not distinguish between slum areas from the other residential areas. Slum areas will be automatically included in sample if they exist. So, these data are not representative for the slum population of urban areas, who are probably more likely to suffer from anemia. While the data are designed to be nationally representative, it is possible that there is some degree of bias in the sampling that might see slum residents underrepresented in the sample. However, we cannot prove it to be a potential source of bias since there is no identifier of slum area in the data. If we had such an identifier, we could compare the estimates by post-stratification. Despite these limitations we believe that our findings help illuminate the association between socioeconomic, demographic, and health variables with anemia in a large PreSAC population in the developing world.

Table 3 Factors associated with anemia among 6–59 months aged children in Bangladesh

Variables	Simple Logistic Regression			Multivariable Logistic Regression		
	OR	95 % CI	P-value	OR	95 % CI	P-value
Household characteristics						
Number of HH members						
≤4	1			-	-	-
5-8	1.05	0.87-1.28	0.582	-	-	-
≥9	0.99	0.76-1.28	0.923	-	-	-
Number of under-5 children						
One	1			-	-	-
More than one	1.01	0.85-1.20	0.907	-	-	-
Number of living children						
1	1					
2	0.80	0.65-0.99	0.043	1.01	0.78-1.31	0.929
3	0.89	0.69-1.14	0.351	1.13	0.81-1.56	0.473
>3	0.92	0.72-1.18	0.499	1.19	0.81-1.74	0.381
Toilet facilities						
Improved	1			1		
Non-improved	1.34	1.13-1.59	<0.001	1.03	0.83-1.27	0.811
Water source						
Improved	1			1		
Non-improved	2.30	1.25-4.44	<0.01	2.48	1.28-5.02	<0.01
Wealth index						
Poor	1			1		
Middle	0.76	0.61-0.93	<0.01	0.74	0.57-0.95	0.018
Rich	0.56	0.45-0.69	<0.001	0.66	0.48-0.92	0.013
Parental characteristics						
Maternal age (*years*)						
<20	1			1		
20-29	0.50	0.38-0.66	<0.01	0.76	0.54-1.07	0.122
30-39	0.46	0.34-0.63	<0.01	0.71	0.46-1.10	0.123
≥40	0.52	0.30-0.90	0.019	0.68	0.34-1.38	0.286
Maternal education						
No education	1.78	1.22-2.61	<0.01	1.23	0.71-2.14	0.468
Primary	1.86	1.30-2.67	<0.01	1.15	0.69-1.92	0.589
Secondary	1.72	1.21-2.46	<0.01	1.10	0.70-1.75	0.670
Higher	1			1		
Father's education						
No education	1.45	1.09-1.94	0.010	1.02	0.66-1.56	0.943
Primary	1.73	1.30-2.30	<0.001	1.25	0.84-1.85	0.276
Secondary	1.47	1.10-1.96	<0.01	1.24	0.86-1.80	0.252
Higher	1			1		
Maternal anemia						
Anemic	1.93	1.62-2.29	<0.001	1.80	1.49-2.18	<0.001
Not anemic	1			1		
Mother's BMI						

Table 3 Factors associated with anemia among 6–59 months aged children in Bangladesh *(Continued)*

<18.5 kg/m²	1.43	1.19-1.72	<0.001	1.07	0.86-1.33	0.554
≥18.5 kg/m²	1			1		
Child's characteristics						
Sex of children						
Male	1			-	-	-
Female	0.92	0.78-1.09	0.320	-	-	-
Age of the children *(months)*						
6-23 months	3.31	2.73-4.02	<0.001	3.01	2.38-3.81	<0.001
24-59 months	1			1		
Size of children at birth						
Large	1			-	-	-
Average	0.89	0.69-1.13	0.341	-	-	-
Small	0.89	0.66-1.20	0.448	-	-	-
Continuous breastfeeding						
No	1			1		
Yes	2.13	1.78-2.55	<0.001	1.18	0.95-1.47	0.143
Diarrhea in last 2 weeks						
No	1			-	-	-
Yes	1.20	0.83-1.75	0.328	-	-	-
Fever in last 2 weeks						
No	1			1		
Yes	1.28	1.07-1.52	<0.01	1.13	0.93-1.37	0.229
Stunting						
No (HAZ ≥ −2 SD)	1			1		
Yes (HAZ < −2 SD)	1.41	1.19-1.68	<0.001	1.38	1.13-1.69	<0.01
Under-weight						
No (WAZ ≥ −2 SD)	1			-	-	-
Yes (WAZ < −2 SD)	1.10	0.92-1.31	0.306	-	-	-
Wasting						
No (WHZ ≥ −2 SD)	1			-	-	-
Yes (WHZ < −2 SD)	0.96	0.76-1.21	0.723	-	-	-
Community characteristics						
Place of residence						
Urban	1			1		
Rural	1.21	1.01-1.46	0.039	0.93	0.74-1.17	0.517
Division						
Barisal	1			1		
Chittagong	0.77	0.56-1.07	0.120	0.72	0.50-1.05	0.087
Dhaka	0.64	0.46-0.89	<0.01	0.63	0.43-0.92	0.016
Khulna	0.83	0.58-1.19	0.309	0.97	0.64-1.45	0.865
Rajshahi	0.68	0.48-0.97	0.035	0.74	0.49-1.10	0.135
Rangpur	0.97	0.69-1.38	0.878	0.94	0.64-1.40	0.769
Sylhet	0.66	0.47-0.91	0.012	0.61	0.41-0.89	0.011

Conclusions

In summary, our analysis highlights concerning continuing public health challenge presented by anemia in a PreSAC population in Bangladesh. This study explores the factors associated with anemia. This study supports the value of population-based interventions such as micronutrient supplementation, food fortification and nutrition education to improve the situation that should be instituted. The findings of the study will assist the government of Bangladesh and policy makers to take necessary steps and design proper interventions that target children aged under-5, and their parents. However, further study is needed to understand the specific set of determinants of anemia among children in Bangladesh.

Competing interests
The authors declare that they have no competing interests.

Authors' contribution
JR Khan conceptualized the study, synthesized the analysis plan, performed the statistical analysis, and drafted first version of manuscript. N Awan helped to conceptualize the analysis plan, interpret the findings and participated in critical review of the manuscript. F Misu helped to synthesize the analysis plan and to interpret the findings. All authors helped to write the manuscript. All authors read and approved the final manuscript.

Acknowledgement
The authors acknowledge the contribution of BDHS, NIPORT, MEASURE DHS and ICF International teams for their efforts to collect data and to open access the data set. The authors also acknowledge Dr Olav Muurlink for his editorial review of the manuscript.

Author details
[1]Centre for Nutrition and Food Security, International Centre for Diarrhoeal Disease Research, Bangladesh (icddr, b), Dhaka, Bangladesh. [2]Institute of Statistical Research and Training, University of Dhaka, Dhaka, Bangladesh. [3]Department of Agricultural Statistics, Bangladesh Agricultural University, Mymensingh, Bangladesh.

References
1. Worldwide prevalence of anemia 1993–2005. WHO global database on anemia. Geneva: World Health Organization; 2008.
2. McLean E, Cogswell M, Egli I, Wojdyla D, De Benoist B. Worldwide prevalence of anaemia, WHO vitamin and mineral nutrition information system, 1993–2005. Public Health Nutr. 2009;12(4):444–54.
3. Iron deficiency anaemia: assessment, prevention and control. Geneva, World Health Organization; 2001.
4. Brabin BJ, Premji Z, Verhoeff F. An analysis of anemia and child mortality. J Nutr. 2001;131:636S–48S.
5. McCann JC, Ames BN. An overview of evidence for a causal relation between iron deficiency during development and deficits in cognitive or behavioral function. Am J ClinNutr. 2007;85(4):931–45.
6. Sachdev H, Gera T, Nestel P. Effect of iron supplementation on mental and motor development in children: systematic review of randomized controlled trials. Public Health Nutr. 2005;8:117–32.
7. Chaparro C, Oot L, Sethuraman K. Overview of the Nutrition Situation in Four Countries in South and Central Asia. Washington, DC: FHI 360/FANTA; 2014.
8. Villalpando S, Shamah-Levy T, Ramírez-Silva CI, Mejía-Rodríguez F, Rivera JA. Prevalence of anemia in children 1 to 12 years of age: results from a nationwide probabilistic survey in Mexico. SaludPublica Mex. 2003;45(4Suppl):S490–98.
9. Cornet M, Le Hesran JY, Fievet N, Cot M, Personne P, Gounoue R, et al. Prevalence of and risk factors for anemia in young children in southern Cameroon. Am J Trop Med Hyg. 1998;58(5):606–11.
10. Fleming AF, Werblinska B. Anaemia in childhood in the guinea savanna of Nigeria. Ann Trop Paediatr. 1982;2(4):161–73.
11. Rashid M, Flora MS, Moni MA, Akhter A, Mahmud Z. Reviewing Anemia and iron folic acid supplementation program in Bangladesh- a special article. Bangladesh Med J. 2010; 39(3). DOI:http://dx.doi.org/10.3329/bmj.v39i3.9952.
12. BBS/UNICEF. Anemia prevalence survey of Urban Bangladesh and Rural Chittagong Hill Tracts 2003. Dhaka, Bangladesh: Bangladesh Bureau of Statistics, Statistics Division, Ministry of Planning, Government of the Peoples Republic of Bangladesh UNICEF; 2004.
13. International Centre for Diarrheal Disease Research Bangladesh (icddr,b), United Nations Children's Fund (UNICEF), Global Alliance for Improved Nutrition (GAIN), and Institute of Public Nutrition. National Micronutrients Status Survey 2011–12: Final Report. Dhaka, Bangladesh: Centre for Nutrition and Food Security, icddr,b; 2013.
14. National Institute of Population Research and Training (NIPORT), Mitra and Associates, ICF International. Bangladesh Demographic and Health Survey 2011. Dhaka: Bangladesh and Calverton, Maryland, USA: NIPORT, Mitra and Associates, ICF International; 2013.
15. Helen Keller International. Bangladesh: the burden of anaemia in rural Bangladesh: the need for urgent action. In: Nutritional Surveillance Project bulletin no 16. Dhaka, Bangladesh: Helen Keller International; 2006.
16. Neumann CG, Gewa C, Bwibo NO. Child nutrition in developing countries. Pediatr Ann. 2004;33(10):658.
17. Kotecha PV. Nutritional anemia in young children with focus on Asia and India. Indian J Community Med. 2011;36(1):8.
18. Ayoya MA, Ngnie-Teta I, Séraphin MN, Mamadoultaibou A, Boldon E, Saint-Fleur JE, et al. Prevalence and risk factors of anemia among children 6–59 Months Old in Haiti. Anemia. 2013;2013:502968.
19. Uddin MKI. Prevalence of anaemia in children of 6 months to 59 months in narayanganj, bangladesh. J Dhaka Med Col. 2010;19(2):126–30.
20. Karr M, Alperstain G, Cuser JC, Mira M. Iron status and anaemia in preschool children in Sydney. Aust NZ J Pub Health. 1996;20(6):618–22.
21. Ngnie-Teta I, Receveur O, Kuate-Defo B. Risk factors for moderate to severe anemia among children in Benin and Mali: insights from a multilevel analysis. Food & Nutrition Bulletin. 2007;28(1):76–89.
22. Adish AA, Esrey SA, Gyorkos TW, Johns T. Risk factors for iron deficiency anaemia in preschool children in northern Ethiopia. Public Health Nutr. 1999;2(3):243–52.
23. Konstantyner T, Oliveira TCR, AguiarCarrazedoTaddei JA. Risk factors for Anaemia among Brazillian infants from the 2006 National Demographic Health Survey. Anaemia. 2012;2012:850681.
24. Assis AM, Barreto ML, Gomes GSS, Prado MS, Santos NS, Santos LMP, et al. Childhood anemia: prevalence and associated factors in Salvador, Bahia, Brazil. Cad Saude Publica. 2004;20(6):1633–41.
25. Leite MS, Cardoso AM, Coimbra Jr CE, Welch JR, Gugelmin SA, Lira PCI, et al. Prevalence of anemia and associated factors among indigenous children in Brazil: results from the First National Survey of Indigenous People's Health and Nutrition. Nutr J. 2013;12:69. doi:10.1186/1475-2891-12-69.
26. Souza LG, Santos RV, Carvalho MS, Pagliaro H, Flowers NM, Coimbra Jr CEA. Demography and health of the Xavante Indians from Central Brazil. Cad SaudePublica. 2011;27(10):1891–905. http://dx.doi.org/10.1590/S0102-311X2011001000003.
27. McSweeney K, Arps SA. A "demographic turnaround": the rapid growth of indigenous populations in lowland South America. Lat Am Res Rev. 2005;40(1):3–29.
28. Osório MM, Lira PI, Ashworth A. Factors associated with Hb concentration in children aged 6–59 months in the state of Pernambuco, Brazil. Br J Nutr. 2004;91(2):307–15.
29. Allen LH. Biological mechanisms that might underlie iron's effects on fetal growth and preterm birth. J Nutr. 2001;131(2S-2):581S–9S.
30. Scholl TO. Iron status during pregnancy: setting the stage for mother and infant. Am J ClinNutr. 2005;81(5):1218S–22S.
31. Singh MB, Fotedar R, Lakshminarayana J, Anand PK. Studies on the nutritional status of children aged 0–5 years in a drought-affected desert area of Western Rajasthan, India. Public Health Nutr. 2006;9(8):961–7.
32. Muniz PT, Castro TG, Araújo TS, Nunes NB, da Silva-Nunes M, Hoffmann EH, et al. Child health and nutrition in the Western Brazilian Amazon:

population-based surveys in two counties in Acre State. Cad SaudePublica. 2007;23(6):1283–93.

33. Singh RK, Patra S. Extent of anaemia among preschool children in EAG States, India: a challenge to policy makers. Anemia.2014. doi:http://dx.doi. org/10.1155/2014/868752.

34. De Pee S, Bloem MW, Sari M, Kiess L, Yip R, Kosen S. The high prevalence of low haemoglobin concentration among Indonesia infants aged 3–5 months is related to maternal anaemia. J Nutr. 2002;132(8):2215–21.

35. Beresford CH, Neale RJ, Brooks OG. Iron absorption and pyrexia. Lancet. 1971;297(7699):568–72.

Permissions

The contributors of this book come from diverse backgrounds, making this book a truly international effort. This book will bring forth new frontiers with its revolutionizing research information and detailed analysis of the nascent developments around the world.

We would like to thank all the contributing authors for lending their expertise to make the book truly unique. They have played a crucial role in the development of this book. Without their invaluable contributions this book wouldn't have been possible. They have made vital efforts to compile up to date information on the varied aspects of this subject to make this book a valuable addition to the collection of many professionals and students.

This book was conceptualized with the vision of imparting up-to-date information and advanced data in this field. To ensure the same, a matchless editorial board was set up. Every individual on the board went through rigorous rounds of assessment to prove their worth. After which they invested a large part of their time researching and compiling the most relevant data for our readers.

The editorial board has been involved in producing this book since its inception. They have spent rigorous hours researching and exploring the diverse topics which have resulted in the successful publishing of this book. They have passed on their knowledge of decades through this book. To expedite this challenging task, the publisher supported the team at every step. A small team of assistant editors was also appointed to further simplify the editing procedure and attain best results for the readers.

Apart from the editorial board, the designing team has also invested a significant amount of their time in understanding the subject and creating the most relevant covers. They scrutinized every image to scout for the most suitable representation of the subject and create an appropriate cover for the book.

The publishing team has been an ardent support to the editorial, designing and production team. Their endless efforts to recruit the best for this project, has resulted in the accomplishment of this book. They are a veteran in the field of academics and their pool of knowledge is as vast as their experience in printing. Their expertise and guidance has proved useful at every step. Their uncompromising quality standards have made this book an exceptional effort. Their encouragement from time to time has been an inspiration for everyone.

The publisher and the editorial board hope that this book will prove to be a valuable piece of knowledge for researchers, students, practitioners and scholars across the globe.

List of Contributors

Henk F. van der Molen and Monique H. W. Frings-Dresen
Coronel Institute of Occupational Health, Academic Medical Center, University of Amsterdam, P.O. Box 22660 1100 DD Amsterdam, The Netherlands

Aalt den Herder, Jan Warning and Henk F. van der Molen
Arbouw, P.O. Box 213 3840 AE Harderwijk, The Netherlands

Paola Rebora, Laura Antolini and Maria Grazia Valsecchi
Center of Biostatistics for Clinical Epidemiology, School of Medicine and Surgery, University of Milano-Bicocca, via Cadore 48, 20900 Monza, Italy

David V. Glidden
Department of Epidemiology and Biostatistics, University of California, San Francisco, California

Johan Israelsson
Department of Internal Medicine, Division of Cardiology, Kalmar County Hospital, SE-39185 Kalmar, Sweden
Department of Medical and Health Sciences, Division of Nursing Science, Linköping University, SE-58185 Linköping, Sweden
Kalmar Maritime Academy, Linnaeus University, SE-39182 Kalmar, Sweden

Gisela Lilja
Department of Clinical Science, Division of Neurology, Lund University, Lund, Sweden
Department of Neurology and Rehabilitation Medicine, Skane University Hospital, SE-22185 Lund, Sweden

Anders Bremer
Faculty of Caring Science, Work Life and Social Welfare and the Centre for Prehospital Research, University of Borås, SE-50190 Borås, Sweden
Division of Emergency Medical Services, Kalmar County Hospital, SE-39185 Kalmar, Sweden

Jean Stevenson-Ågren
Information School, University of Sheffield, Regent Court, 211 Portobello Street, Sheffield S1 4DP, England
eHealth Institute, Linnaeus University, SE-39182 Kalmar, Sweden

Kristofer Årestedt
Center for Collaborative Palliative Care, Linnaeus University, SE-39182 Kalmar, Sweden
Department of Medical and Health Sciences, Division of Nursing Science, Linköping University, SE-58185 Linköping, Sweden

Jessy Z'gambo and Charles Michelo
Department of Public Health, Epidemiology & Biostatistics Unit, School of Medicine, University of Zambia, Lusaka, Zambia

Yorum Siulapwa and Jessy Z'gambo
Department of Public Health, Environmental Health Unit, School of Medicine, University of Zambia, Lusaka, Zambia

Ju Yeon Park, Deok Ryun Kim, Soon Ae Kim, Ayan Dey, Thomas F. Wierzba and Mohammad Ali
International Vaccine Institute, Seoul, South Korea

Bisakha Haldar, Aiyel Haque Mallick, Ranjan Kumar Nandy, Dipika Sur, Suman Kanungo and Byomkesh Manna
National Institute of Cholera and Enteric Diseases, Kolkata, India

Dilip Kumar Paul, Saugata Choudhury and Shushama Sahoo
B.C. Roy Post Graduate Institute of Pediatric Sciences, Kolkata, India

Thomas F. Wierzba
PATH, Washington, DC, USA

Mohammad Ali
Johns Hopkins Bloomberg School of Public Health, Baltimore, USA

E. Anne Lown, Patricia A. McDaniel and Ruth E. Malone
Department of Social and Behavioral Sciences, School of Nursing, University of California, San Francisco, CA 94143-0612, USA

Adrien Roussot, Jonathan Cottenet and Catherine Quantin
Service de Biostatistique et d'Informatique Médicale (DIM), CHRU Dijon, Dijon 21000, France
Université de Bourgogne, Dijon 21000, France

Maryse Gadreau
Laboratoire d'Economie de Dijon, Université de Bourgogne, UMR 6307 CNRS, INSERM U1200, Dijon, France

Maurice Giroud and Yannick Béjot
Registre des AVC dijonnais, EA4184, CHRU, Univ de Bourgogne, Dijon, France

Catherine Quantin
INSERM, CIC 1432, Dijon, France
Clinical Epidemiology/Clinical Trials Unit, Clinical Investigation Center, Dijon University Hospital, Dijon, France
Biostatistics, Biomathematics, Pharmacoepidemiology and Infectious Diseases (B2PHI), Univ. Bourgogne Franche-Comté, Inserm UMR 1181, Dijon 21000, France

Monica D. Ramirez-Andreotta
Department of Soil, Water, and Environmental Science, University of Arizona, 1177 E Fourth Street, Rm. 429, Tucson, Arizona, USA

Julia Green Brody
Silent Spring Institute, Newton, MA, USA

Paloma I. Beamer, Nathan Lothrop, Monica D. Ramirez-Andreotta and Miranda Loh
Mel and Enid Zuckerman College of Public Health, University of Arizona, Tucson, AZ 85721, USA

Miranda Loh
Institute of Occupational Medicine, Edinburgh, UK

Phil Brown
Department of Sociology and Anthropology and Department of Health Sciences, Northeastern University, Boston, MA, USA

Heidi Weberruß, Birgit Böhm and Renate Oberhoffer
Institute of Preventive Pediatrics, Technische Universität München, Georg-Brauchle-Ring 60/62, Campus D, 80992 Munich, Germany

Robert Dalla Pozza, Heinrich Netz and Raphael Pirzer
Department of Pediatric Cardiology, Ludwig-Maximilians-University, Marchioninistraße 15, 81377 Munich, Germany

Sing Yu Moorcraft, Cheryl Marriott, Clare Peckitt, David Cunningham, Ian Chau, Naureen Starling, David Watkins and Sheela Rao
The Royal Marsden NHS Foundation Trust, London, UK
The Royal Marsden NHS Foundation Trust, Sutton, UK

Ruth A. Ashton
Malaria Consortium, London, UK

Richard Reithinger, Ruth A. Ashton and Simon J. Brooker
Faculty of Infectious and Tropical Diseases, London School of Hygiene & Tropical Medicine, London, UK

Takele Kefyalew, Zelalem Kebede and Gezahegn Tesfaye
Malaria Consortium Ethiopia, Addis Ababa, Ethiopia

Esey Batisso and Tessema Awano
Malaria Consortium Southern Nations, Nationalities and People's Regional State sub-office, Hawassa, Ethiopia

Tamiru Mesele
Southern Nations, Nationalities and People's Regional State Health Bureau, Hawassa, Ethiopia

Sheleme Chibsa
President's Malaria Initiative, U.S. Agency for International Development, Addis Ababa, Ethiopia

Richard Reithinger
RTI International, Washington, DC, USA

Al Motavalli
Department of Anaesthesia, The Royal Victorian Eye & Ear Hospital, 32 Gisborne St, East Melbourne, VIC 3002, Australia

Debra Nestel
HealthPEER, Faculty of Medicine, Nursing and Health Sciences, Monash University, Melbourne, VIC, Australia

Andrée Gamble
Health Science & Biotechnology Department, Holmesglen Institute, Chadstone, Victoria, Australia

Margaret Bearman
HealthPEER - Health Professions Education and Educational Research, Monash University, Melbourne, Victoria, Australia

Debra Nestel
Simulation Education in Healthcare, School of Rural Health, HealthPEER, Faculty of Medicine, Nursing and Health Sciences, Monash University, Melbourne, Victoria, Australia
Graduate Programs in Surgical Education, University of Melbourne, Parkville, Victoria, Australia

Mahama Saaka
University for Development Studies, School of Allied Health Sciences, P O Box 1883, Tamale, Ghana

Asamoah Larbi
International Institute of Tropical Agriculture (IITA), P O Box 6, Tamale, Ghana

Sofo Mutaru
Ghana Health Service, Tamale, Northern Region, Ghana

Irmgard Hoeschle-Zeledon
International Institute of Tropical Agriculture (IITA), PMB 5320, Oyo Road, Ibadan, Nigeria

Stephanie O'Regan and Leonie Watterson
Sydney Clinical Skills and Simulation Centre, Royal North Shore Hospital, Level 6 Kolling Building, Reserve Rd, St Leonards, NSW 2065, Australia

Elizabeth Molloy and Debra Nestel
Health Professions Education and Educational Research (HealthPEER), Faculty of Medicine, Nursing and Health Sciences, Monash University, Building 13C, Office G09, Clayton Campus, Victoria 3800, Australia

Carine J. M. Doggen, Marlies Zwerink and Rolf E. Egberink
Department of Health Technology and Services Research (HTSR), MIRA institute for Biomedical Technology and Technical Medicine, University of Twente, RA 5252, PO Box 217, 7500 AE, Enschede, The Netherlands

Hanneke M. Droste and Paul J. A. M. Brouwers
Department of Neurology, Medisch Spectrum Twente, Enschede, The Netherlands

Gert K. van Houwelingen
Department of Cardiology, Thoraxcentrum Twente, Medisch Spectrum Twente, Enschede, The Netherlands

Fred L. van Eenennaam
Ambulance Oost, Hengelo, The Netherlands

Rolf E. Egberink
Regional Network for Emergency Care, Acute Zorg Euregio, Enschede, The Netherlands

Marjo J. E. Campmans-Kuijpers and Joline W. J. Beulens
Julius Center for Health Sciences and Primary Care, University Medical Center Utrecht, P.O. Box 85500 3508 GA Utrecht, The Netherlands

Cecile Singh-Povel and Jan Steijns
FrieslandCampina, Amersfoort, The Netherlands

Jahidur Rahman Khan
Centre for Nutrition and Food Security, International Centre for Diarrhoeal Disease Research, Bangladesh (icddr, b), Dhaka, Bangladesh

Nabil Awan
Institute of Statistical Research and Training, University of Dhaka, Dhaka, Bangladesh

Farjana Misu
Department of Agricultural Statistics, Bangladesh Agricultural University, Mymensingh, Bangladesh

Printed in the USA
CPSIA information can be obtained
at www.ICGtesting.com
JSHW051444221024
72173JS00006B/1569